D0166216

Statistical Applications for Health Information Management

Carol E. Osborn, PhD, RHIA

Health Information Management and Systems Division
The Ohio State University
Columbus, Ohio

AN ASPEN PUBLICATION®
Aspen Publishers, Inc.
Gaithersburg, Maryland
2000

Library of Congress Cataloging-in-Publication Data

Osborn, Carol E.
Statistical applications for health information management/Carol E. Osborn.
p.   cm.
Includes bibliographical references and index.
ISBN 0-8342-1243-9
1. Health—Information services—Statistical methods. I. Title.
RA394.O83 2000
362.1'068'4—dc21
00-021793

Orders: (800) 638–8437
Customer Service: (800) 234-1660

About Aspen Publishers • For more than 40 years, Aspen has been a leading professional publisher in
a variety of disciplines. Aspen's vast information resources are available in both print and electronic
formats. We are committed to providing the highest quality information available in the most appropriate format for our customers. Visit Aspen's Internet site for more information resources, directories,
articles, and a searchable version of Aspen's full catalog, including the most recent publications:
www.aspenpublishers.com
Aspen Publishers, Inc. • The hallmark of quality in publishing
Member of the worldwide Wolters Kluwer Group.

Editorial Services: Stephanie Neuben
Library of Congress Catalog Card Number: 00-021793
ISBN: 0-8342-1243-9

Printed in the United States of America

1 2 3 4 5

To my husband, Richards, for his love,
support, and infinite patience.

Table of Contents

Preface

This text was written specifically for health information management students enrolled in baccalaureate degree programs and for practicing health information management professionals. This text focuses on applying statistical techniques to problems in health care. Because the focus is on application, it is assumed that the student has had a previous course in probability theory and the normal distribution.

This text is set up so that students can either use the Aspen Publishers, Inc., Web site that supports this book or input the data for each problem using their own statistical software. It is not the intent of this book to teach the student how to use SPSS, Microsoft Excel, or any other type of statistical package or electronic spreadsheet. They are included in this text as examples; I am not endorsing any of these products. My goal in writing this book was to introduce students and professionals to how statistical techniques can be used to describe and make inferences from health care data. There are many statistical books available on the market, but none is directed specifically to the health information management profession. Also, because there are other texts that introduce the student to traditional hospital statistics such as average length of stay and total inpatient service days, they are not covered in this text.

The home page for *Statistical Applications for Health Information Management* is:
www.aspenpublishers.com/books/osborn

Acknowledgments

I want to thank my colleague, Melanie Brodnik, PhD, RHIA, for her unending support in allowing me to complete this project.

Many thanks also go to Larry Sachs, PhD, for reviewing the text and offering suggestions for improvement.

I would also like to thank the "unknown" reviewers who made many helpful suggestions for improving this work.

CHAPTER 1

Commonly Used Frequency Measures in Health Care

KEY TERMS	Variable	Morbidity rates
	Frequency distribution	Incidence rate
	Rate	Prevalence rate
	Ratio	Point prevalence rate
	Proportion	Risk ratios
	Dichotomous variables	Relative risk
	Confounding factor	Odds ratio
	Mortality rates	Attributable risk
	Crude death rate	Kaplan Meier survival analysis
	Age-specific death rate (ASDR)	
	Age-adjusted death rate	
	Standard mortality ratio (SMR)	
	Race-specific death rate	
	Sex-specific death rate	
	Cause-specific death rate	
	Case fatality rate	
	Proportionate mortality ratio (PMR)	
	Maternal mortality rate	
	Neonatal mortality rate	
	Postneonatal mortality rate	
	Infant mortality rate	

LEARNING OBJECTIVES

At the conclusion of this chapter, you should be able to:

1. Define key terms.
2. Calculate measures of morbidity, mortality, and risk of disease for health care facilities and communities.
3. Identify variables that affect morbidity and mortality rates over time.
4. Adjust measures of morbidity and mortality by both the direct and indirect methods of standardization.

5. After adjustment, compare health care facility mortality/morbidity rates with community, state, and/or national rates.
6. Calculate risk of disease between groups.
7. Conduct survival analysis for tumor registries and clinical trials.

It is often said that hospitals and other types of health care facilities are data rich but information poor. There are many types of databases within the facility—disease, operative, and physician's index, to name a few. It is the job of the health information management professional to turn the data contained in these databases into information that can be used by physicians, administrators, and other interested parties. The health information management professional can become an invaluable member of the health care team by providing data that are presented in a meaningful way and by presenting data that have been analyzed to serve a specific medical or clinical need. Some typical questions might be:

- What are the top 25 medical and top 10 surgical diagnosis-related groups (DRGs) for inpatient discharges from our facility?
- Which medical/surgical services admit the most patients?
- Is the average length of stay (ALOS) for these DRGs significantly different from the national ALOS for these DRGs?
- How do our charges compare with national charges? How does our reimbursement compare with our charges?
- What geographical area does the health care facility serve?
- How many patients were admitted to the facility by payer? What is the number of inpatient service days by payer? What are the average charges by payer?
- How do lengths of stay (LOSs) compare by physician?
- How many patients acquired nosocomial infections?

In the course of this text, we will answer these questions. We will learn how to use descriptive statistics to describe patient populations, how to analyze clinical data for significant differences and relationships, and how to present data in graphic form. Our mission is to collect, analyze, and interpret clinical information for both clinical and administrative health care decision makers.

We will begin our discussion of clinical data analysis by reviewing morbidity and mortality measures that are often used to describe patient and community populations.

INTRODUCTION TO FREQUENCY DISTRIBUTIONS

In health care, we deal with vast quantities of clinical data. Since it is very difficult to look at data in raw form, data are summarized into frequency distributions. A **frequency distribution** shows the values that a variable can take and the number of observations associated with each value. A **variable** is a characteristic or property that may take on different values. Height, weight, sex, and third-party payer are examples of variables.

For example, suppose we are studying the variable patient LOS in the pediatric unit. To construct a frequency distribution, we first list all the values that LOS can take, from the lowest observed value to the highest. We then enter the number of observations (frequencies) corresponding to a given LOS. Table 1–1 illustrates what the resulting frequency distribution looks like. Notice that all values for LOS between the lowest and highest are listed, even though there may not be any observations for some of the values. Each column of the distribution is properly labeled; the total is given in the bottom row. We can also display a frequency distribution by categories into which a variable may fall. Table 1–2 shows a frequency distribution for the number of patients discharged from Critical Care Hospital by religion, a variable composed of categories. The proportion for each category is also displayed in the table. The sum of the proportions for each category is equal to 1.0. We will examine frequency distributions in greater detail in Chapter 4.

Table 1–1 Frequency Distribution for Patient Length of Stay (LOS), Pediatric Unit

LOS in Days	No. of Patients
1	2
2	2
3	0
4	6
5	6
6	11
7	6
8	5
9	3
10	1
Total	42

Table 1–2 Frequency Distribution of Number of Patients Discharged from Critical Care Hospital by Religion, July 20xx

Religion	No. of Discharges	Proportion
Protestant	422	.48
Catholic	315	.36
Jewish	20	.02
Other	127	.14
Total	884	1.00

RATIOS, PROPORTIONS, AND RATES

Variables often have only two possible categories, such as alive or dead, or male or female. Variables having only two possible categories are called dichotomous. The frequency measures used with **dichotomous variables** are ratios, proportions, and rates. All three measures are based on the same formula:

$$\text{ratio, proportion, rate} = x/y \times 10^n$$

In this formula, x and y are the two quantities being compared, and x is divided by y. 10^n is read as "10 to the nth power." The size of 10^n may equal, for example, 1, 10, 100, or 1,000, depending on the value of n:

$$10^0 = 1$$
$$10^1 = 10$$
$$10^2 = 10 \times 10 = 100$$
$$10^3 = 10 \times 10 \times 10 = 1,000$$

Ratios

In a **ratio**, the values of a variable, such as sex (x = female, y = male), may be expressed so that x and y are completely independent of each other, or x may be included in y. For example, the sex of patients discharged from a hospital could be compared in either of two ways:

Female/male or x/y
Female/(male + female) or $x/(x + y)$

In the first option, x is completely independent of y, and the ratio represents the number of female discharges compared to the number of male discharges. In the second option, x is a proportion of the whole, $x + y$. The ratio represents the number of female discharges compared to the total number of discharges. Both expressions are considered ratios.

How then would you calculate the female-to-male ratio for a hospital that discharged 457 women and 395 men during the month of July? The procedure for calculating a ratio is outlined in Exhibit 1–1.

Exhibit 1–1 Calculation of a Ratio: Discharges for July 20xx

1. Define x and y.
   x = number of female discharges
   y = number of male discharges
2. Identify x and y.
   $x = 457$
   $y = 395$
3. Set up the ratio x/y.
   457/395
4. Reduce the fraction so that either x or y equals 1.
   1.16/1

There were 1.16 female discharges for every male discharge.

Proportions

A **proportion** is a particular type of ratio. A proportion is a ratio in which x is a portion of the whole, $x + y$. In a proportion, the numerator is always included in the denominator. Exhibit 1–2 outlines the procedure for determining the proportion of hospital discharges for the month of July that were female.

Exhibit 1–2 Calculation of a Proportion: Discharges for July 20xx

1. Define x and y.
   x = number of female discharges
   y = number of male discharges
2. Identify x and y.
   $x = 457$
   $y = 395$
3. Set up the proportion
   $x/(x + y)$.
   457/(457 + 395) = 457/852
4. Reduce the fraction so that either x or $x + y$ equals 1.
   0.54/1.00

The proportion of discharges that were female is 0.54.

Rates

Rates are a third type of frequency measure. In health care, rates are often used to measure an event over time and are sometimes used as performance improvement measures. The basic formula for a rate is

$$\frac{\text{No. of cases or events occurring during a given time period} \times 10^n}{\text{No. of cases or population at risk during same time period}}$$

In inpatient facilities, there are many commonly computed rates. In computing the Caesarean section rate, we count the number of Caesarean sections (C-sections) performed during a given period of time; this value is placed in the numerator. The number of cases or population at risk is the number of women who delivered during the same time period; this number is placed in the denominator. By convention, inpatient hospital rates are calculated as the rate per 100 cases ($10^n = 10^2 = 10 \times 10 = 100$) and are expressed as a percentage. The method for calculating the hospital C-section rate is presented in Exhibit 1–3.

Exhibit 1–3 Calculation of C-Section Rate for July 20xx

> For the month of July, 23 C-sections were performed; during the same time period, 149 women delivered. What is the C-section rate for the month of July?
>
> 1. Define the variable of interest (numerator) and population or number of cases at risk (denominator).
>   Numerator: total number of C-sections performed in July
>   Denominator: total number of women who delivered in July, including C-sections
> 2. Identify the numerator and denominator.
>   Numerator: 23
>   Denominator: 149
> 3. Set up the rate.
>   23/149
> 4. Divide the numerator by the denominator, and multiply by 100 ($10^n = 10^2$).
>   (23/149) x 100 = 15.4%.
>
> The C-section rate for the month of July is 15.4%.

The Glossary of Healthcare Terms[1] presents many of the formulas for calculating these rates. However, once we understand the underlying structure for these computations, we do not always have to rely on rote memorization of them.

POPULATION-BASED MORTALITY MEASURES

As the profession of health information management moves into integrated health care delivery systems and assumes more prominence in managed care organizations, it becomes more important to be familiar with community-based mortality and morbidity data. This type of information is often used in planning health services, such as number of inpatient facilities, type of outpatient facilities, and number or size of managed care plans for a given community, as well as for developing managed care contracts with hospitals and physicians.

Crude Death Rate

The **crude death rate** is a measure of the actual or observed mortality in a given population. Crude rates apply to a population without regard to characteristics of the population, such as the distribution of age or sex. The crude death rate is the starting point for further development of adjusted rates. It measures the proportion of a population that has died during a specific period of time, usually one year, or the number of deaths per 1,000 in a community for a given period of time. The crude death rate is calculated as follows below (the midinterval population is the estimated population of a given community at the midpoint of the time frame under study):

$$\frac{\text{Total deaths during a given time interval}}{\text{Estimated midinterval population}} \times 10n = \text{deaths}/10n$$

In calculating the crude death rate, the power of n is usually equal to the value that will result in a value greater than 1. This allows for easier interpretation of the rate—a death rate of less than 1 per 100 is not very meaningful. For example, the 1999 midyear population of Anytown, USA, is 1,996,355; 275 deaths occurred in 1999. The power of n that will result in a whole number is 4; $10^4 = 10 \times 10 \times 10 \times 10 = 10,000$. The crude death rate is calculated as follows:

$$(275 \times 10,000)/1,996,355 = 2,750,000/1,996,355 = 1.38 \text{ deaths per } 10,000$$

When analyzing crude death rates, or any type of rate, it is important to remember that these events do not occur in a vacuum. When analyzing any data set, we need to remember that the data do not stand alone but reflect trends in the environment. Trends in death rates can be influenced by three variables: time, place, and person. Examples of time, place, and person variables are outlined in Exhibit 1–4.

An example of how trended data may be affected by time, place, and person variables is presented in Figure 1–1. The line graph shows that the number of newly diagnosed acquired immune deficiency syndrome (AIDS) cases steadily increased from 1983 to 1992; then a rather dramatic increase occurred in 1993, which was then followed by a return to previous levels in 1994 and 1995. What happened in 1993 that resulted in such a large increase in the number of newly diagnosed AIDS cases?

Exhibit 1–4 Variables Affecting Trends in Community Morbidity and Mortality Rates

- Time
  - Revisions in International Classification of Diseases, 9th Revision (ICD-9) coding of death certificates
  - Improvements in medical technology
  - Earlier detection and diagnosis of disease
- Place
  - Changes in environments
  - International and intranational differences in medical technology and the use of medical technology
  - Diagnostic practices of physicians
  - Variation in physician practice patterns by region
- Person
  - Age
  - Sex
  - Ethnicity
  - Social habits (smoking, diet, alcohol)
  - Genetic background
  - Emotional and mental characteristics

Figure 1–1 AIDS Cases Diagnosed in Ohio by Year, 1983–1995. *Source:* Reprinted from *Prevention Monthly*, Vol. 19, No. 3, p. 6, 1996, Ohio Department of Health.

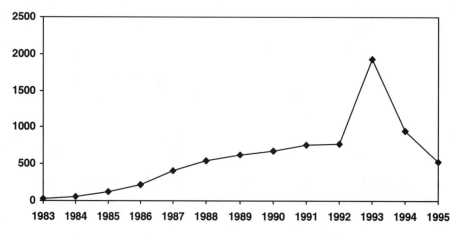

This is an example of how the time variable can affect the number of cases diagnosed. In 1993, the case definition of AIDS changed so that individuals who were human immunodeficiency virus (HIV) positive were designated as having full-blown AIDS at an earlier point in the progression of their disease. In 1993, the case definition was expanded to include HIV-positive cases with low CD4 counts, pulmonary tuberculosis, and recurrent pneumonia as AIDS qualifying conditions. The result was that a large number of HIV-positive individuals who already had one of these conditions suddenly qualified as AIDS cases.

Now let's return to our discussion of the crude death rate. Crude rates do not allow for valid comparisons across populations because of differences in the populations—primarily age. This is because age is the most important variable that influences mortality. To illustrate, let's compare two hypothetical crude mortality rates for the states of Arizona (10.9/1,000) and Alaska (4.4/1,000). The conclusion drawn from a comparison of the crude mortality rates is that the death rate is 148% higher in Arizona than in Alaska: (10.9 – 4.4)/4.4. However, the discrepancy is due largely to the age differences in the populations of Arizona and Alaska. In general, the population in Arizona is older than the population in Alaska. Without adjusting the rate, one might erroneously conclude that the Alaskan population was healthier than the population of Arizona. In this example, the comparison is confounded by age. **Confounding factor** is a general term used to describe the effect of a third variable on the estimate of risk of a health outcome.

Confounding occurs when a third factor related to outcome is differentially distributed across the levels (or categories) of a variable of interest. When this happens, we must take measures to separate the effect of the **confounding variable**—in this case, age—from the effect of the variable of interest. We may accomplish this by selecting subjects to be compared so that they are matched with respect to the confounding variables or by using statistical adjustments during analysis to remove the effect of the confounding variable. For example, review the data in Table 1–3. Analysis of the data reveals that the overall crude rate between blacks and whites is similar but that the age-specific death rate for blacks is higher than the rates for whites in every group. Why is there such a contradiction? It is because the 1995 population of the state of Alabama consisted of old whites and young blacks —32.6% of the white population was 24 years old or younger, and 45.0% of the black population was 24 years old or younger.

Table 1–3 Age-Specific Death Rates per 1,000 Population by Race, Alabama, 1995

Race	Crude Rate	<1 Yr.	1–4 Yr.	5–14 Yr.	15–24 Yr.	25–44 Yr.	45–64 Yr.	≥65 Yr.
White	10.08	7.14	0.42	0.27	1.10	1.93	7.73	52.30
Black	10.03	15.20	0.98	0.52	1.66	3.79	13.51	61.20

Source: Data from Centers for Disease Control and Prevention, CDC Wonder Data Base, http://wonder.cdc.gov.

Age-Specific Death Rates

In Table 1–3, we see the **age-specific death rates** (ASDR) for both whites and blacks. The ASDR is calculated as follows:

$$\frac{\text{No. of deaths in the age group of interest}}{\text{Estimated midperiod population in the age group of interest}} \times 10n$$

Age-Adjusted Death Rates

Age-adjusted death rates are used when there are differences in the age distribution for the populations that are being compared. In Table 1–4, you can see that the population proportions for each age group vary slightly by race. For example, the proportion of whites that are older than age 65 is 0.142 (14.2%), and the proportion of blacks that are older than 65 is 0.099 (9.9%). When we adjust the crude rate for age, we are constructing a summary rate that is free of age bias. In Table 1–4, the ASDR for each age group is expressed as a percentage. There are two methods for adjusting the crude death rate—direct and indirect. We will first discuss the direct method of standardization.

Table 1–4 Calculation of Crude Death Rate, Alabama, 1995

Age Group	(a) White Pop.	(b) Pop. Prop.	(c) Deaths	(d) ASDR (c/a) x 100	(d) Black Pop.	(e) Pop. Prop.	(f) Deaths	(g) ASDR (f/d) x 100
<1	39,759	0.013	284	0.71	19,868	0.018	302	1.52
1–4	159,202	0.051	67	0.04	78,863	0.072	77	0.10
5–14	391,255	0.126	104	0.03	191,320	0.175	100	0.05
15–24	423,303	0.136	465	0.11	202,525	0.185	336	0.17
25–44	948,788	0.305	1,834	0.19	323,950	0.296	1,228	0.38
45–64	704,351	0.227	5,445	0.77	170,728	0.156	2,307	1.35
65+	442,471	0.142	23,142	5.23	108,396	0.099	6,634	6.12
Total	3,109,129	1.000	31,341	1.01	1,095,650	1.000	10,984	1.00

Crude Death Rate = 1.01/100   Crude Death Rate = 1.00/100

Source: Data from Centers for Disease Control and Prevention, CDC Wonder Data Base, http://wonder.cdc.gov.

Direct Standardization

To age-adjust the crude death rates, we compare the two groups being studied to a standard population. We then apply the ASDRs for each group to this standard population. As an example, we will use the data in Table 1–4 to standardize the crude death rates for whites and blacks in the state of Alabama. The crude death rate for whites is 1.01 per 100, and the crude death rate for blacks is 1.00 per 100. The difference between the crude rates is not significant.

To calculate the standardized rate, we first calculate the ASDR for each age group in the two populations. We then combine the populations for each age group. By multiplying ASDR for each group by the combined population, we can obtain the expected number of deaths for each group as if the population for each age group were the same. For example, for the age group from 1 to 4 years, we add 159,202 and 78,863 to obtain a total of 238,065. We then multiply the combined population total for each age group by the ASDR to obtain the expected number of deaths for each age group in each of the populations being compared.

Thus, the groups are compared on an equal basis. The expected death rate for each population is calculated as follows:

Group	Age	Total Population
White	1–4	238,065
Black	1–4	238,065

ASDR	Expected No. of Deaths
.0004	95.2
.0010	238.1

After we have calculated the expected number of deaths for each age group in each population, we sum the expected number of deaths in each population group, as in Table 1–5. For whites the total number of expected deaths is 39,348.4, and for blacks the total is 52,862.7. The expected number of deaths for each population group is then divided by the combined population. The result is that the standardized age-adjusted death rate for blacks is slightly higher (1.26%) than that for whites (0.94%).

Table 1–5 Calculation of Adjusted Death Rate—Direct Standardization

Age Group	(a) Total Population	(b) ASDR Whites	(c) Expected No. of Deaths (a x b)	(d) ASDR Blacks	(e) Expected No. of Deaths (a x d)
<1	59,627	.0071	423.4	.0152	906.3
1–4	238,065	.0004	95.2	.0010	238.1
5–14	582,575	.0003	174.8	.0005	291.3
15–24	625,828	.0011	688.4	.0017	1,063.9
25–44	1,272,738	.0019	2,418.2	.0038	4,836.4
45–64	875,079	.0077	6,738.1	.0135	11,813.6
65+	550,867	.0523	28,810.3	.0612	33,713.1
Total	4,204,479	.0708	39,348.4	.0100	52,862.7

Standardized Age-Adjusted Rate = 0.94%
(39,348.4/4,204,779)

Standardized Age-Adjusted Rate = 1.26%
(52,862.7/4,204,779)

Source: Data from Centers for Disease Control and Prevention, CDC Wonder Data Base, http://wonder.cdc.gov.

Even though the standardized adjusted rate is not "real," it allows researchers to make better comparisons between groups. Although the crude rates are virtually the same, the adjusted rates indicate that mortality among blacks is slightly higher than that for whites. Without adjustment, we would make the assumption that there was no difference in mortality between the two groups. An adjusted rate informs us that this may not necessarily be the case.

Indirect Standardization

The indirect method of standardization is used when ASDRs are not available or when the population that we wish to compare is small, as when we are comparing hospital inpatients to much larger populations. When using this method, we use standard rates obtained from some population and apply them to our population of interest. The basic steps for indirect standardization appear in Exhibit 1–5. In our hypothetical example, we compare 1995 Utah hospital discharges that resulted in death due to pneumonia to the number of hospital discharges that resulted in death due to pneumonia in Salt Lake County, Utah.

Exhibit 1–5 Basic Steps for Indirect Standardization

1. Determine the standard mortality rates for pneumonia in the state of Utah for the age groups of interest.
2. Multiply the ASDR for the state of Utah (column c) times the number of county discharges in each age category to obtain the expected number of deaths for each category (columns c × d = column f) in Salt Lake County, Utah.
3. Sum the number of expected deaths.
4. Compute the standard mortality ratio (SMR), which compares the number of actual or observed deaths to the number of expected deaths. In Table 1–6, the number of actual or observed deaths is 86, and the number of expected deaths is 76.93.
5. Multiply the SMR by 100. The SMR is interpreted as a percentage lesser or greater than that of the standard population.

Table 1–6 Mortality Rates Due to Pneumonia (ICD-9 Codes 480–486.9), 1995, Ages 35+, State of Utah versus Salt Lake County, Utah

	State of Utah			Salt Lake County, Utah		
Age	(a) Utah Discharges	(b) No. of Deaths	(c) ASDR (b x 100)/a	(d) County Discharges	(e) Observed Deaths	(f) Expected Deaths (c x d)
35–45	366	7	1.91	154	3	2.94
45–54	392	9	2.30	162	2	3.73
55–64	522	22	4.21	197	9	8.29
65–74	940	53	5.64	322	27	18.16
75+	1,874	133	7.10	617	45	43.81
	4,094	224	5.47	1,452	86	76.93

Source: Reprinted from Utah Inpatient Hospital Discharge Data Set, http://hlunix.ex.state.ut.us/had.

In our calculations in Table 1–6, we see that the overall mortality rate due to pneumonia in the state of Utah is 5.47% and that the mortality rate in Salt Lake County is 5.92% [(86 x 100)/1,452]. Salt Lake County had 9.07 more deaths than what was expected on the basis of the standard rates for the state of Utah; therefore, the expected mortality rate is 5.30% [(76.93 × 100)/1,452]. To make the comparison to the standard rates, we calculate a **standard mortality ratio** (SMR). The SMR compares the actual number of deaths in the group under study (Salt Lake County) to the expected number of deaths based on the standard population rates that were applied to the study group. For the data in Table 1–6, the SMR is calculated as

$$SMR = \frac{\text{Observed death rate}}{\text{Expected death rate}} = \frac{0.0592}{0.0530} =$$
$$1.12 \times 100 = 112\%$$

If the calculated SMR is equal to 100, the number of observed deaths is the same as the number of expected deaths. If the SMR is greater than 100, the number of observed deaths is greater than the number of expected deaths; conversely, the interpretation of the SMR is that Salt Lake County's pneumonia death rate is 12% greater than that for the state of Utah. Stated another way, the death rate is 12% greater than what would be expected on the basis of the **mortality rates** due to pneumonia for the entire state of Utah.

In summary, rates are adjusted to remove the effect of the confounding factor for which the adjustment has been made—in this case, age. However, it is always necessary to calculate the crude rate because this represents the actual event. An adjusted rate is used for comparative purposes; adjusted rates do not reveal the underlying raw data that are shown by the crude rates.

Race- and Sex-Specific Death Rates

Mortality rates may be calculated for any variable of interest, such as race or sex, using the same basic formula specified for calculating the crude death rate. In general, men have higher mortality rates than women. In 1995, the sex-specific rate was 9.2 per 1,000 for men and 8.6 per 1,000 for women. It would be misleading to review the **sex-specific death rates** without review of the individual age-specific rates. Table 1–7 indicates that the death rate for men is significantly higher for every age group. If we want to determine why the death rate of men is higher than that for women, we can compare causes of death by sex and age group. For example, in the combined age groups from 15 to 44 years, the death rate for men is higher than that for women because accidental death is the leading cause of death for men in these age groups. Sex-specific diseases may account for the differences in the death rates for other age groups, such as prostate cancer in men and breast cancer in women. Calculating the age-specific rates and sex-specific rates can help us better understand what is taking place in the health care environment.

Table 1–7 Gender-Specific Death Rates, United States, 1995

Age Group	Men			Women			ASDR
	Population	Deaths	Rate/ 1,000	Population	Deaths	Rate/ 1,000	
0–4	10,051,688	20,231	2.013	9,590,943	15,745	1.642	1.83
5–14	19,528,541	5,219	0.267	18,605,947	3,377	0.182	0.23
15–24	18,352,070	25,777	1.405	17,594,565	8,467	0.481	0.95
25–34	20,431,915	41,826	2.047	20,441,224	15,919	0.779	1.41
35–44	21,061,683	70,131	3.330	21,406,036	32,139	1.501	2.41
45–54	15,181,651	90,922	5.989	15,897,109	52,078	3.276	4.60
55–64	10,044,058	142,290	14.167	11,087,026	93,222	8.408	11.15
65–74	8,342,094	274,001	32.846	10,417,069	206,889	19.861	25.63
75–84	4,329,706	319,408	73.771	6,815,274	332,769	48.827	58.52
85+	1,016,875	182,823	179.789	2,611,279	378,436	144.924	154.70
	128,340,281	1,172,628	9.137	134,466,472	1,139,041	8.471	8.80

Source: Data from Centers for Disease Control and Prevention, CDC Wonder Data Base, http://wonder.cdc.gov.

Cause-Specific Death Rates

The **cause-specific death rate** is the death rate due to a specified cause. It may be stated for an entire population or for any age, sex, or race. The numerator is the number of deaths due to a specified cause and the denominator is the size of the population at midyear. It is usually expressed in terms of a rate per 100,000 ($10^n = 10^5 = 100,000$). The formula is

$$\frac{\text{Deaths assigned to a specified cause}}{\text{during a given time interval} \times 100,000}{\text{Estimated midinterval population}}$$

Table 1–8 presents the cause-specific death rates for males and females. The cause-specific death rate for pneumonia in the population aged 65 or older is 210.85 per 100,000. The cause-specific rates for each age group are consistently higher for men than for women. This may lead us to investigate why men are more susceptible to pneumonia than women. In reviewing the rates in Table 1–6, we can also see that the death rate increases with age for both men and women.

Table 1–8 Cause-Specific Mortality Rates Due to Pneumonia (ICD-9 Codes 480–486.9), Age 65+, United States, 1995

Age Group	Men			Women			
	Population	Deaths	Rate/ 100,000	Population	Deaths	Rate/ 100,000	ASDR
65–74	8,342,094	6,223	74.60	10,417,069	1,358	13.04	40.41
75–84	4,329,706	13,154	303.81	6,815,274	12,696	186.29	231.94
85+	1,016,875	13,000	1,278.43	2,611,279	24,275	929.62	1,027.38
	13,688,675	32,377	236.52	19,843,622	38,329	193.62	210.85

Source: Data from Centers for Disease Control and Prevention, CDC Wonder Data Base, http://wonder.cdc.gov.

Case Fatality Rate

The **case fatality rate** or killing power of a disease measures the probability of death among the diagnosed cases of a disease. The higher the ratio, the more virulent the infection. It is most often used as a measure in acute infectious disease. The case fatality rate is not useful in chronic disease because such diseases have a longer and more variable course.

The formula for the case-fatality rate is

$$\frac{\text{No. of deaths due to a disease during a given time interval} \times 100}{\text{No. of cases of the disease in the same time interval}}$$

Proportionate Mortality Ratio

The **proportionate mortality ratio** (PMR) describes the proportion of all deaths for a given time interval that are due to a specific cause. Each cause is expressed as a percentage of all deaths, and the sum of all the causes is 1.00 (100%). The PMR is not a mortality rate, since the denominator is all deaths, not the population in which the deaths occurred. Its formula is:

$$\frac{\text{No. of deaths due to a disease during a given time interval} \times 100}{\text{No. of deaths from all causes in the same time interval}}$$

The PMR is often used to make comparisons between and within age groups and occupational groups as well as for the general population. The PMR for pneumonia appears in Table 1–9.

Table 1–9 Proportionate Mortality Ratios for Pneumonia (ICD-9 Codes 480–486.9), United States, 1995

Age Group	Pneumonia Deaths	All Deaths	PMR/100
0–4	634	35,976	1.76
5–14	121	8,596	1.41
15–24	201	34,244	0.59
25–34	621	57,745	1.08
35–44	1,466	102,270	1.43
45–54	2,061	143,000	1.44
55–64	3,427	235,512	1.46
65–74	10,657	480,890	2.22
75–84	25,850	652,177	3.96
85+	37,275	561,259	6.64
	82,313	2,311,669	3.56

Source: Data from Centers for Disease Control and Prevention, CDC Wonder Data Base, http://wonder.cdc.gov.

Maternal Mortality Rate

The **maternal mortality rate** measures deaths associated with pregnancy. Pregnancy often places a woman at risk for medical problems that would not usually be encountered in the nonpregnant state, such as hemorrhage or toxemia of pregnancy. Pregnancy also complicates chronic conditions such as diabetes mellitus and heart disease. In some women, pregnancy precipitates gestational diabetes. The rate is calculated only for deaths that are related to pregnancy; thus, if a pregnant woman is killed in an automobile accident, the death is not considered a pregnancy-related death.

The numerator is the number of deaths assigned to causes related to pregnancy during a given time period; the denominator is the number of live births reported during the same period. Because the maternal mortality rate is usually very small, it is usually expressed as the number of deaths per 100,000 live births.

Rates of Infant Mortality

There are three rates of infant mortality, all of which are based on age. Of the three, the infant mortality rate is the most commonly used measure for comparing health status between nations. All three rates are expressed in terms of the number of deaths per 1,000.

Neonatal Mortality Rate

The neonatal period is defined as the period from birth up to but not including 28 days of age. The numerator is the number of deaths of infants under 28 days of age during a given time period; the denominator is the total number of live births reported during the same period. The **neonatal mortality rate** may be used as an indirect measure of the quality of prenatal care and/or the mother's prenatal behavior (e.g., tobacco, alcohol, and drug use).

Postneonatal Mortality Rate

The postneonatal period is the time period from 28 days of age up to but not including one year of age. The numerator is the number of deaths among children from age 28 days up to but not including one year of age during a given time period; the denominator is the total number of live births reported less the number of neonatal deaths during the same period. The **postneonatal mortality rate** is often used as an indicator of the quality of the infant's home environment.

Infant Mortality Rate

In effect, the **infant mortality rate** is a summary of the neonatal and postneonatal mortality rates. The numerator is the number of deaths among children under one year of age; the denominator is the number of live births reported during the same period. Table 1–10 provides a summary of these rates.

Table 1–10 Frequently Used Mortality Measures

Measure	Numerator (x)	Denominator	10^n
Crude death rate	Total no. of deaths reported during a given time interval	Estimated midinterval population	1,000 or 10,000
Cause-specific death rate	Total no. of deaths due to a specific cause during a given time interval	Estimated midinterval population	100,000
Proportionate mortality ratio	Total no. of deaths due to a specific cause during a given time interval	Total no. of deaths from all causes during the same time interval	100 or 1,000
Case fatality rate	Total no. of deaths assigned to a specific disease during a given time interval	Total no. of cases of the disease during the same time interval	100
Neonatal mortality rate	No. of deaths under 28 days of age during a given time interval	No. of live births during the same time interval	1,000
Postneonatal rate	No. of deaths from 28 days up to and not including one year of age, during a given time interval	No. of live births during the same time interval less neonatal deaths	1,000
Infant mortality rate	No. of deaths under one year of age during a given time interval	No. of live births during the same time interval	1,000
Maternal mortality rate	No. of deaths assigned to pregnancy-related causes during a given time interval	No. of live births during the same time interval	100,000

Source: Adapted from *Principles of Epidemiology: An Introduction to Applied Epidemiology and Biostatistics*, pp. 100 and 116, 1992, U.S. Department of Health and Human Services, Public Health Service.

FREQUENTLY USED MEASURES OF MORBIDITY

Some commonly used measures to describe the presence of disease in a community or a specific location, such as a nursing home, are incidence and prevalence rates. Disease can be illness, injury, or disability, and measures can be further elaborated into specific measures of age, sex, race, or other characteristics of a particular population.

Incidence Rate

The **incidence rate** is the commonly used measure for comparing frequency of disease in populations. Populations are compared using rates instead of raw numbers because rates adjust for differences in the size of the populations. The incidence rate expresses the probability or risk of illness in a population over a period of time. The formula for calculating the incidence rate is:

$$\frac{\text{Total no. of new cases of a specific disease during a given time interval} \times 10^n}{\text{Total population at risk during the same time interval}}$$

For the incidence rate, the denominator represents the population from which the case in the numerator arose, such as a nursing home, school, or company. For 10^n, a value is selected so that the smallest rate calculated results in a whole number.

Prevalence Rate

The **prevalence rate** is the proportion of persons in a population that have a particular disease at a specific point in time or over a specified period of time. The formula for calculating the prevalence rate is

$$\frac{\text{All new and preexisting cases of a specific disease during a given time interval} \times 10^n}{\text{Total population during the same time period}}$$

Incidence and prevalence rates are often confused. The rates differ in which cases are included in the numerator. The numerator of the incidence rate is new cases occurring during a given time period; the numerator of the prevalence rate is all cases present during a given time period. In comparing the two, you can see that the incidence rate includes only individuals whose illness began during a specified period of time; whereas the numerator for the prevalence rate includes all individuals ill from a specified cause, regardless of when the illness began. A case is counted in prevalence until the individual recovers. Exhibit 1–6 presents an example of incidence and prevalence rates in a nursing home.

Exhibit 1–6 Calculation of Incidence and Prevalence Rates of *Klebsiella pneumoniae* at the Manor Nursing Home, Month of January

---

At Manor Nursing Home, 10 new cases of *Klebsiella pneumoniae* occurred in January. For the month of January there were a total of 17 cases of *Klebsiella pneumoniae*. The facility had 250 residents during January.

What are the incidence and prevalence rates for *Klebsiella pneumoniae* during January?

Incidence Rate

1. Identify the variable of interest (numerator) and population at risk (denominator).

   Numerator: Total no. of new cases of *Klebsiella pneumoniae* in January
   Denominator: Total no. of nursing home residents in January

2. Identify the numerator and denominator.

   Numerator: 10
   Denominator: 250

3. Set up the rate.

   10/250

4. Divide the numerator by the denominator and multiply by 100 ($10^n = 10^2$)

   $(10/250) \times 100 = .04 = 4.0\%$

   The incidence rate for *Klebsiella pneumoniae* for the month of January is 4.0%.

Prevalence Rate

1. Identify the variable of interest (numerator) and population at risk (denominator).

   Numerator: total no. of cases of *Klebsiella pneumoniae* in January
   Denominator: total no. of nursing home residents in January

2. Identify the numerator and denominator.

   Numerator: 17
   Denominator: 250

3. Set up the rate.

   17/250

4. Divide the numerator by the denominator and multiply by 100 ($10^n = 10^2$). $(17/250) \times 100 = .068 = 6.8\%$

   The prevalence rate for *Klebsiella pneumoniae* for the month of January is 6.8%.

At times we may be interested in tracking prevalence rates more closely—for example, tracking *Klebsiella pneumoniae* on a daily basis. We can do this by calculating the point prevalence rate. The **point prevalence rate** is the number of cases of a specific disease at a specific point in time. The point prevalence rate is more narrow in its time frame than the general prevalence rate. Table 1–11 displays the point prevalence rates for each day during one week in January.

For a summary of morbidity measures, see Table 1–12.

Table 1–11 Point Prevalence Rates of *Klebsiella pneumoniae* for the Manor Nursing Home, Week of January 3

	Sun	*Mon*	*Tues*	*Wed*	*Thurs*	*Fri*	*Sat*
No. of cases	10	12	14	13	15	16	16
No. of residents	250	250	250	250	250	250	250
Point prevalence rate	4.0%	4.8%	5.6%	5.2%	6.0%	6.4%	6.4%

Table 1–12 Frequently Used Measures of Morbidity

Measure	*Numerator*	*Denominator*
Basic formula for computing rates	No. of events occurring during a given time interval	No. of cases or population at risk during the same time interval
Incidence rate	Total no. of new cases of a specific disease during a given time interval	Total population at risk during the same time interval
Prevalence rate	All new and preexisting cases of a specific disease during a given time interval	Total population during the same time interval
Relative risk	Risk for exposed group	Risk for unexposed group
Relative risk using incidence rates	Incidence rate for group of primary interest	Incidence rate for comparison group
Attributable risk	Risk for exposed group minus risk for unexposed group	Risk for exposed group

Source: Data from *Principles of Epidemiology: An Introduction to Applied Epidemiology and Biostatistics*, 1992, U.S. Department of Health and Human Services, Public Health Service.

RELATIVE MEASURES OF DISEASE FREQUENCY

Risk Ratio/Relative Risk

Relative risk (RR) is a ratio that compares the risk of disease or other health event between two groups. What we are comparing is the actual risk of illness between the two groups. In calculating relative risk, we are using the actual rates of illness for each group to make the comparison. The two groups may be differentiated by demographic variables, such as sex or race, or by exposure to a suspected risk factor.

The group of primary interest is labeled as the *exposed* group, and the comparison group is labeled the *unexposed* group. The exposed group is placed in the numerator, and the unexposed group is placed in the denominator:

$$\frac{\text{Risk for exposed group}}{\text{Risk for unexposed group}}$$

A risk ratio of 1.0 indicates that the risk is identical in both groups; a risk ratio greater than 1.0 indicates that the risk is greater for the numerator group; and a risk ratio of less than 1.0 indicates that the risk is less for the numerator group.

As an example, we can compare the risk of death due to pneumonia in men versus women in Michigan in 1995. First, the collected data are summarized in a two-by-two table. *Two-by-two* refers to two variables, each with two categories, as shown in Table 1–13.

Table 1–13 Relative Risk of Death Due to Pneumonia, Women versus Men Aged 75 to 84, State of Michigan, 1995

Sex	Death Due to Pneumonia		Total
	Yes	No	
Men	240	299,405	299,645
	(a)	(b)	(a + b)
Women	155	370,696	370,851
	(c)	(d)	(c + d)

Risk of illness among men:
$a/(a + b) = 240/(240 + 299{,}405) = .0008$
Risk of illness among women:
$c/(c + d) = 155/(155 + 370{,}696) = .0004$
Risk ratio, men to women: $.0008/.0004 = 2$
Thus, the risk of death due to pneumonia among men aged 75 to 84 is two times greater than the risk of death due to pneumonia in women in the same age group.

Source: Data from Centers for Disease Control and Prevention, CDC Wonder Data Base, http://wonder.cdc.gov.

To determine the risk of death among men, we compare the total number of men who died from pneumonia ($a = 240$) to the total number of men in the group of interest ($a + b = 240 + 299{,}405$). The same procedure is followed to determine the risk of death due to pneumonia among women. The two ratios are then compared to determine the RR of death due to pneumonia among men as compared to women. A summary of these calculations appears in Table 1–13. Note that even though the risk of death among men is 2 times greater than the risk of death among women, the RR in each group is rather small, 0.08% and 0.04% respectively.

Table 1–14 Lung Cancer Data

Cigarettes/Day	Death Rate/1,000/Year
0	0.07
1–14	0.57
15–24	1.39
25+	2.27

Rate ratios:
1–14 cigarettes/day to nonsmokers:
  0.57/0.07 = 8.1
15–24 cigarettes/day to nonsmokers:
  1.39/0.07 = 19.9
25+ cigarettes/day to nonsmokers:
  2.27/0.07 = 32.4
Thus, the risk is 8.1 times greater for those who smoke 1 to 14 cigarettes per day than for nonsmokers; 19.9 times greater for those who smoke 15 to 24 cigarettes per day than for nonsmokers; and 32.4 times greater for those who smoke 25+ cigarettes per day than for nonsmokers.

Source: Adapted from *Principles of Epidemiology: An Introduction to Applied Epidemiology and Biostatistics*, p. 95, 1992, U.S. Department of Health and Human Services, Public Health Service.

Instead of using the risk ratios to compare risks between groups, we can use actual rates to make the same comparisons. In Table 1–14, hypothetical mortality rates are used to compare the risk of death due to lung cancer by number of cigarettes smoked per day.

Using the same procedure, we can compare the risk of stroke between men who smoke and men who do not smoke. In this example, we are trying to determine if there is a greater risk of stroke among men who smoke than among men who do not smoke. The statistic is called "relative risk using incidence rates" and is calculated as

$$\frac{\text{Incidence rate for group of primary interest}}{\text{Incidence rate for comparison group}}$$

The data for this example are presented in Table 1–15. Notice that these ratios represent only RR, or the possibility of acquiring an illness, in comparison to another group.

Table 1–15 Twelve-Year Risk of Stroke among Male Smokers and Nonsmokers

Smokers	Stroke		Total
	Yes	No	
Yes	171	3,264	3,435
No	117	4,320	4,437
Total	288	7,584	7,872

Risk of stroke among smokers:
171/3,435 = .049
Risk of stroke among nonsmokers:
117/4,437 = .026
Risk of stroke of male smokers to male non-smokers: .049/.026 = 1.88
Thus, the risk of stroke is 1.88, or almost two times greater in men who smoke than men who do not smoke.

Odds Ratio

The **odds ratio** (OR) is another relative measure of occurrence of illness. The odds in favor of a particular event are defined as the frequency with which the event occurs divided by the frequency with which it does not occur. Estimates of RR and the OR are both used to measure the strength of the association between exposure and disease. The OR is an estimate of RR. It is calculated from data obtained from retrospective studies where actual incidence rates are not calculated.

To calculate the OR, a two-by-two table is first constructed as shown in Table 1–16. Exhibit 1–7 displays the calculation of the odds ratio using the data from Table 1–15. The results indicate that the odds of having a stroke is 1.93 times greater in men who smoke than in men who do not smoke.

Table 1–16 Two-by-Two Table for Odds Ratio

	Disease	
Risk Factor	Cases	Non-cases
Present	a	b
Absent	c	d

Odds ratio = $(a \times d)/(b \times c)$, where a = number of persons with disease and with exposure of interest, b = number of persons without disease and with exposure of interest, c = number of persons with disease but without exposure of illness, and d = number of persons without disease and without exposure of interest.

$a + c$ = total persons with disease (cases)

$b + d$ = total persons without disease (controls)

Exhibit 1–7 Procedure for Calculating Odds Ratio (OR)

$$OR = \frac{a}{b} \div \frac{c}{d}$$

$$= \frac{a \times d}{b \times c}$$

$$OR = \frac{171 \times 4,320}{3,264 \times 117}$$

$$= 1.93$$

The probability of having a stroke is 1.93 times greater in men who smoke than in men who do not smoke.

The interpretation of the OR is similar to that for RR. If the exposure is not related to the diagnosis, the OR will equal 1; if the exposure is positively related to the disease, the OR will be greater than 1; and if the exposure is negative, the OR will be less than 1.

We could also apply this same ratio, or any others, to the acute care setting. An outcomes evaluator learns that patients on the surgical unit were exposed to the *E. coli* bacterium. Data were collected for two weeks to determine if the odds for obtaining *E. coli* infection were greater for patients on the surgical units than for patients hospitalized on the medical unit. The data are displayed in Table 1–17. As you can see from the calculations for the OR, the odds or probability of obtaining an *E. coli* infection is 2.68 times greater for a patient hospitalized on the surgical unit than for a patient hospitalized on a medical unit.

Table 1–17 *E. coli* Infections of Medical and Surgical Patients

Hospital Unit	Nosocomial Infection		Total
	Yes	No	
Surgical unit	20	628	648
Medical unit	10	842	852
Total	30	1,470	1,500

The odds ratio is calculated as follows:
$$OR = (a \times d)/(b \times c) = (20 \times 842)/(10 \times 628) = 2.68$$

When the health outcome is uncommon, the OR approximates the RR. Using the same data from Table 1–17, we can determine the RR as follows:

$$\frac{\text{Risk of infection on surgical unit: } 20/648 = .031}{\text{Risk of infection on medical unit: } 10/852 = .012}$$

Risk of infection on surgical unit compared to medical unit: $.031/.012 = 2.58$

As you can see, the results for both the OR and the RR are similar, 2.68 and 2.58 respectively.

Attributable Risk

The **attributable risk** (AR) is a measure of the impact of a disease or other causative factor on a population. With this calculation, we assume that the occurrence of the disease in a group not exposed to the risk factor represents the baseline or expected risk for that disease; any risk above that level in the exposed group is attributed to exposure to the risk factor. Basically, the assumption is that the disease will occur in some individuals even without exposure to a given risk factor. The AR measures the additional risk of illness as a result of an individual's exposure to the risk factor.

With AR, we attempt to answer the question "How much of the disease that occurs can be attributed to a certain exposure?" and subsequently, "How much of the risk of disease can we prevent if we eliminate the exposure to the risk factor in question?"

$$\frac{\text{(Risk for exposed group)} - \text{(risk for unexposed group)}}{\text{Risk for exposed group}}$$

$$\times\ 100$$

Using the lung cancer data from Table 1–14, we calculate the attributable proportion as outlined in Exhibit 1–8.

Exhibit 1–8 Calculation of Attributable Proportion

1. Identify the exposed group rate.
   Lung cancer death rate for smokers of 1–14 cigarettes per day = 0.57 per 1,000 per year
2. Identify the unexposed group rate.
   0.07 per 1,000 per year
3. Calculate the attributable proportion.

$$\frac{0.57 - 0.07}{0.57} \times 100 = 87.7$$

The conclusion from the calculation of the attributable proportion is that 87.7% of the lung cancer cases are due to or attributed to smoking 1 to 14 cigarettes per day. Approximately 12% (1.00 − .877) of the cases in this group would have occurred without exposure to the risk factor—in this case, cigarettes. By carrying out the calculations for the remaining two groups, we can see that the AR increases with the number of cigarettes smoked per day.

$$\text{AR 15–24 cigarettes/day} = [(1.39 - 0.07)/1.39] \times 100 = 95.0\%$$

$$\text{AR 25+ cigarettes/day} = [(2.27 - 0.07)/2.27] \times 100 = 96.9\%$$

Approximately 5% and 3%, respectively, of the individuals in these two groups would have acquired the disease regardless.

KAPLAN MEIER SURVIVAL ANALYSIS

Many individuals within the health information management profession are employed in tumor registries or in the capacity of assisting researchers in analyzing data from clinical trials. In clinical trials, the researcher is interested in determining whether a specific medical or surgical intervention improves survival for a particular condition. A major criterion in measuring the success of a clinical trial is the survival time of individuals undergoing the experimental treatment. There are several methods for analyzing survival rates, but we will limit the discussion to the Kaplan Meier method, a type of life table analysis, since it is most often used in analysis of data collected from clinical trials. **Kaplan-Meier survival analysis** requires a dichotomous outcome such as survival/death or improvement/no improvement.

The major reason for using the Kaplan Meier method is that it takes into account some of the problems commonly encountered when conducting prospective studies. Calculating survival rates is often complicated by the fact that patients are lost to follow-up after completion of the clinical trial. The Kaplan Meier method compensates for subjects who are lost to follow-up or who choose to withdraw from the study. To conduct an accurate survival analysis, we need to know

- reason for patients' withdrawal from the study (i.e., death, loss to follow-up, or censorship)
- date of withdrawal from study (i.e., date of death, date patient last seen alive or lost to follow-up, or date withdrawn alive or censored)

When survival time is censored, the subject is alive at the time of analysis or was alive at the time of analysis or when last seen. Survival times tagged with a "+" indicate that they are censored.

Table 1–18 presents some hypothetical data for 10 patients in a clinical trial for treatment of bladder cancer. The survival times, in months (column 1), for each patient are rank ordered from lowest to highest.

Each row in Table 1–18 represents an interval. The first row is the first study interval. An interval is a death-free time period. So row 1, column 6, represents a death-free time period

Table 1–18 Hypothetical Data on Survival Times for Bladder Cancer Patients

(1) Survival Time Mo.	(2) No. Living Prior to Subject's Death	(3) No. Living after Subject's Death	(4) # Lost to Follow-Up	(5) p_x	(6) Interval for p_x (Mo.)	(7) p_x at End of Interval
—	—	—	—	1.000	0 to <23	1.000
23	10	9	—	0.900	23 to <34	0.900
34	9	8	—	0.889	34 to <37	0.800
37	8	7	—	0.875	37 to <41	0.700
40+			1	—	—	—
41	6	5	—	0.833	41 to <42	0.583
42	5	4	—	0.800	42 to <43	0.466
43	4	3	—	0.750	43 to <45	0.350
45	3	2	—	0.667	45 to <47	0.233
47	2	1	—	0.500	47 to <48	0.117
48+	1	1	1	1.000	>48	0.117

+ Patient censored, lost to follow-up, or withdrawn alive.

of less than 23 months. This is interpreted as meaning that the probability (p_x) of surviving up to but less than 23 months is 1.000 (10/10). The p_x of the first interval is always 1.000 because the first death ends the first interval. The occurrence of a death ends one death-free interval and begins another.

Column 1 in Table 1–18 indicates the survival time, in months, for each subject. Two patients were lost to follow-up, as indicated by "+"—one at 40 months and one at 48 months. Patients lost to follow-up are not included in the calculations of survival rates. Columns 2, 3, and 4 indicate the number surviving before and after each death and the number lost to follow-up during that interval. Column 5 is the proportion of patients surviving the interval and is obtained by dividing the proportion surviving from the beginning of the interval— from the time of the previous death to just before the next death. For example, for the interval "23 to <34," 10 patients were alive at the start of the interval, and 9 were alive at the end. To obtain p_x, divide 9 by 10 to obtain 0.900.

Column 6 is the death-free period—that is, the time of the last death to the time of the next death. Column 7, p_x, is proportion of subjects surviving from the beginning of the study to the end of the interval. The p_x is obtained by multiplying the p_x values of all the intervals up to and including the row of interest. For the survival time of 34 months, p_x is obtained by multiplying $1.000 \times 0.900 \times 0.889 = 0.800$. Based on the calculations in Table 1–18, the probability of surviving 48 months is 0.117.

We can use SPSS (Statistical Package for the Social Sciences) to conduct the Kaplan Meier survival analysis. SPSS is a microcomputer statistical package that we will use throughout this text to solve statistical problems. For the Kaplan Meier survival analysis, two columns on the data sheet need to be completed. The first column indicates the survival time in months, for each case; the second column indicates whether the survival time is censored. This can be accomplished by assigning "1" for uncensored survival times and "2" for censored survival times under the "Define Variable" selection. An example of the SPSS data sheet appears in Exhibit 1–9.

Exhibit 1–9 SPSS Data Sheet for Survival Data

Survival Time (Mo.)	Status
23.00	Uncensored
34.00	Uncensored
37.00	Uncensored
40.00	Censored
41.00	Uncensored
42.00	Uncensored
43.00	Uncensored
45.00	Uncensored
47.00	Uncensored
48.00	Censored

After completing the data sheet, select "Survival" and then "Kaplan Meier" under the "Statistics" menu. The output, including the survival graph, appears in Figure 1–2. Note that the SPSS printout provides only the p_x (cumulative survival)—the probability of surviving to the end of the interval.

Figure 1–2 SPSS Output for Kaplan Meier Survival Analysis

Survival Analysis for MONTHS (survival time in months)

Time	Cumulative Status	Standard Survival	Cumulative Error	Number Events	Remaining
23.00	Uncensored	.9000	.0949	1	9
34.00	Uncensored	.8000	.1265	2	8
37.00	Uncensored	.7000	.1449	3	7
40.00	Censored			3	6
41.00	Uncensored	.5833	.1610	4	5
42.00	Uncensored	.4667	.1658	5	4
43.00	Uncensored	.3500	.1602	6	3
45.00	Uncensored	.2333	.1431	7	2
47.00	Uncensored	.1167	.1092	8	1
48.00	Censored			8	0

Number of Cases: 10   Censored: 2 (20.00%)   Events: 8

	Survival Time	Standard Error	95% Confidence Interval
Mean:	40.43 (Limited to 48.00)	2.27	(35.98, 44.89)
Median:	42.00	1.42	(39.21, 44.79)

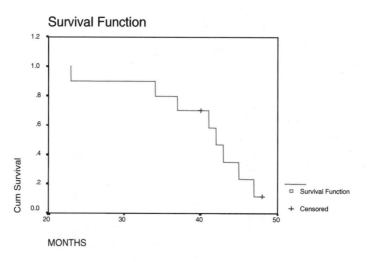

Survival Function

SPSS provides a summary of the number of cases included in the analysis, including the number of censored cases. The confidence intervals for the mean and median survival times also are provided. We will discuss confidence intervals in Chapter 5.

The graph depicts the cumulative survival rate for the group under study. Time, in months, is displayed on the x axis, and proportion surviving is displayed on the y axis.

CONCLUSION

In this chapter, we have discussed rates, ratios, and proportions in the form of mortality and morbidity rates and RR. Facility-based morbidity and mortality rates may be compared with community/state/national rates after adjustment. We may adjust rates by either the direct or the indirect method. Crude rates are important for internal analysis or other noncomparative purposes.

We also reviewed various ratios that are used to measure frequency of disease. Using the various risk ratios and the OR, we can compare risk of certain diseases and causes of morbidity between groups.

Last, we discussed one method commonly used for survival analysis—the Kaplan Meier method. Survival analysis is a tool often used in tumor registries and when analyzing results of clinical trials.

NOTE

1. Hanken, M.A., and K.A. Waters. 1994. *Glossary of healthcare terms*. Chicago: American Health Information Management Association.

ADDITIONAL RESOURCES

Centers for Disease Control. CDC Wonder Data Base. http://wonder.cdc.gov

Elston, R., and W. Johnson. 1987. *Essentials of biostatistics*. Philadelphia: F.A. Davis Co.

Gordis, L. 1996. *Epidemiology*. Philadelphia: W.B. Saunders.

Jekel, J.F., et al. 1996. *Epidemiology, biostatistics and preventive medicine*. Philadelphia: W.B. Saunders.

Kahn, H., and C. Sempos. 1989. *Statistical methods in epidemiology*. New York: Oxford University Press.

Morton, R., et al. 1989. *A study guide to epidemiology and biostatistics*. Gaithersburg, MD: Aspen Publishers, Inc.

Mosby's Medical, Nursing, and Allied Health Dictionary. 4th ed. 1994. St. Louis, MO: C.V. Mosby.

Ohio Department of Health. 1996. *Prevention Monthly* 19, no. 3:6.

U.S. Department of Health and Human Services, Public Health Service. 1992. *Principles of epidemiology: An introduction to applied epidemiology and biostatistics*. (1992).

Utah Inpatient Hospital Discharge Data Set. http://hlunix.ex.state.ut.us/had

Appendix 1–A

Exercises for Solving Problems

KNOWLEDGE QUESTIONS

1. Define the key terms listed at the beginning of this chapter.

2. Describe the differences and similarities between rates, ratios, and proportions.

3. Outline the procedure for age-adjusting crude mortality rates by the direct standardization method.

4. Describe the differences between the direct and indirect standardization methods of adjusting mortality and morbidity rates.

5. Describe the differences between neonatal mortality rate, postneonatal mortality rate, and infant mortality rate.

6. Describe the difference between incidence and prevalence rates.

MULTIPLE CHOICE

For questions 1 and 2, refer to the following table:

Age Group	Population	No. of Deaths
<30	15,000	20
30–65	17,000	55
>65	6,000	155

1. What is the crude mortality rate?
   a. 230
   b. 6.1 per 1,000
   c. 8.6 per 1,000
   d. 6.1 per 10,000

2. The age-specific death rate for the over-65 age group is:
   a. 155
   b. 25.8 per 1,000
   c. 1.55 per 10,000
   d. 25.8 per 10,000

PROBLEMS

1. Review the hypothetical data in the Table 1–A–1 and answer the questions below:
   a. What is the ratio of male neonates with infection to female neonates with infection?
   b. What proportion of neonates lived?
   c. What proportion of neonates with infection who were delivered vaginally died? What proportion who were delivered by C-section died?
   d. What is the case fatality rate for neonates with infection for the month of June?
   e. What is the relative risk of death for neonates with dyspnea compared to neonates with fever?

Table 1–A–1 Neonatal Infections, Critical Care Hospital, June 19xx

DOB	Sex	Delivery Type	Delivery Site	Outcome	Admitting Symptoms
6/2	F	Vaginal	Del. rm.	Lived	Dyspnea
6/2	M	C-section	Oper. rm.	Lived	Fever
6/8	F	Vaginal	Emer. rm.	Died	Dyspnea
6/8	F	Vaginal	Del. rm.	Lived	Fever
6/11	F	C-section	Oper. rm.	Lived	Pneumonia
6/14	F	C-section	Oper. rm.	Lived	Fever
6/14	M	Vaginal	Del. rm.	Lived	Fever
6/15	F	C-section	Oper. rm.	Lived	Fever
6/15	M	C-section	Oper. rm.	Died	Pneumonia
6/16	M	Vaginal	Del. rm.	Lived	Fever
6/18	M	Vaginal	Del. rm.	Died	Dyspnea

Source: Adapted from *Principles of Epidemiology: An Introduction to Applied Epidemiology and Biostatistics*, p. 74, 1992, U.S. Department of Health and Human Services, Public Health Service.

2. Review the data in Table 1–A–2 and answer the questions below.
   a. What is the case fatality rate for AIDS for the years 1981 through 1994?
   b. The midyear population for the state of Ohio in 1994 was 11,140,950. What is the incidence rate for AIDS for 1994?

Table 1–A–2 AIDS Cases in Ohio, 1981–1995

Year of Diagnosis	Total No. of New Cases	Cases Dead
1981	2	2
1982	7	7
1983	27	25
1984	58	56
1985	120	113
1986	211	198
1987	401	374
1988	540	482
1989	631	537
1990	682	577
1991	763	644
1992	775	587
1993	1935	908
1994	947	259
1995	259	63

Source: Reprinted from *Prevention Monthly*, Vol. 19, No. 3, p. 6, 1996, Ohio Department of Health.

3. Review the data in Table 1–A–3 and answer the questions below.
   a. What is the male-to-female ratio for AIDS in Ohio? In the United States?
   b. Out of the total number of AIDS cases in Ohio, what proportion are women? Of the total cases in the United States, what proportion are women?
   c. What proportion of the total AIDS cases in Ohio are ages 30 to 39? What proportion in the United States are ages 30 to 39?
   d. Calculate the proportion of AIDS cases in Ohio by race. Calculate the proportion of AIDS cases in the United States by race.
   e. How do the above ratios and proportions, Ohio versus United States, compare?

Table 1–A–3 Ohio and U.S. AIDS Cases by Age, Race, and Sex, 1981–1996

Demographics	Total Ohio	Total U.S.
Age		
<13	90	6,611
13–19	52	2,184
20–29	1,650	87,293
30–39	3,561	216,833
40–49	1,725	115,769
50+	690	48,205
Race		
White	5,136	228,644
Black	2,368	160,148
Hispanic	243	82,910
Other	21	5,197
Sex		
Male	7,041	408,874
Female	727	68,021

Source: Reprinted from *Prevention Monthly*, Vol. 19, No. 3, p. 11, 1996, Ohio Department of Health.

4. Complete the columns in Table 1–A–4.
   a. Compute the age-specific death rates for whites and blacks.
   b. Compute the 1995 overall crude death rate for the state of Ohio and the crude death rates for whites and blacks.
   c. Compute the 1995 age-adjusted death rates for whites and blacks in the state of Ohio using the standardized method.
   d. Is there a difference between the age-adjusted mortality rates for whites and blacks? If so, explain the reason for the discrepancy.

Table 1–A–4 Age-Specific Mortality Rates, State of Ohio, 1995

Age	(a) White Pop.	(b) Deaths	(c) White ASDR	(d) Black Pop.	(e) Deaths	(f) Black ASDR	(g) Comb. Pop. Total	(h) Expected No. of Deaths, Whites (g x c)	(i) Expected No. of Deaths, Blacks (g x f)
<1	129,185	940		22,802	399				
1–4	512,043	177		98,498	55				
5–9	665,727	131		112,686	33				
10–14	688,172	154		106,745	40				
15–19	676,178	428		104,773	136				
20–24	655,443	523		96,644	160				
25–34	1,440,473	1,452		183,586	437				
35–44	1,585,681	2,896		191,776	763				
45–54	1,194,694	4,861		121,726	1,000				
55–64	842,359	9,311		90,682	1,664				
65–75	762,331	20,739		73,786	2,718				
75–84	453,272	28,437		35,096	2,399				
85+	146,246	24,180		11,069	1,676				
Total	9,751,804	94,229		1,249,869	11,480				

Source: Data from Centers for Disease Control and Prevention, CDC Wonder Data Base, http://wonder.cdc.gov.

5. Calculate the odds ratio for the data in Table 1–13 on page 22. Interpret the results.

6. At Critical Care Hospital, the complication rate for hip replacement surgery is 8.96%. The relevant statistics appear in Table 1–A–5. The administrative staff at the hospital is concerned that the hospital complication rate does not compare favorably with the overall complication rate of all patients with hip replacement surgery in the county. The complication rate for the county is 5.5%. The county complication rate for patients age 65 or older is 8.0%; for those under age 65, the complication rate is 3.0%. Using the indirect method of standardization, calculate the complication rate for the hospital that has been adjusted for age.

Table 1–A–5 Critical Care Hospital, Complication Rates, Hip Replacement Surgery

Age Group	No. of Patients	No. of Patients with Complications	Complication Rate
≥65	170	17	10.0%
<65	42	2	4.76%
Total	212	19	8.96%

7. The overall mortality rate for patients who have had a cerebrovascular accident (CVA) is 15.8% at CGH. You have been asked to compare the hospital's mortality rate to that of the state. Using the data provided in Table 1–A–6, calculate the age-adjusted death rate and the standard mortality ratio (SMR) for the hospital, using the indirect method of standardization. Explain the results.

Table 1–A–6 Mortality Rates for CVAs, State versus City General Hospital

Severity of Illness	State Mortality Rate	Hospital Discharges for CVA	Observed Deaths	Expected Deaths
1	4.2	55	2	
2	5.9	116	8	
3	7.8	195	20	
4	20.9	147	29	
5	34.6	62	32	
		575	91	

INTERNET ACTIVITY

An important skill for the health information management professional is the ability to search the Internet for information. This can be particularly useful when one is searching for comparative information. This activity is designed to provide experience working with an on-line interactive database and to provide experience analyzing and summarizing the results of data queries.

Instructions

1. The Utah Department of Health has an on-line interactive database that is available for public use. The database is constructed from the Uniform Hospital Discharge Data Set (UHDDS). Information on DRGs and ICD-9-CM codes (International Classification of Diseases, 9th revision, Clinical Modification) can be obtained through queries. The public data set contains data for the years since 1992. The Web site address is hlunix.hl.state.ut.us/hda

2. Once at the site, click "Descriptive Statistics." This should take you to the Utah Hospital Discharge Query System. The Utah External Injury Data System will also be accessed.

3. Answer the questions that follow. An alternative Web site is the Centers for Disease Control and Prevention's data sets at http://wonder.cdc.gov

Questions

1. For the diagnosis of acute myocardial infarction, ICD-9-CM category 410:
   a. Prepare tables that display the number of discharges by year, 1992 through 1997, and by gender.
   b. Prepare a line graph that displays the number of deaths by gender for the years 1992 through 1997.
   c. Prepare a table that displays the number of discharges by age for 1997.
   d. Prepare a bar graph that displays the average length of stay by gender for the years 1992 through 1997.
   e. Prepare a line graph that displays the median charges by year, 1992 through 1997.
   f. Discuss your findings.

2. How many patients with coronary atherosclerosis, ICD-9-CM category 414, had a coronary artery bypass graft (CABG) procedure, ICD-9-CM procedure category 36?
   a. Display the results in both a table and a bar or line graph by year, 1992 through 1997, and by gender.
   b. Construct a bar graph that displays average length of stay by year and gender for patients with coronary atherosclerosis and CABG procedure.
   c. Discuss your findings.

3. Determine the number of patient discharges with pathological fractures, ICD-9-CM code 733.1, by year, 1992 through 1997, and by gender. You are interested in patients aged 65 years and over. Prepare a line graph displaying the number of discharges by year and by gender. Discuss your findings.

4. In table form, how many patients were discharged, by year, 1992 through 1997, and by gender, with malignant neoplasms of the trachea, bronchus, and lung? Use the selection option that is available on the database. Prepare a bar or line graph that displays the number of patients who expired from these illnesses. The graph should display the results by year and by gender. Briefly discuss the results. In discussing your results, what caution should you make to the reader with regard to your findings?

5. For ICD-9-CM code 185, for the years 1992 through 1997:
   a. Prepare a bar graph or pie chart, by third-party payer, of all men discharged with a diagnosis of prostate cancer.
   b. Prepare a bar graph that displays the number of men, by age group, discharged with prostate cancer.
   c. Discuss your findings.

6. For patients discharged with pneumonia during the years 1992 through 1997 (use the selection option that is available on the database):
   a. Prepare a table that reports the average length of stay for patients discharged with pneumonia by year and by gender. Include only patients who are aged 65 years and older.
   b. Prepare a bar or line graph to display your results.
   c. Discuss your findings.

7. Use the External Injury Data System to determine the number of patients discharged, by gender, who were involved in motor vehicle accidents for the years 1992 through 1997. Prepare a bar graph illustrating the number of patients who expired by year and by gender. Discuss your findings.

8. Determine the number of patients whose cause of death was homicide for the years 1992 through 1997 by age group and by sex. Construct a bar graph displaying the number of patients who expired, by year and by sex.

CHAPTER 2

Graphic Display of Data

KEY TERMS	Tables	Bar charts	Pie chart
	Table shell	Grouped bar chart	Histogram
	Box head	Stacked bar chart	Frequency polygon
	Stub	100% component bar chart	Line graph
	Cell		Scatter diagram
	Note		
	Source		

LEARNING OBJECTIVES

At the conclusion of this chapter, you should be able to:

1. Define key terms.
2. Determine which graphic technique is appropriate for the type of information to be conveyed.
3. Determine the appropriate graphic techniques for the various scales of measurement.
4. Outline the essential components of tables.
5. Correctly prepare tables for one, two, three, and/or four variables.
6. Outline the principles for construction of bar charts and pie charts.
7. Differentiate between the following types of bar charts: one-variable bar chart, grouped bar charts, stacked bar charts, and 100% component bar charts.
8. Correctly prepare bar charts and pie charts.
9. Correctly prepare the following types of graphs: histograms, frequency polygons, line graphs, and scatter diagrams.
10. Differentiate between histograms and bar charts.
11. Differentiate between frequency polygons and line graphs.

The purpose of tables, charts, and graphs is to summarize and display data clearly and effectively. They are all means of summarizing quantities of information to the reader. Tables, charts, and graphs offer the opportunity to analyze data sets and to explore, under-

40

stand, and present distributions, trends, and relationships in the data. The primary purpose of tables, charts, and graphs is to communicate information about the data to the user.

Whether the graphic technique used is a table, chart, or graph, it should

- display the data
- allow the viewer to think about what the data convey
- avoid distortion of the data
- encourage the reader to make comparisons
- reveal data at several levels, from a broad overview to the fine detail
- serve a reasonably clear purpose: description, exploration, tabulation, or decoration
- be closely related to the statistical and verbal descriptions of the data set

CONSTRUCTION OF TABLES

A **table** is an orderly arrangement of values that groups data into rows and columns. Almost any type of quantitative information can be grouped into tables. For example, we can use tables to display frequencies for such vital statistics as morbidity rates or hospital admission and discharge data. Tables are useful for demonstrating patterns and other kinds of relationships. They also serve as a basis for more visual displays of data, such as graphs and charts, where some of the detail may be lost.

Because tables generally do not capture the interest of the reader, they should be used sparingly. In addition, it is often difficult to see trends in data that are presented in a table.

Table Shells

Although data cannot be analyzed until they have been collected, it is useful to prepare a **table shell** that shows how the data will be organized and displayed. It also helps one work through the data collection process in advance to ensure that once the data have been collected they can be analyzed in the manner desired. The basic shell for construction of tables appears in Exhibit 2–1. Table shells are tables that are complete except for the data.

In summary, a table should be self-explanatory, even if it is taken out of its original context. A table should convey all the information necessary for the reader to understand the data. Check the table to be sure that

- It is a logical unit.
- It is self-explanatory. Ask yourself if the table can stand on its own if photocopied and removed from its context.
- All sources are specified.
- Headings are specific and understandable for every column and row.
- Row and column totals are checked for accuracy.
- Cells are not left blank; enter "0" or "–".
- Categories are mutually exclusive and exhaustive.

Consideration should also be given to alignment of data in tables. Guidelines for aligning text include the following: align text in a table to the left; text that serves as a column label

Exhibit 2–1 Table Shell

TITLE Box Head		Sex					
		Male		Female		Total	
	Age	No.	%	No.	%	No.	%
Stub		Row Variable→→		→→→→		→→	
	<45			Column Variable			
	45–54			↓			
	55–64			↓			
	65–74			↓			
	75+			↓			

Note:

Source: Adapted from *Self-Instructional Manual for Cancer Registries, Book 7: Statistics and Epidemiology for Cancer Registries*, p. 23, U.S. Department of Health and Human Services, Public Health Service, National Institutes of Health, National Cancer Institute.

may be centered; numeric values should be aligned to the right; and if the numeric values contain decimals, they should be decimal aligned. Some word-processing and microcomputer statistical software programs have features that assist in the formatting of tables. The essential components of a table are outlined in Exhibit 2–2.

A One-Variable Table

The most basic table is a frequency distribution with just one variable. The first column shows the values or categories of the variable represented by the data, such as age or sex. The second column shows the number of persons or events that fall into each category. A third column may be added to show the percentage of persons or events in each category. Because of rounding, column totals for percentages often add up to 99.9% or 100.1%. Even when this occurs, the total given should be 100.0%, with a footnote explaining that the difference is due to rounding. An example of a one-variable table, which displays some hypothetical admissions data, is presented in Table 2–1. The variable is sex, which is divided into two mutually exclusive categories, male and female. The "Table Auto Format" feature in Microsoft Word 1997 was used to format the table.

Two- and Three-Variable Tables

We can use tables to display data that have more than one variable. Data can be tabulated to show counts by two or three variables, such as age and sex. A two-variable table that is

Exhibit 2–2 Essential Components of Tables

TITLE	The title should be as complete as possible and should clearly relate the content of the table. It should answer the following questions:

- What are the data? (e.g., counts, percentages)
- Who? (e.g., white females with breast cancer; black males with lung cancer)
- Where are the data from? (e.g., hospital, state, community)
- When? (e.g., year, month)

For example: Site Distribution by Age and Sex of Cancer Patients upon First Admission to General Hospital

BOX HEAD	The box head contains the captions or column headings. The heading of each column should contain as few words as possible but should explain exactly what the data in the column represent.
STUB	The row captions are known as the stub. Items in the stub should be grouped to facilitate interpretation of data. For example, group ages into five-year intervals.
CELL	The box formed by the intersection of a column and a row
Optional Items: NOTE	Anything in the table that cannot be understood by the reader from the title, box head, or stub should be explained by notes. Notes contain numbers, preliminary or revised numbers, or explanations for any unusual numbers. Definitions, abbreviations, and/or qualifications for captions or cell names should be footnoted. A note usually applies to a specific cell(s) within the table, and a symbol, such as ** or #, may be used to key the cell to the note. If several notes are required, it is better to use small letters than to use symbols or numbers. Note numbers may be confused with the numbers within the table.
SOURCE	If data from a source outside your research are used, the exact reference to the source should be given. Indicating the source lends authenticity to the data and allows the reader to locate the original source if more information is needed.

Source: Adapted from *Self-Instructional Manual for Cancer Registries, Book 7: Statistics and Epidemiology for Cancer Registries*, p. 24, U.S. Department of Health and Human Services, Public Health Service, National Institutes of Health, National Cancer Institute.

Table 2–1 XYZ Hospital Admissions by Sex, 1999

Sex	No.	%
Male	30	60.0%
Female	20	40.0%
Total	50	100.0%

cross-tabulated is usually called a two-by-two contingency table. In Table 2–2, "lung cancer patients" are classified on two variables, race and sex; race is the row variable, and sex is the column variable. Contingency tables, which will be discussed in greater detail in Chapter 9, are often used in calculating measures of association such as chi square.

Table 2–2 Lung Cancer Patients by Race and Sex, General Hospital, 1985–1989

| Race | Sex | | Total |
	Male	Female	
White	316	204	520
Black	35	15	50
Total	351	219	570

Source: Reprinted from *Self-Instructional Manual for Cancer Registries, Book 7: Statistics and Epidemiology for Cancer Registries*, p. 32, U.S. Department of Health and Human Services, Public Health Service, National Institutes of Health, National Cancer Institute.

Tables 2–3 and 2–4 are examples of data classified on three and four variables. Because tables classifying data on more than two variables can be quite confusing to the reader, they should be avoided if at all possible.

Table 2–3 Lung Cancer Patients by Sex and Male-to-Female Ratio for Whites and Blacks by Age, General Hospital, 1985–1989

Race and Age	Male	Female	M/F Ratio	Total
White				
<45	20	20	1.0	40
45–54	36	30	1.2	66
55–64	92	66	1.4	158
65–74	112	50	2.2	162
75+	56	38	1.5	94
Subtotal	316	204	1.5	520
Black				
<45	2	—	0.0	2
45–54	6	4	1.5	10
55–64	14	6	2.3	20
65–74	10	4	2.5	14
75+	3	1	3.0	4
Subtotal	35	15	2.3	50
Total	351	219	1.6	570

Source: Reprinted from *Self-Instructional Manual for Cancer Registries, Book 7: Statistics and Epidemiology for Cancer Registries*, p. 32, U.S. Department of Health and Human Services, Public Health Service, National Institutes of Health, National Cancer Institute.

Table 2–4 Frequency Distribution of Leukemia Cases by Chronicity, Morphology, Race, and Sex, University Hospital, 1985–1989

Chronicity and Morphology	Black			White			Grand Total
	Male	Female	Total	Male	Female	Total	
Acute							
Acute lymphocytic	35	45	80	631	461	1,092	1,172
Acute myelocytic	46	45	91	631	539	1,170	1,261
Monocytic	29	28	57	451	407	858	915
Acute, NOS	44	13	57	451	328	779	1,064
Total acute	154	131	285	2,164	1,735	3,899	4,184
Chronic							
Chronic lymphocytic	96	64	160	1,444	740	2,184	2,344
Chronic myelocytic	67	53	120	812	670	1,482	1,602
Leukemia, NOS	3	3	6	90	144	234	240
Total chronic	166	120	286	2,346	1,554	3,900	5,086
Grand Total	320	251	571	4,510	3,289	7,799	9,270

Note: NOS, not otherwise specified.

Source: Reprinted from *Self-Instructional Manual for Cancer Registries, Book 7: Statistics and Epidemiology for Cancer Registries,* p. 33, U.S. Department of Health and Human Services, Public Health Service, National Institutes of Health, National Cancer Institute.

In a three-way classification table, it sometimes becomes quite challenging to arrange the data in a readable format. A multidimensional relationship must be shown in a two-dimensional space. In Table 2–3, we have expanded the classification of the lung cancer data to include not only race and sex but also age. The row categories are divided by age. In Table 2–4, a four-way table, leukemia cases are classified by chronicity (acute or chronic), morphology (tissue type), race, and sex.

CHARTS

Graphs and charts of various types are the best means for presenting data for quick visualization of relationships. Graphs and charts emphasize the main points and analyze and clarify relationships between variables that may otherwise remain elusive.

Regardless of the type of graph or chart that is being prepared, several principles of construction should be followed. First, it is important to avoid distortion of the data. To avoid distortion, the representation of numbers on the graph should be directly proportional to the numerical quantities that are being represented on the graph. It is also important to consider proportion and scale. Graphs should accommodate the eye in that they should emphasize the horizontal. It is also easier for the eye to read along the horizontal axis from left to right. Graphs should be greater in length than they are in height. The three-quarter high rule is a useful guide: the height (*y* axis) of the graph should be three-fourths the length (*x* axis) of the graph. It is also easier for the eye to read along the horizontal axis from left to right. A longer horizontal axis helps to point out the causal variable in more detail. Other helpful hints in preparing graphs or charts include spelling out abbreviations in a note so that misunderstandings are avoided; using colors to help understand groupings that may appear in the graph; and using both upper- and lowercase letters in titles, as the use of all capital letters can be unfriendly to the eyes. Guidelines for construction of a bar chart are summarized in Exhibit 2–3.

Exhibit 2–3 Guidelines for Constructing a Bar Chart

When constructing a bar chart, keep the following points in mind:

- Arrange the bar categories in a natural order, such as alphabetical order, order by increasing age, or an order that will produce increasing or decreasing bar lengths.
- The bars may be positioned vertically or horizontally.
- All bars should be of the same width.
- The length of the bars should be in proportion to the frequency of the event.
- Avoid using more than three bars (categories) within a group of bars.
- Leave a space between adjacent groups of bars but not between bars within a group.
- Code different variables by differences in bar color, shading, cross-hatching, etc. Include a legend that interprets your code.

Source: Adapted from *Principles of Epidemiology: An Introduction to Applied Epidemiology and Biostatistics*, p. 251, 1992, U.S. Department of Health and Human Services, Public Health Service.

There are many types of charts. We will first discuss the construction of charts for data that fall into categories.

Bar Charts

One-Variable Bar Chart

We can use **bar charts** to display data for one or more variables. Bar charts are appropriate for displaying data that are categorical. The simplest bar chart is the one-variable bar chart. Each category of the variable is represented by a bar. In Figure 2–1, the bar represents one variable, hospital operating margin, which is placed in categories by years—1981 through 1991. There is one bar representing hospital operating margin for each of the 11 years in the bar chart.

The length or height of each bar is proportional to the number of persons or events in the category. The presentation of the information in this bar chart makes it easy to see at a glance that hospital operating margin was the greatest in 1985 and the least in 1988.

Figure 2–1 Hospital Operating Margins in Percentages, 1981–1991. *Source:* Reprinted from *Medicare and the American Health Care System: Report to the Congress*, p. 68, 1993, Prospective Payment Assessment Commission.

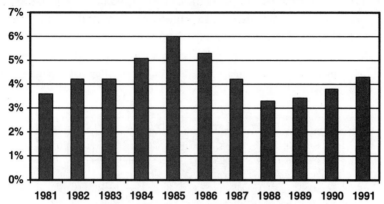

Bar charts may be drawn either horizontally or vertically. Figure 2–2 presents the same information that appears in Figure 2–1, but in a horizontal format. Personal preference determines the format used.

Figure 2–2 Hospital Operating Margins in Percentages, 1981–1991. *Source:* Reprinted from *Medicare and the American Health Care System: Report to the Congress*, p. 68, 1993, Prospective Payment Assessment Commission.

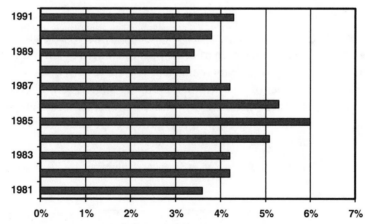

It is not uncommon to confuse a bar chart with a histogram. A bar chart is used to display data that fall into groups or categories, whereas histograms are used to illustrate frequency distributions of continuous variables. In a bar chart, the bars that represent the categories of the variables are separated, whereas in a histogram the bars are joined. A **histogram** is used to display the frequency distribution of a continuous variable, such as age. A bar chart is used to display the frequency distribution of a variable that is discrete with noncontinuous categories such as race or sex.

Computer software makes it easy to present bar charts in either two-dimensional or three-dimensional form. When bars are presented in three-dimensional form, it is sometimes difficult for the reader to estimate the true height of the bar. In a 3-D bar chart, the back edges of the bar appear higher than the front edge, as in Figure 2–3. To make sure that the reader correctly interprets the bar, label the data points at a point on the bars, as in Figure 2–3.

Figure 2–3 Hospital Operating Margins in Percentages, 1981–1991. *Source:* Reprinted from *Medicare and the American Health Care System: Report to the Congress*, p. 68, 1993, Prospective Payment Assessment Commission.

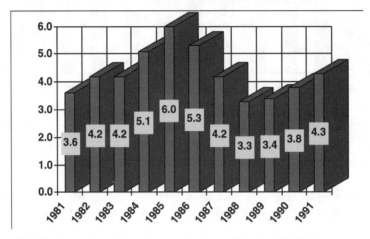

Grouped Bar Charts

A **grouped bar chart** is used to display information from tables containing two or three variables. An example of a grouped bar chart can be demonstrated by the variable sex, which has two categories: male and female. Bars within a group are usually joined; in this case, the grouping is by year. The number of bars within a grouping should be limited to three. There must also be a legend to indicate what categories the bars represent. In viewing the grouped bar chart in Figure 2–4, we can easily see that proportionately, more women than men were admitted to the hospital for the years 1995 and 1996.

Figure 2–4 Percentage of Hospital Admissions by Sex

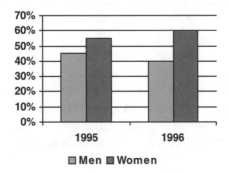

Stacked Bar Charts

In a **stacked bar chart**, bar segments for each data category are stacked like building blocks on top of one another to form a single bar. In a stacked bar chart, the bar represents the total number of cases that occurred in a category; the segments of the bar represent the frequency of cases within the category. As an example, the data that appear in Table 2–5 are presented as a stacked bar chart in Figure 2–5. Each bar in the stacked bar chart represents the

Table 2–5 Number of Cancer Cases, for Leading Non–Sex-Specific Sites by Sex, First Diagnosed by City Hospital, 1990

Primary Site	Male	Female	Total
Oral cavity/pharynx	94	67	161
Larynx	47	12	59
Bronchus/lung	117	83	200
Stomach	31	21	52
Colon/rectum	84	65	149
Gallbladder	50	23	73
Bladder	58	20	87
Kidney	57	24	81
Hodgkin's disease	48	47	95
Leukemia	65	60	125
Total	651	431	1,082

Source: Reprinted from *Self-Instructional Manual for Cancer Registries, Book 7: Statistics and Epidemiology for Cancer Registries*, p. 45, U.S. Department of Health and Human Services, Public Health Service, National Institutes of Health, National Cancer Institute.

Figure 2–5 Number of Cancer Cases, for Leading Non–Sex-Specific Sites by Sex, First Diagnosed by City Hospital, 1990. *Source:* Reprinted from *Self-Instructional Manual for Cancer Registries, Book 7: Statistics and Epidemiology for Cancer Registries*, p. 45, U.S. Department of Health and Human Services, Public Health Service, National Institutes of Health, National Cancer Institute.

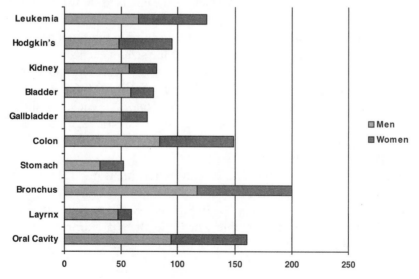

total number of cancer cases for a specific primary site; the bar segments represent the number of males and the number of females affected within the total number of cases.

Stacked bar charts should be used with caution, since they are very difficult to interpret. The stacked components of the bars do not rest on a flat baseline. What this means is that where one category of the variable ends, the next begins. Each category rides the bumps of those below it. Stacked bar charts can be difficult to interpret because, except for the bottom category, the categories do not rest on a flat baseline.

From the stacked bar graph in Figure 2–5, it can be readily seen that men are affected more often than women. But the exact number of cases for women in each category is difficult to determine. Stacked bar charts are deceptive, so they are often used to exaggerate or hide information.

100% Component Bar Charts

The **100% component bar chart** is a variant of the stacked bar chart. In a 100% bar chart, all of the bars are of the same height and show the variable categories as percentages of the total rather than the actual values. Each bar is much like its own pie chart. A set of 100% bar charts can be used instead of multiple pie charts. This is more advantageous because it is easier to make comparison between bars than between pies.

Figure 2–6 presents the same information that appears in Figure 2–5. The stacked bars for each year represent 100% of the various types of cancer cases by sex. Each category of the sex variable is represented in terms of a percentage, in one bar. As you can see, it is much more difficult to determine the actual percentage of cases for each sex that were treated at City Hospital.

Pie Charts

A **pie chart** is an easily understood chart in which the sizes of the slices show the proportional contribution of each part of the pie. We can use pie charts to show the component parts of a single group or variable. To calculate the size of each slice of the pie, first determine the proportion of the pie to be represented by each slice. Multiply the proportion by 360—the total number of degrees in a circle. The result will be the size of each slice in degrees.

In the pie chart in Figure 2–7, one slice of the pie, stage II, represents 50% of the cases or 50% of the pie. Within the pie chart, this slice of the pie equals 180° (360° × .50 = 180°). Two categories of the pie, stages III and IV, represent 15% of the cases each, and the size of their respective slices is 54° (360° × .15 = 54°); one category of the pie, stage I, represents 20% of the cases, which is equivalent to 72° (360° × .20 = 72°). The sum of the degrees for each slice of the pie is 360° (180° + 54° + 54° + 72° = 360°).

The pie chart in Figure 2–7 demonstrates how the whole pie is divided into segments. By convention, the largest slices of the pie begin at 12 o'clock, as in Figure 2–7. The slices of the pie should be arranged in some logical order. In Figure 2–8, the stage I category appears in the 12 o'clock position. This is an example where pie slices are arranged according to a logical or conventional order rather than according to magnitude.

Figure 2–6 Percentage of Cancer Cases for Leading Non–Sex-Specific Sites by Sex. *Source:* Reprinted from *Self-Instructional Manual for Cancer Registries, Book 7: Statistics and Epidemiology for Cancer Registries*, p. 45, U.S. Department of Health and Human Services, Public Health Service, National Institutes of Health, National Cancer Institute.

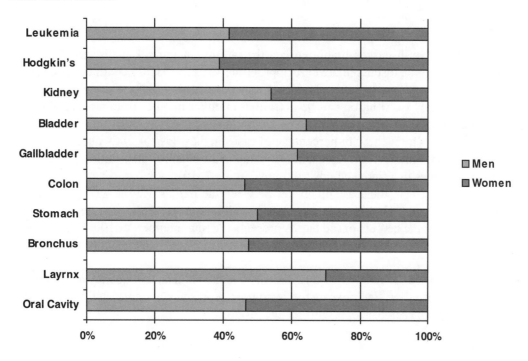

Figure 2–7 Percentage Distribution of Invasive Cervical Cancer Cases by Stage, Women's Hospital, 1990–1991, Ordering by Magnitude of Groupings

Figure 2–8 Percentage Distribution of Invasive Cervical Cancer Cases by Stage, Women's Hospital, 1990–1991, Ordering by Sequences of Stages

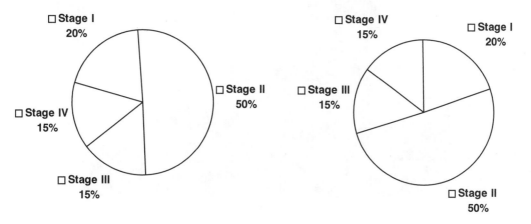

It is not recommended to use pie charts to compare multiple distributions because they are not optimal for comparing components for more than one group. When components of more than one group are to be compared, a 100% component bar chart should be used.

Histograms

Thus far we have discussed graphing data that are in categorical or discrete form. The techniques that will be discussed next are appropriate for data that are continuous in nature.

A histogram is appropriate for displaying a frequency distribution for one continuous variable. The frequency distribution can be presented in either number or percentage form. A histogram consists of a series of bars, each having as its base one class interval and as its height the number (frequency) or percentage of cases in that class. A class interval is a type of category; a class interval can represent one value in a frequency distribution (Figure 2–9) or a group of values in a frequency distribution (Figure 2–10).

In this type of graph, there are no spaces between the bars, since the data points represented are continuous. That is, a data point may fall anywhere in the area covered by the graph. The sum of the heights of the bars represents the total number, or 100% of the cases. When the distribution of the data needs to be emphasized more than the actual values, use a histogram.

An example where the class interval represents a single value in a frequency distribution is displayed in Figure 2–9. Each bar of the histogram represents a single age, in contrast to Figure 2–10, where each bar represents an age group.

Figure 2–9 Age on Admission to Pediatric Unit

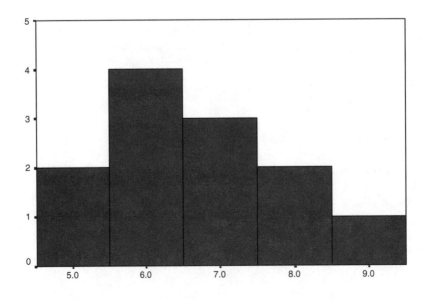

Figure 2–10 Number of Malignant Tumors of Bone and Soft Tissue by Age Group at Diagnosis, Cases First Diagnosed at University Hospitals, 1990. *Source:* Reprinted from *Self-Instructional Manual for Cancer Registries, Book 7: Statistics and Epidemiology for Cancer Registries*, p. 48, U.S. Department of Health and Human Services, Public Health Service, National Institutes of Health, National Cancer Institute.

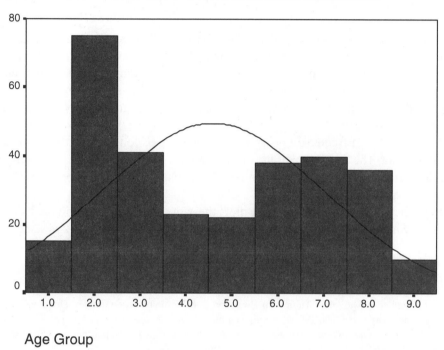

Age Group

Age at diagnosis for soft tissue tumors is the variable represented in the histogram in Figure 2–10. The values at the bottom of the x axis represent the following age groups:

Value	Age Group	Midpoint of Class Interval
1	0–9	4.5
2	10–19	14.5
3	20–29	24.5
4	30–39	34.5
5	40–49	44.5
6	50–59	54.5
7	60–69	64.5
8	70–79	74.5
9	80–89	84.5

In the histogram, it is clear that the most frequent age group in which tumors of bone and soft tissue are diagnosed is age 10–19. The distribution of age at diagnosis is not normal, as indicated by the superimposed normal curve. We will discuss the normal distribution and the normal curve in Chapter 5.

Frequency Polygons

A **frequency polygon** may be used as an alternative to the histogram. Like a histogram, a frequency polygon is a graph of a frequency distribution. To construct a frequency polygon, simply join the midpoints at the top of each bar in the histogram (4.5, 14.5, 24.5, etc.). The advantage of the frequency polygon over the histogram is that several frequency polygons can be plotted on the same graph for comparison purposes. Frequency polygons also are easy to interpret.

When constructing a frequency polygon, make the x axis longer than the y axis to avoid distorting the data. The frequency of the observations is always placed on the y axis, and the scale of the variables under study is placed on the x axis. Frequency values are plotted at the midpoint of each class interval.

The frequency polygon in Figure 2–11 plots the same data that appear in the histogram in Figure 2–10. Since the x axis represents the total distribution, the line always starts and ends with zero.

Figure 2–11 Number of Malignant Tumors of Bone and Soft Tissue by Age Group at Diagnosis, Cases First Diagnosed at University Hospitals, 1990. *Source:* Reprinted from *Self-Instructional Manual for Cancer Registries, Book 7: Statistics and Epidemiology for Cancer Registries*, p. 48, U.S. Department of Health and Human Services, Public Health Service, National Institutes of Health, National Cancer Institute.

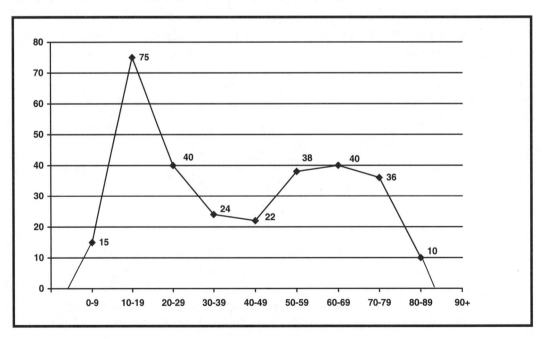

The frequency polygon tells us that age at diagnosis reaches its peak in age group 10 to 19, falls steadily until ages 40 to 49, and again increases slightly from ages 40 to 79 before falling again. A frequency polygon presents this pattern with more clarity than the histogram.

Line Graphs

A **line graph** is often used to display time trends and survival curves. The *x* axis shows the unit of time from left to right, and the *y* axis measures the values of the variable being plotted. A line graph does not represent a frequency distribution.

A line graph consists of a line connecting a series of points on an arithmetic scale. Like all graphs, it should be designed so that it is easy to read. The selection of proper scales, complete and accurate titles, and informative legends is important. If a graph is too long and narrow, either vertically or horizontally, it has an awkward appearance and may exaggerate one aspect of the data. The trend in per capita health care spending is displayed in Figure 2–12.

The line graph is especially useful when there are a large number of values to be plotted, that is, when you have a continuous variable with an unlimited number of possible points. It also allows the presentation of several sets of data on one graph.

Either actual numbers or percentages may be used on the *y* axis of the line graph. Use percentages on the *y* axis when more than one distribution is to be shown on one graph. A percentage distribution allows comparisons between groups where the actual totals are different.

If more than one set of data is plotted on the same graph, different types of lines (solid or broken) should be used to distinguish between the lines. The number of lines should be kept to a minimum—a line graph can soon become too cluttered. Each line should be identified in a legend or on the graph itself.

Figure 2–12 Adjusted per Capita Health Care Spending, Selected Years, 1975–1994. *Source:* Reprinted from *Medicare and the American Health Care System: Report to the Congress*, p. 14, 1993, Prospective Payment Assessment Commission.

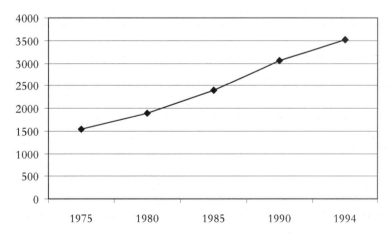

There are two kinds of time-trend data: (1) point data, which reflect an instant in time, and (2) period data, which cover an average or total over a specified period of time, such as a year or five-year time frame. In point data, the scale marker on the x axis indicates a particular point in time, such as one, two, or three years of survival. On the other hand, in plotting of period data, the horizontal scale lines are used to indicate the interval limits, and the values are plotted at the midpoint at each interval. For example:

Year of Diagnosis	Midpoint of Interval
1980–1984	1982
1985–1989	1987
1990–1994	1992

Table 2–6 presents an example of point data that are graphed in Figure 2–13. Other examples are presented in Table 2–7 and Figure 2–14.

Table 2–6 Relative Survival Rates by Year of Diagnosis for Kidney Cancer Surveillance, Epidemiology, and End Results Reporting (SEER), 1980–1984

Years of Survival	1980	1981	1982	1983	1984
1	72.3	67.9	70.5	71.8	73.2
2	62.9	58.2	60.5	63.2	65.4
3	58.9	53.4	55.2	58.5	61.5
4	56.1	50.8	52.3	55.6	58.4
5	55.3	48.3	50.0	54.0	56.1

Source: Reprinted from *Self-Instructional Manual for Cancer Registries, Book 7: Statistics and Epidemiology for Cancer Registries*, p. 53, U.S. Department of Health and Human Services, Public Health Service, National Institutes of Health, National Cancer Institute.

Figure 2–13 Relative Survival Rates by Year of Diagnosis for Kidney Cancer Surveillance, Epidemiology, and End Results Reporting (SEER), 1980–1984. *Source:* Reprinted from *Self-Instructional Manual for Cancer Registries, Book 7: Statistics and Epidemiology for Cancer Registries*, p. 53, U.S. Department of Health and Human Services, Public Health Service, National Institutes of Health, National Cancer Institute.

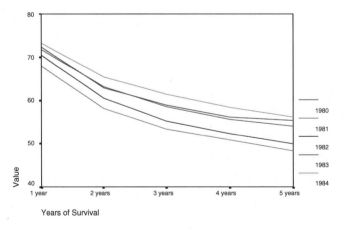

Table 2–7 Five-Year Survival Rates for Kidney Cancer by Stage for Patients Diagnosed 1974–1976, 1977–1978, and 1979–1984

Year of Diagnosis	Midpoint of Interval	Survival Rate		
		Localized	Regional	Distant
1974–1976	1975	80	71	28
1977–1978	1977.5	84	71	29
1979–1984	1981.5	85	74	31

Source: Reprinted from *Self-Instructional Manual for Cancer Registries, Book 7: Statistics and Epidemiology for Cancer Registries*, p. 55, U.S. Department of Health and Human Services, Public Health Service, National Institutes of Health, National Cancer Institute.

Figure 2–14 Five-Year Relative Survival Rates for Kidney Cancer by Stage, for Patients Diagnosed 1974–1976, 1977–1978, and 1974–1984. *Source:* Reprinted from *Self-Instructional Manual for Cancer Registries, Book 7: Statistics and Epidemiology for Cancer Registries*, p. 55, U.S. Department of Health and Human Services, Public Health Service, National Institutes of Health, National Cancer Institute.

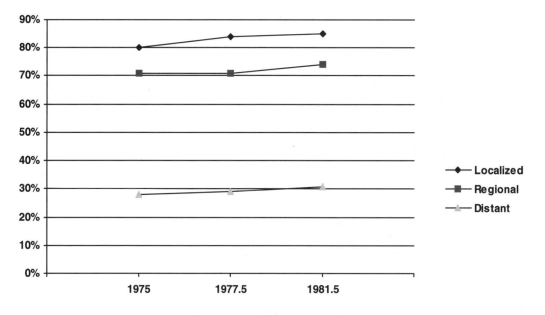

Scatter Diagrams

A **scatter diagram**, or scatter plot, is a graphic technique used to display the relationship between two continuous variables. One variable is plotted on the x axis and the other is plotted on the y axis. To create a scatter diagram, there must be a pair of values for every person, group, or other entity in the data set, one value for each variable. Each pair of values is plotted by placing a point on the graph where the two values intersect.

To interpret a scatter diagram, analyze the overall pattern of the plotted points. Plotted points that appear to fall in a straight line indicate a linear relationship between x and y, whereas widely scattered points indicate no relationship between *x* and *y*. Table 2–8 presents hypothetical data of test scores and the grade point averages of 10 students. Figure 2–15 is a scatter plot that depicts the relationship between the two variables, test scores (x) and grade point average (y).

The scatter diagram in Figure 2–15 indicates a strong linear relationship between the variables test scores and grade point average. Scatter diagrams are used to assist in interpretation

Table 2–8 Test Scores and Grade Point Averages of 10 Students

Student	Test Score (X)	GPA (Y)
1	24	1.5
2	61	3.5
3	30	1.7
4	48	2.7
5	60	3.4
6	32	1.6
7	19	1.2
8	22	1.3
9	41	2.2
10	46	2.7

Figure 2–15 Scatter Diagram of Test Scores and Grade Point Average

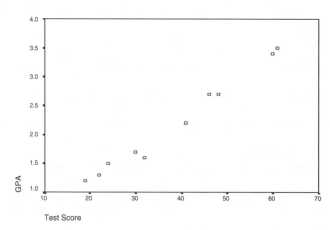

of inferential statistics such as correlation and linear regression. We will discuss these topics in Chapter 8.

CONCLUSION

Tables, charts, and graphs are effective methods of summarizing data and displaying data in a clear, concise format. Tables are often used to display data, and they may be used to display data about one or more variables. An advantage of tables is that large amounts of data may be displayed and summarized, as in a four-way table. However, if too much information is included in a table, it can be confusing to the reader.

Bar charts or graphs are often used for displaying categorical data, but they are appropriate for data that are continuous in nature. Bar charts allow for quick visualization of the variable of interest. Relationships between two variables are also easily seen in a bar chart. Bar charts may take the form of a simple bar chart, a grouped bar chart, a stacked bar chart, or a 100% component bar chart. The form selected should be appropriate to the data and easily interpreted by the reader.

Pie charts are useful for displaying the parts of a whole. For example, we could display the proportion of patients admitted by third-party payer, or the proportion of burn patients admitted by severity of burn. Pie charts should be used to display proportions of one nominal-level variable; pie charts are not appropriate for comparing distributions of two or more variables.

Histograms and frequency polygons are used to display the frequency distribution of one continuous variable. Histograms and frequency polygons represent 100% of the cases in a frequency distribution; the shape of the distribution can be easily seen in these two types of graphs.

Line graphs are used to display trends in data; they are also used in survival analysis. A line graph consists of a line connecting a series of points on an arithmetic scale. To avoid distortion in the data, the graph should not be too long or too narrow. When constructing bar graphs and line graphs, the three-quarters–high rule should be used as a guide to avoid data distortion. Either actual numbers or percentages may be displayed in a line graph.

ADDITIONAL RESOURCES

Al-Assaf, A.F., and J.A. Schmele, eds. 1993. *The textbook of total quality management.* Delray Beach, FL: St. Lucie Press. 124–125.

Duncan, R.C., et al. 1983. *Introductory biostatistics for the health sciences.* Albany, NY: Delmar Publishers. 56.

Jones, G.E. 1995. *How to lie with charts.* San Francisco: Cybex, Inc.

Longo, D., and D. Bohr, eds. 1991. *Quantitative methods in quality management.* Chicago: American Hospital Association. 10–11.

Moore, D. 1979. *Statistics: Concepts and controversies.* San Francisco: W.H. Freeman & Co. 100–129.

Nunnally, J. 1978. *Psychometric theory.* New York: McGraw-Hill. 3–5.

Prospective Payment Assessment Commission. 1993. *Medicare and the American health care system. Report to the Congress.* Washington, DC.

Prospective Payment Assessment Commission. 1996. *Medicare and the American health care system. Report to the Congress.* Washington, DC.

Self instructional manual for cancer registries, Book 7: Statistics and epidemiology for cancer registries. U.S. Department of Health and Human Services, Public Health Service, National Institutes of Health, NIH Publication No. 94-3766. 1994.

Tufte, E.R. 1983. *The visual display of quantitative information.* Chelshire, CT: Graphics Press. 13.

U.S. Department of Health and Human Services, Public Health Service. 1992. *Principles of epidemiology: An introduction to applied epidemiology and biostatistics.* Atlanta, GA: USDHHS.

Weisberg, H.F. 1992. *Central tendency and variability.* Newbury Park, CA: Sage Publications. 4.

Appendix 2–A

Exercises for Solving Problems

KNOWLEDGE QUESTIONS

1. Define the key terms listed at the beginning of this chapter.

2. The purpose of a table, chart, or graph is to communicate information to the data user. What questions should be considered to accomplish this objective?

3. What questions should be answered in the title of a table, chart, or graph?

4. What points should be considered when constructing a bar chart?

5. Describe the differences between a stacked bar chart and a 100% component bar chart.

6. Differentiate between a bar chart and a histogram.

MULTIPLE CHOICE

1. You want to graph the average length of stay by sex and service for the month of April. The best choice is a:
   a. bar graph
   b. histogram
   c. line graph
   d. pie chart

2. You want to graph the number of deaths due to prostate cancer for the years 1990 to 1999. The best choice is a:
   a. frequency polygon
   b. histogram
   c. line graph
   d. pie chart

3. A pie chart may be used to display the:
   a. average length of stay by year
   b. percentage of discharges by third-party payer
   c. number of discharges per year and third-party payer
   d. number of patients discharged by sex and service

4. A histogram may be used to display:
   a. discharges by age
   b. discharges by third-party payer
   c. discharges by service
   d. discharges by sex

5. You want to display the number of discharges by sex and service for 1999. The best choice is a:
   a. bar chart
   b. cluster line graph
   c. histogram
   d. line graph

PROBLEMS

Prepare the appropriate charts and graphs for the following problems. Include a title for each and identify the data source when indicated.

1. The admissions data in Table 2–A–1 compare actual admissions by hospital service with the budgeted number of hospital admissions for the month of January for Critical Care Hospital. Using computer graphic software, construct a bar chart that compares budgeted admissions with actual admissions. Write a short summary of the results.

Table 2–A–1 Admissions Report for January

Hospital Service	Budgeted Admissions	Actual Admissions
Medicine	769	728
Surgery	583	578
OB/GYN	440	402
Psychiatry	99	113
Physical medicine and rehab.	57	48
Other adult	178	191
Newborn	312	294

2. Using the data in Table 2–A–2, prepare a pie chart for January patient days by service for Critical Care Hospital.

Table 2–A–2 Patient Days by Service

Service	Patient Days
Medicine	4,436
Surgery	4,036
OB/GYN	1,170
Psychiatry	1,223
Phys. med. and rehab.	1,318
Other adult	688
Newborn	1,633

3. Table 2–A–3 contains length-of-stay data by service for the month of January for Critical Care Hospital. Construct a stacked bar chart that compares actual average length of stay with the budgeted average length of stay.

Table 2–A–3 Average Length of Stay (ALOS) by Services

Service	Budgeted ALOS	Actual ALOS
Medicine	6.39	6.09
Surgery	7.23	6.98
OB/GYN	3.22	2.91
Psychiatry	11.56	10.82
Physical medicine	22.98	27.46
Other adult	3.93	3.60
Newborn	4.97	5.55

4. Organize the following statistics for the month of January into a table.

Critical Care Cancer Research Institute Statistics for January

Discharges
    Medicine   198
    Surgery   152
    Gynecology   74
    Otolaryngology   48
Average Length of Stay
    Medicine   6.6
    Surgery   6.2
    Gynecology   4.4
    Otolaryngology   6.0
Discharge Service Days
    Medicine   1,313
    Surgery   947
    Gynecology   328
    Otolaryngology   290

5. Exhibit 2–A–1 displays the lengths of stay for 80 patients at the Critical Care Cancer Research Institute. Construct a histogram of these data.

Exhibit 2–A–1 Lengths of Stay for 80 Patients

1	2	3	5	6	10	13	16
1	2	3	5	6	10	13	17
1	2	3	5	6	10	13	17
1	2	4	5	6	10	14	17
1	2	4	5	8	11	14	18
1	2	4	5	8	11	14	19
1	2	4	5	8	11	14	19
1	2	4	6	8	11	15	20
2	3	4	6	8	12	15	20
2	3	5	6	9	12	16	20

6. The Health Care Financing Administration (HCFA) issued a report indicating per capita national health care spending for the years 1990 to 1994. Construct a line graph of these data.

Year	Per Capita Spending
1990	3,051
1991	3,160
1992	3,323
1993	3,418
1994	3,510

Source: Reprinted from *Medicare and the American Health Care System: Report to the Congress*, p. 14, 1993, Prospective Payment Assessment Commission.

7. In the same report, HCFA reported national health care spending by sector for selected years. Construct a line graph that compares spending by sector.

National Health Care Spending, by Sector,
Selected Years (in Billions)

Year	Hospital	Nursing Home Facilities	Health	Physicians
1975	52.6	8.7	0.6	23.9
1980	102.7	17.6	2.4	45.2
1985	168.3	30.7	5.6	83.6
1990	256.4	50.9	13.1	146.3
1994	338.5	72.3	26.2	189.4

Source: Reprinted from *Medicare and the American Health Care System: Report to the Congress*, p. 15, 1993, Prospective Payment Assessment Commission.

Chapter 3

Introduction to Measurement

KEY TERMS

Measurement
Validity
   Content validity
   Construct validity
   Criterion-related validity
Sensitivity
Specificity
Predictive Value
Reliability
   Stability
   Internal consistency
   Interrater agreement

Kappa coefficient
Timeliness
Scales of measurement
   Nominal
   Ordinal
   Ratio
   Interval
Continuous variable

LEARNING OBJECTIVES

At the conclusion of this chapter, you should be able to:

1. Define key terms.
2. Relate the importance of validity and reliability to the measurement process.
3. Differentiate between the following aspects of validity: content, construct, and criterion related.
4. Differentiate between the following aspects of reliability: stability, internal consistency, and interrater agreement.
5. Determine the sensitivity, specificity, and predictive value of a test.
6. Compare and contrast the following scales of measurement: nominal, ordinal, ratio, and interval.
7. Classify variables to the scales of measurement.
8. Identify variables as either discrete or continuous.

WHAT IS MEASUREMENT?

In the daily operations of any organization, whether in business, manufacturing, or health care, data are collected for decision making. To be effective, decision makers must have confidence in the data collected. Confidence requires that the data collected be accurate, timely, and reliable. Assurance of these aspects of data quality is what the **measurement** process is about.

Our discussion of analysis of clinical data in health care begins with the topic of measurement. We cannot accurately collect, analyze, and make conclusions regarding clinical data without an understanding of the measurement process. In measurement, we are concerned with measuring an attribute or property of a person, object, or event according to a particular set of rules. In some cases, measurement may be direct, as when we are using a yardstick to measure the property "width of a desk" (object). However, in health care we do not always have the ability to measure persons, objects, or events directly. For example, "quality of care" cannot be measured directly with a yardstick or any other measuring device. Consequently, an indirect measure must be developed.

Whether we are dealing with direct or indirect measures, the result of the measurement process is numbers, and there must be a set of rules for assigning numbers to the objects being measured. The measurement process requires rigorous definition of what will be collected and the method by which it will be collected so that the resulting numbers will be meaningful, accurate, and informative. The advantage of standardizing the process is that the results are the same regardless of who is doing the data collection. The resulting uniformity also allows for comparisons between and within institutions. Through measurement, one creates data that can be analyzed using statistical techniques and that can be presented as meaningful information. Through the measurement process, we can transform data into information.

To illustrate, consider the process by which the data for the Caesarean section (C-section) rate is collected. The C-section rate is often used as a performance indicator for hospital obstetric services, especially by managed care plans. A low C-section rate is desirable, since C-sections are more expensive than vaginal deliveries. The first step in the process is to define C-section rate, the event to be measured. Now we must consider the properties that characterize this event—in other words, what data will be collected. The procedure for measuring this event is presented in Exhibit 3–1. As you can see, calculation of the C-section rate is a straightforward process.

However, quantifying some of the performance indicators of the Joint Commission on Accreditation of Healthcare Organizations (Joint Commission) is not always so easily accomplished. Since some performance indicators cannot be directly measured, we must use some attribute that is considered to represent the presence or absence of the attribute of interest—an indirect measure. As an analogy, consider the personal attribute of intelligence. Intelligence is a personal attribute that cannot be directly measured with a yardstick or with any type of device; instead it is indirectly measured through a standardized IQ test, which consists of questions that are assumed to be representative of intelligence.

Exhibit 3–2 outlines the procedure for collecting data on the performance indicator "acute myocardial infarction (AMI) mortality." AMI mortality is a performance indicator that measures outcome. The occurrence of this event is considered an indicator of an undesirable outcome and should be avoided. But in calculating the mortality rate, we must first decide who will be counted. Do we count everyone who had an AMI? Do we count only those

Exhibit 3–1 Measurement of Caesarean Section Rate

Caesarean Section Rate (event):
    The ratio during any given time period of surgical deliveries (Caesarean sections) to the total number of deliveries.
Data To Be Collected (Properties):
    1. Total number of Caesarean sections performed for a given period
    2. Total number of deliveries for the period
Data Sources:
    1. Medical records of discharged obstetrical patients for the period
    2. Daily discharge reports for the period
    3. Disease and operations indexes of the International Classification of Disease, 9th Revision, Clinical Modification (ICD-9-CM)
    4. Labor and delivery room logs
Calculation:

$$\frac{\text{Total no. of Caesarean sections for period}}{\text{Total no. of deliveries for same period}} \times 100$$

Exhibit 3–2 Example of Measurement of a Joint Commission Quality Indicator

Measure: Acute Myocardial Infarction (AMI) Mortality (Event)

Type of Measure: Outcome

Rationale: Inpatient mortality for AMI is a performance indicator that can help a facility to evaluate outcomes related to the inpatient episode or delay factors prior to the inpatient episode that affect the inpatient outcome.

Data To Be Collected (Properties):
    Total number of inpatient discharges identified as having a principal diagnosis classified to ICD-9-CM subcategory 410.x1 for a specified time frame.

Data Sources:
    1. Medical records of discharged patients with principal diagnosis of 410.x1 for the period
    2. ICD-9-CM disease indexes identifying cases with principal diagnosis of 410.x1
    3. Statistical reports identifying number of cases discharged from diagnosis-related groups (DRGs) 121, 122, and/or 123

Calculation:

$$\frac{\text{Total no. of inpatient deaths with principal diagnosis of AMI (ICD-9 code 410.xx) for the period} \times 100}{\text{Total no. of inpatients discharged with principal diagnosis of AMI (ICD-9 code 410.xx) for the period}}$$

Source: © Joint Commission: *National Library of Healthcare Indicators.* Oakbrook Terrace, IL: Joint Commission on Accreditation of Healthcare Organizations, 1997, 124. Reprinted with permission.

admitted for AMI? Do we count those who had an AMI after admission? Standardization of the process helps ensure that everyone is counting the same type of cases. As you can see in Exhibit 3–2, we are interested in counting only patients who have a principal diagnosis of AMI. This occurrence, to be measured, must be rigorously defined, and procedures for data collection must be strictly followed.

VALIDITY

Accuracy in measurement cannot happen without **validity**. The measuring instrument, whether a ruler, an IQ test, or a survey instrument, is considered valid if it measures what it is intended to measure and for the intended purpose. A ruler or scale is a direct measure. In health care, because we cannot measure quality with yardsticks and scales, quality is often assessed through indirect measures.

As an example, the Joint Commission performance measure "diabetes short-term complications" is displayed in Exhibit 3–3. The stated focus of this measure is on "ambulatory care-sensitive admissions for diabetes." The developers of this performance measure state that this indicator may be used as a "proxy measure for . . . access to primary and preventive health care services."[1] Thus, this performance measure is serving as an indirect measure for access to a certain type of ambulatory care. Inpatient discharges are serving as the proxy measure.

To implement this performance measure, we must now ask what qualifies as a short-term diabetic complication. Is each health care facility free to define what qualifies as a diabetic complication? Are both Type I and Type II diabetics to be included? What about complications of gestational diabetes? It should become obvious that if we are to have valid data, qualifying complications must be rigorously defined. Without rigorous definition of the measure, consistent, comparable data will not result from the data collection process, and confidence in the information will be lost. There are many types of validity, but we will limit our discussion to three: content, construct, and criterion-related validity.

Content validity is the adequacy of the sample or the number of items used to represent the content area being measured. It is the extent to which the instrument makes sense in terms of the property or attribute being measured. This is often referred to as content validity. For example, if we are interested in assessing an individual's competency in ICD-9-CM coding, a sample of 10 items from the vast domain of coding guidelines and principles is inadequate. It is not logical that 10 items could adequately measure an individual's ability to apply ICD-9-CM guidelines and principles to all body systems. By its very nature, content validity is a matter of judgment and is evaluated by a panel of experts.

Construct validity is the ability of an instrument to measure the selected property or attribute of interest. How do we know that an intelligence test actually measures intelligence or that a survey instrument on patient satisfaction actually measures patient satisfaction? Construct validity is considered to be the link between theory and the property/attribute under study. A statistical technique of factor analysis is often used to evaluate construct validity. In our example of diabetes short-term complications, how do we know that the identified complications are representative of lack of access to ambulatory care?

Exhibit 3–3 Joint Commission Performance Measure—Diabetes Short-Term Complications

Measure: Diabetes short-term complications

Focus of Measure: Ambulatory care–sensitive (ACS) admissions for diabetes

Type of Measure: Process

Rationale: Adequate and timely preventive primary and outpatient ambulatory care may prevent hospitalizations for such chronic conditions as asthma, congestive heart failure, and diabetes. Similarly, effective outpatient treatment of acute conditions such as pneumonia and cellulitis may prevent complications requiring hospitalizations. Such preventable hospitalizations are known as access or ACS admissions.

Numerator Statement: Number of discharges with short-term complications per 100 adult discharges with diabetes.

Data Sources:
1. Medical records of discharged patients with principal diagnosis of diabetes mellitus (ICD-9-CM codes 250.02, 250.03, 250.1x, 250.2x, 250.3x) for the period
2. ICD-9-CM disease indexes identifying cases with principal or secondary diagnosis of diabetes mellitus (250.xx)
3. UB-92 billing forms

Calculation:

$$\frac{\text{Total no. of inpatients discharged with principal}}{\text{diagnosis of 250.02, 250.03, 250.1x, 250.2x, 250.3x} \times 100}{\text{All nonmaternal discharges, 18 years of age or older,}\atop\text{with diabetes for the period}}$$

Testing:
　　Reliability: No
　　Validity: No
　　Relevance: Yes

Source: © Joint Commission: *National Library of Healthcare Indicators.* Oakbrook Terrace, IL: Joint Commission on Accreditation of Healthcare Organizations, 1997, 74. Reprinted with permission.

In **criterion-related validity**, we are applying a known criterion or gold standard to the measurement instrument. It is assessed by correlating the measure of interest with an external criterion that is known to measure the property of interest. Criterion-related validity can be either concurrent or predictive. An example of criterion-related validity that is predictive is the Scholastic Achievement Test. This test is used to predict the success of an individual in the first year of college. Linear regression may be used to evaluate predictive validity.

SENSITIVITY, SPECIFICITY, AND PREDICTIVE VALUE OF A MEASURE

Sensitivity, **specificity**, and **predictive value** are aspects of data accuracy. They assist in evaluating the validity of a measure, especially the indirect performance indicators that are often used in health care. A measure is sensitive to the extent that it identifies every case in which the property of interest is truly present (cell a, Table 3–1). If the measure is not sensitive, it will not detect the property of interest when it is present (cell c). Specificity is the aspect of measurement that results in exclusion of cases when the property of interest is truly absent (cell d). If the measurement is not specific, it will falsely detect the property of interest when it is not present (cell b). The accuracy of a test or measure is dependent upon the number of false positives and false negatives that occurs as a result of using the measure. If the test is accurate, the number of false positives and false negatives will be low. The predictive value is the proportion of positive tests that are truly positive (a/a + b). The predictive value of a positive test increases as sensitivity and specificity increase.

Table 3–1 Assessing Sensitivity and Specificity of a Measure

	True Situation Event		
Test/Measure	Performance Indicator Present	Performance Indicator Absent	Total
Positive	a	b	a + b
Negative	c	d	c + d
Total	a + c	b + d	a + b + c + d

Sensitivity: $a/(a + c)$
Specificity: $d/(b + d)$
Predictive value: $a/(a + b)$: the predictive value of a positive
                   $c/(c + d)$: the predictive value of a negative
There are four possible outcomes, represented by the four cells:
Cell a: true positives—the variable of interest is present and the measure reveals its presence.
Cell b: false positives—the measure indicates the variable of interest to be present, but it is incorrect.
Cell c: false negatives—the variable of interest is present, but the measure does not reveal it.
Cell d: true negatives—the variable of interest is absent, and the measure indicates that it is absent.

Source: Adapted from R. Morton, J.R. Hebel, and R.J. McCarter, *A Study Guide to Epidemiology and Biostatistics*, p. 66, © 1989, Aspen Publishers, Inc.

To determine the specificity and sensitivity of a proposed measure, a pilot test of the measure may be conducted, with the results displayed in a table such as the one displayed in Table 3–1. In this table, the rows represent the true situation—the presence or absence of the performance indicator. The columns represent the possible results of the measure for the performance indicator of interest. The test is positive when it tells us that the performance indicator is present and negative when it tells us that the performance indicator of interest is not present.

A test is accurate to the extent that it does not result in false positives and false negatives. A large number of false positives will lead to the unnecessary examination of cases where no problem exists. In time, this will lead to the loss of the data's credibility. A large number of false negatives can result in overlooking cases that actually contain the performance indicator of interest.

An example may help clarify assessment of sensitivity and specificity. A quality improvement team wants to evaluate the performance measure on diabetic short-term complications because it has not been tested for reliability and validity by the Joint Commission (Exhibit 3–3). The team knows in advance that diabetes with the specified complications, such as ketoacidosis and uncontrolled diabetes, was the reason for admission in 20 cases. How effective is our test in identifying these 20 cases? The results of the pilot test are displayed in Table 3–2.

Table 3–2 Assessing Sensitivity and Specificity of Admission for Diabetes with Specified Complication

Admission for Diabetes with Specified Complication	Specified Complication Present		
	Yes	*No*	*Total*
Yes	15	10	25
No	5	70	75
Total	20	80	100

In this example, diabetes mellitus with the specified complications occurred in 20 cases ($a + c = 15 + 5$). The measure correctly identified 15 of the 20 cases; thus, the sensitivity for the measure is .75 ($a/(a + c)$). The test incorrectly identified 10 patients as having the problem. These are false positives. The test correctly identified 70 of the 80 cases that had no problem; thus the specificity is .88 [$d/b + d = 70/(10 + 70)$]. The test also failed to identify 5 cases where there were problems; these are false negatives.

Validity is the extent to which a measure actually measures a property or attribute one wants to measure. In this example, the measure correctly identified 15 of the 25 cases in which the diabetic complication was present; thus, the predictive value is .60 [$a/a + b = 15/(15 + 10)$]. The test correctly measures the property of interest 60% of the time.

Sensitivity, specificity, and predictive value quantify the accuracy of the quality measure. With a sensitivity of .75, the measure misses 25% of the cases in which we are interested. The predictive value is .60; thus, 40% of the time the measure tells us that there may be a problem with performance when there is none. In this example, the measure is not highly accurate.

RELIABILITY

Error is integral to the measurement process, whether it is the measurement of weight, height, or blood pressure. Even when measurement is made as accurately as the instrument allows and all procedures are followed, repeated measures do not always give exactly the same results. This is because error is a component of all measurement. But an instrument that is reliable will tend to have results that are consistent with each other over repeated trials.

A measurement process is said to be reliable if repeated measurements over time on the same property or attribute give the same or approximately the same results. A yardstick is reliable because it will provide approximately the same result every time an object is measured, regardless of who is doing the measuring. An example of an unreliable measuring device is a scale that gives widely different weights each time the same object is measured.

Measures should also be unbiased. A measurement process is unbiased if it does not systematically overstate or understate the true value of the attribute/property being measured. An example of a biased but reliable measure is a scale that consistently measures weight 10 pounds less than the actual weight. An unbiased measure is correct on average.

There are three aspects of **reliability**: stability, internal consistency, and interrater agreement. **Stability**, or test-retest reliability, is the extent to which the same results are obtained on repeated applications. Stability is evaluated by administering the instrument to the same group on two separate occasions—hence the name *test-retest reliability*. A reliability coefficient is calculated from the two sets of scores. The reliability coefficient ranges from 0 (no reliability) to 1.0 (perfect reliability).

Internal consistency measures the extent to which the items on the measurement instrument are homogeneous, or consistent with one another. Internal consistency is measured by Cronbach's alpha, which is often referred to as coefficient alpha. Coefficient alpha also has a range of 0.0 to 1.0; an instrument should have a minimum coefficient alpha of .70 for acceptability.

Interrater agreement is the extent to which results are in agreement when different individuals administer the same instrument to the same individuals or groups. This is an important concept in coding. If we have four coders assigning codes to peripheral vascular disease due to insulin-dependent diabetes mellitus, we want all four coders to come up with the same codes. Interrater agreement should be 100%. The kappa statistic is used to assess interrater agreement. This statistic is limited, however, because it requires that the responses be dichotomous. In the coding example, the codes would be evaluated as either right or wrong.

In using kappa, we are interested in determining the extent of agreement, not disagreement, between raters. Kappa is obtained by the following formula:

$$\kappa = A_O - A_E / N - A_E$$

where A_O is the number of observations that are in agreement and A_E is the number of observations in agreement expected by chance alone.

A_O is obtained by summing the table diagonals ($A_O = a + d$), and the percentage of agreement is obtained by A_O/N. A_E is obtained by multiplying the row total times the column total and dividing by the grand total, as follows:

$$A_E = \sum_{i=1}^{k} \text{(row marginal) (column marginal)}/N$$

The range for the **kappa coefficient** is −1.0 to +1.0. A negative value indicates that the proportion of agreement that resulted from chance is greater than the proportion of observed agreement. High positive values of kappa indicate strong interrater agreement.

Let us now consider an example where two raters have been asked to evaluate the accuracy of a simple random sample of 200 medical records that have been coded. The coded charts were evaluated as right or wrong. The results appear in Table 3–3.

Table 3–3 Results of Coding Assessments by Two Raters

	Rater 2		
Rater 1	Right	Wrong	Total
Right	80	20	100
Wrong	25	75	100
Total	105	95	200

To obtain the number of observations that are in agreement between the two raters, A_O, the diagonals are summed: $80 + 75 = 155$. The percent agreement between the two raters is 77.5% (155/200). The number of observations in agreement that is expected by chance, A_E, is obtained by

$$A_E = \sum_{i=1}^{k} \text{(row marginal)(column marginal)}/N$$
$$= (100)(105)/200 + (100)(95)/200$$
$$= 52.5 + 47.5$$
$$= 100$$
$$\kappa = (A_O - A_E)/(N - A_E)$$
$$= (155 - 100)/(200 - 100) = .55$$

The interpretation of kappa is that the obtained agreement of 77.5% is approximately 55% greater than what would be achieved by chance alone. Interpretation of the kappa statistic is as follows:

$\kappa < .20$ negligible
$.20 \leq \kappa < .40$ minimal
$.40 \leq \kappa < .60$ fair
$.60 \leq \kappa < .80$ good
$\kappa \geq .80$ excellent

In our example, the obtained kappa coefficient, .55, indicates that the raters obtained fair agreement in their assessment of the sample of coded records.

In summary, a measure is reliable if (1) the same individual measures the same attribute at another time and achieves the same result, (2) the individual applies the measure consistently on all attributes, and (3) several individuals reach the same result when measuring the same attribute.

TIMELINESS

A critical aspect of data quality is **timeliness**. One must consider whether the data are collected and available within a useful time frame. Does the collected information represent the current condition of the patient or state of the organization? Data collected today are more critical and useful to the decision maker than data collected yesterday or two weeks ago. The value of collected data decreases with time.

For data to be accurate, the measure creating the data must be rigorously defined. A common failure in the measurement process is to undertake the measurement process without a clear definition of what is to be measured, who will use the resulting information, and how the information will be used for making decisions. The measurement process must begin with a strong commitment to identifying the information needs of those who will be using the information.

SCALES OF MEASUREMENT

As stated previously, all measurement results in a number. To properly assign numbers to the measurement results, one must understand the **scales of measurement**. Understanding the differences in the scales of measurement is also critical to make appropriate use of graphic displays of data, to correctly select statistical techniques for data analysis, and to facilitate data entry.

Nominal Scale

The **nominal** scale is the lowest level of measurement. In the nominal scale, measures are organized into categories; there is no recognition of order within these categories. Examples of categories on the nominal scale of measurement are sex, religion, and third-party payer. To facilitate computer analysis, numbers are assigned to nominal variable—for example, male $= 1$, female $= 2$. The numbers assigned to the various categories carry no numerical weight; the numbers merely serve as labels for the categories.

Statistical summaries of variables on the nominal scale may be prepared through the use of a frequency distribution. On the nominal scale, a frequency distribution would indicate the number of cases falling into each category. Using statistical notation, the frequency distribution would be represented as follows:

$$N = \sum_k f_k$$

where N is the total number of cases, f_k is the frequency within category, and

$\sum_k$ is a summation over all categories k.

As a hypothetical example, consider the nominal variable "method of payment." For initial patient data collection, options may be commercial insurance ($k = 1$), managed care ($k = 2$), Medicare ($k = 3$), Medicaid ($k = 4$), self-pay ($k = 5$), and other ($k = 6$). Thus, there are six categories. A frequency distribution for patients admitted by method of payment is presented in Table 3–4. In our example, the total number of patients admitted during the week of July 23 is 256 (N = 256); and the number of Medicare patients (frequency) who were admitted is 62 (f_3 = 62).

Table 3–4 Number of Patients Admitted by Method of Payment, Week of July 23

Commercial Insurance	Managed Care	Medicare	Medicaid	Self-Pay	Other	Total
75	43	62	55	6	15	256

Sometimes it is useful to show the proportion of cases falling into a category k. This proportion is designated a p_k. A proportion is the number of cases that fall within a particular category divided by the total number of cases and is represented as

$$p_k = f_k/N$$

The proportion of cases falling into each category will sum to 1. Using the same data from Table 3–4, Table 3–5 represents the proportions and cumulative proportions for each category.

Table 3–5 Proportion of Patients Admitted by Method of Payment, Week of July 23

Category	Frequency (f)	Proportion (p)	Cum. Proportion
Commercial insurance	75	.293	.293
Managed care	43	.168	.461
Medicare	62	.242	.703
Medicaid	55	.215	.918
Self-pay	6	.023	.941
Other	15	.059	1.00
Total (N)	256	1.000	

The distribution of a variable into the various categories can also be represented by percentages, which are proportions multiplied by 100. For data that fall on the nominal scale of measurement, frequencies may be represented in tables, charts, and graphs. The most appropriate measure of central tendency for nominal-level data is the mode. For nominal data, the mode tells us the category that has the most observations.

When designing a system of data collection for nominal variables, remember that the categories must be mutually exclusive and exhaustive. That is, each data element can fall into only one category, and all possible categories must be accounted for. It may be appropriate to assign an "other" category, as in the above example, when the number of data elements falling into some possible categories may be too small for data analysis or when the category is not important to the purpose of the data collection.

Ordinal Scale

Some non-numeric scales have an order to their categories; these are called **ordinal** variables. On the ordinal scale, the order of the numbers is meaningful, not the number itself, so the usual arithmetic operations are not meaningful. This is because the intervals or distance between categories are not necessarily equal. It is not appropriate to perform arithmetic operations, such as calculating averages, on ordinal variables.

Examples of ordinal variables are the numbers assigned to indicate class rank, the ordering of adjectives that describe patient condition, and a Likert-type scale that may be used to describe patient satisfaction. These examples are displayed in Table 3–6. A number may be assigned to represent the ordering of the variables. In the case of class rank, we know that an individual classified as a senior has completed more credit hours than a sophomore, but we cannot say that a senior has completed twice as many credit hours as a sophomore. The same is true regarding patient condition. A patient that is in critical condition is not necessarily twice as sick as an individual who is in stable condition. Only the order of the value is meaningful. On this scale, a patient in critical condition is sicker than a patient in guarded condition. The frequency distributions of ordinal variables may be portrayed in the same way as for nominal variables.

Table 3–6 Examples of Ordinal Variables

Class Rank	Patient Condition	Patient Satisfaction
1—Freshman	1—Resting and Comfortable	1—Strongly agree
2—Sophomore	2—Stable	3—Agree
3—Junior	3—Guarded	3—No opinion
4—Senior	4—Critical	4—Disagree
		5—Strongly disagree

Nominal and ordinal variables are considered discrete variables. Discrete variables have gaps between successive values. Diagnosis-related groups (DRGs) are examples of discrete/nominal variables.

Scales for Metric Variables

Metric variables are numeric variables that answer questions of how much or how many. Metric variables fall on one of two scales of measurement: ratio or interval. Arithmetic operations may be performed on ratio- and interval-scale measures.

- *Ratio Scale*. The **ratio** scale is the highest level of measurement. On the ratio scale there is a defined unit of measure, a real zero point, and the intervals between successive values are equal. For example, consider the variable of length. Length has defined units of measurement, such as inches, and a true zero point—0 inches. With a real zero point, statements such as "Mary is twice as tall as Jill" can be made. Multiplication on the ratio scale by a constant does not change its ratio character, but addition of a constant to a ratio measure does. For example, if an older sibling is twice as tall as a younger sibling, and both grow 2 inches, the ratio of their heights is no longer 2:1. But if we multiply their respective heights by 2 (e.g., 60" × 2 and 30" × 2), the ratio between the two heights remains 2:1.
- *Interval Scale*. Measures that fall on the **interval** scale have a defined unit of measurement but do not have a true zero point. The most important characteristic of the interval scale is that the intervals between successive values are equal. On the Fahrenheit scale, the interval between 20°F and 21°F is the same as the interval between 21° and 22°F. But since there is not a true zero on this scale, we cannot say the 40°F is twice as warm as 20°F.

An advantage of metric data is that they can be grouped. Interval and ratio variables are continuous. If a variable is continuous, it may take on fractional values, such as 85.3235°F. With **continuous variables**, there are no gaps between values, since the values progress fractionally. Graphic techniques that may be used to display interval and ratio data include histograms, frequency polygons, and stem and leaf plots. Measures of central tendency that may be reported for interval and ratio data are the mean, median, and mode.

The scale of measurement depends on the method of measurement, not on the attribute being measured. For example, if we score a test by summing the total number of correct answers, the resulting measures fall on the ratio scale. However, if each question is tallied according to the total number who got the question right and the total number who got the question wrong, the measures fall on the nominal scale because the measure falls into one of two categories—"right" or "wrong." When developing measures for any purpose, one must consider on what scale of measurement the collected data will fall so that the appropriate statistical procedures may be selected.

CONCLUSION

Measurement is a process that requires rigorous definition of what is being measured, the data sources, and how the variable measured will be calculated. Several aspects of a measure should be evaluated: validity, reliability, sensitivity, specificity, and predictive value.

The validity of a measure is the extent to which an instrument measures what it is intended to measure. Several aspects of validity were discussed: content validity, construct validity, and criterion-related validity. With content validity, we are interested in determining whether the number of items on an instrument adequately measure the content of interest. With construct validity, we are trying to determine if the items on an instrument actually assess the attribute of interest, such as patient satisfaction. And, with criterion-related validity, we are assessing whether the measure is correlated with an external criterion: for example, whether a rise in serum glutamicoxaloacetic transaminase enzyme levels is correlated with acute myocardial infarction.

Reliability is the extent to which an instrument gives the same results over time or over repeated measures. Several aspects of reliability were discussed: test-retest reliability, internal consistency, and interrater agreement. Test-retest reliability is the extent to which repeated administrations of an instrument provide the same results. Internal consistency is the extent to which the items on an instrument are related to one another. And interrater agreement is the extent to which different individuals who administer the same instrument achieve similar results.

Other critical aspects of a measure are sensitivity, specificity, and predictive value. Sensitivity is the ability of an instrument to detect the property of interest in every case where it exists. Specificity is the ability of an instrument to exclude cases in which the property of interest is truly absent. A test is accurate to the extent that it does not result in false positives and false negatives. Predictive value is the ability of an instrument or test to correctly measure the proportion of positive tests that are truly positive or the proportion of negative tests that are truly negative.

Finally, to understand the measurement process, we must understand the differences in the scales of measurement: nominal, ordinal, interval, and ratio. In the nominal scale of measurement, measures are organized into categories; the nominal scale is the lowest level of measurement. In the ordinal scale of measurement, there is "order" to the categories; the numbers themselves are not meaningful, but the order is. On the interval and ratio scales of measurement, the intervals between successive values are equal. Arithmetic calculations may be performed on interval and ratio measures. The interval scale differs from the ratio scale in that the interval scale does not have a true zero.

NOTE

1. Joint Commission on Accreditation of Healthcare Organizations, *National Library of Health Care Indicators*, Oakbrook Terrace, IL: Joint Commission on Accreditation of Healthcare Organizations, 1997, 74 [Diabetes], 124 [AMI].

ADDITIONAL RESOURCES

Al-Assaf, A.F., and J.A. Schmele, eds. 1993. *The textbook of total quality management.* Delray Beach, FL: St. Lucie Press. 124–125.

Fales, J. 1995. Automatic data collection and productivity. Unpublished lecture.

Hanken, M.A., and K. Waters. 1994. *Glossary of healthcare terms.* Chicago: American Health Information Management Association. 61.

Jekel, J., et al. 1996. *Epidemiology, biostatistics and preventive medicine.* Philadelphia: W.B. Saunders Co.

Joint Commission on Accreditation of Healthcare Organizations. 1997. *Accreditation manual for hospitals.* Oakbrook Terrace, IL: Joint Commission on Accreditation of Healthcare Organizations.

Kane, R.L., ed. 1997. *Understanding health care outcomes research.* Gaithersburg, MD: Aspen Publishers, Inc. 228–229.

Longo, D., and D. Bohr, eds. 1991. *Quantitative methods in quality management.* Chicago: American Hospital Association. 10–11.

Moore, D. 1979. *Statistics: Concepts and controversies.* San Francisco: W.H. Freeman & Co. 100–129.

Nelson, E. 1995. Measuring for improvement: Why, what, when, how, for whom? *Quality Connection* 4, no. 2: 3.

Nunnally, J. 1978. *Psychometric theory.* New York: McGraw-Hill. 3–5.

Osborn, C.E. 1998. Developing instruments for assessment of patient outcomes. *Journal of Rehabilitation Outcomes Measurement* 2, no. 6: 18–25.

U.S. Department of Health and Human Services, Public Health Service. 1992. *Principles of epidemiology: An introduction to applied epidemiology and biostatistics.* Atlanta, GA: USDHHS.

Wan, T.T.H. 1995. *Analysis and evaluation of health care systems.* Baltimore, MD: Health Professions Press. 41–43.

Appendix 3–A

Exercises for Solving Problems

KNOWLEDGE QUESTIONS

1. Define the key terms listed at the beginning of this chapter.

2. Describe the measurement process.

3. Why are validity and reliability requirements of accuracy in the measurement process?

4. Compare and contrast the following aspects of validity: content validity, construct validity, and criterion-related validity.

5. You weighed your dog this morning on your bathroom scale. His weight was 15 lb. You decided to weigh him again in the evening, and his weight had increased to 20 lb. This is most likely what type of measurement error? Explain your answer.

6. Compare and contrast the following measures of reliability: stability, internal consistency, and interrater agreement.

7. Relate the importance of determining the sensitivity, specificity, and predictive value of a screening measure.

8. Define nominal, ordinal, interval, and ratio scales of measurement.

9. What is the difference between a discrete variable and a continuous variable?

MULTIPLE CHOICE

1. You are conducting a study in which "sex" is the property of interest. The variable "sex" falls upon which of the following scales of measurement?
   a. nominal
   b. ordinal
   c. ratio
   d. interval

2. You are interested in the lengths of stay for patients of Dr. Wells for a quality improvement study. The variable "length of stay" falls upon which of the following scales of measurement?
   a. nominal
   b. ordinal
   c. ratio
   d. interval

3. You are assisting Dr. Scorch in his study of burn patients. He wants to classify the number of burn patients by severity of burn: first degree, second degree, or third degree. The variable "severity of burn" falls upon which of the following scales of measurement?
   a. nominal
   b. ordinal
   c. ratio
   d. interval

4. "Severity of burn" is an example of which of the following types of variables?
   a. continuous
   b. discrete
   c. interval
   d. ratio

For questions 5 through 8 refer to the following case:

You have designed a survey instrument with a 5-point Likert-type scale consisting of statements that measure physician satisfaction with health information management services. On the scale, 1 = *strongly agree (SA)* and 5 = *strongly disagree (SD)*.

5. You decide to take an average of the scores for each statement. In this case, you would be treating the data as falling upon which of the following scales of measurement?
   a. nominal
   b. ordinal
   c. ratio
   d. interval

6. After reviewing the results, you decide that the mode might be the more appropriate measure of central tendency for these data. In reporting the mode, you are treating the data as falling upon which of the following scales of measurement?
   a. nominal
   b. ordinal
   c. ratio
   d. interval

7. You have distributed this survey to the physicians five times. You are satisfied that the results are consistent. This aspect of reliability is:
   a. internal consistency
   b. test-retest reliability
   c. interrater reliability
   d. all of the above

8. However, upon careful review of the instrument, you decide that there are not enough items to adequately cover services provided by your department. You are concerned about which of the following types of validity?
   a. content
   b. construct
   c. criterion related
   d. all of the above

9. Which of the following variables would be considered "continuous"?
   a. age
   b. sex
   c. religion
   d. principal diagnosis code

10. Which of the following variables would be considered "discrete"?
    a. age upon admission
    b. patient length of stay
    c. DRG assignment upon discharge
    d. time spent in operating room

11. Both the specificity and sensitivity of a recently developed clinical indicator are .99. This means that:
    a. if the indicator is present, it has a 99% chance of testing positive by the measure
    b. if the indicator is absent, it has a 99% chance of testing negative by the measure
    c. the case has a 99% chance of being correctly classified by the measure
    d. a and b
    e. all of the above

PROBLEMS

1. The hospital readmission rate is often considered an indicator of an undesirable patient outcome. The quality improvement team is interested in reducing the number of readmissions among patients discharged with a principal diagnosis of congestive heart failure (CHF). The team believes that the high readmission rate is due to the difficulty that these patients have in controlling the number of drugs that they typically take. The team believes that by improving patient/family education regarding drug administration, the readmission rate could be reduced. Thus, they have developed the screen "CHF patients taking three or more drugs" to identify these patients before discharge. To evaluate the effectiveness of the measure, the team conducts a study on all CHF patients discharged the previous year. The results appear in Table 3–A–1:

   a. Calculate the sensitivity, specificity, and predictive value for this measure.

   b. On the basis of your results, is this an effective measure? Why or why not?

Table 3–A–1 Readmissions of CHF Patients

No. of Drugs Administered	Readmissions among CHF Patients		Total
	Readmitted	Not Readmitted	
≥3 drugs	200	40	240
<3 drugs	100	900	1,000
Total	300	940	1,240

2. Exhibit 3–A–1 displays selected data elements from the Ohio Cancer Incidence Surveillance System abstract. Identify the scale of measurement for each element, determine if the measure is discrete or continuous, and determine what measure(s) of central tendency may be used for each—mean, median, or mode.

Exhibit 3–A–1 Selected Data Elements from Ohio Cancer Incidence Surveillance System

Data Element	Measurement Scale Discrete/Continuous Variable	Measure of Central Tendency
Zip code		
Gender:		
1 = male		
2 = female		
3 = other hermaphrodite		
4 = transsexual		
9 = unknown		
Age in years at time of diagnosis		
Source of information:		
1 = hospital inpatient/outpatient or clinic		
3 = laboratory only		
4 = physician's office		
5 = nursing home		
6 = autopsy only		
7 = death certificate only		
9 = unknown		
Anatomical site (ICD-O, 2nd edition)		
Laterality at diagnosis:		
0 = not a paired site		
1 = right: origin of primary		
2 = left: origin of primary		
3 = only one side involved, right or left origin unspecified		
4 = bilateral involvement		
9 = paired site, but no information concerning laterality, midline tumor		
Grade:		
1 = well differentiated		
2 = moderately differentiated		
3 = poorly differentiated		
4 = undifferentiated		

Source: Reprinted from State of Ohio Data Abstract Form.

3. At Werethebest Hospital, 34 Caesarean sections were performed during January; at Weresosick Hospital, 54 Caesarean sections were performed during the month of January. During January, Werethebest Hospital had 200 deliveries; Weresosick Hospital had 1,100 deliveries. The national benchmark for the C-section rate is 15%.

   The head of obstetrics at Werethebest Hospital claims that their OB service provides better care than that provided at the rival hospital. Do you agree with this assessment?

4. Develop measures for the following obstetric performance indicators proposed by the Joint Commission. Your measure should include a definition, identification of data sources, and procedures for calculation (formula).
   a. Maternal readmissions within 14 days of delivery
   b. Intrahospital maternal deaths occurring within 42 days postpartum
   c. Patients with excessive maternal blood loss

5. As part of the quality improvement team, you have prepared a report on acute myocardial infarction (AMI) mortality, which is displayed in Table 3–A–2. You query DRG 121, Circulatory Disorders with AMI and Cardiovascular (CV) complications, Discharged Alive; DRG 122, Circulatory Disorders with AMI without CV Complications, Discharged Alive; and DRG 123, Circulatory Disorders with AMI, Expired.
   a. Assess the report below for validity and reliability. What corrections should be made to calculate the AMI mortality rate?
   b. What is the AMI mortality rate?
   c. Review Table 3–A–3, which displays the average length of stay for each DRG. What factors should also be considered when presenting the AMI mortality rate? What is the net AMI mortality rate?

Table 3–A–2 Acute Myocardial Infarctions, DRGs 121, 122, and 123

Principal Diagnosis	DRG 121	DRG 122	DRG 123
410.01	3	1	1
410.11	9	3	4
410.31	2	1	0
410.41	11	11	1
410.61	1	0	0
410.71	66	31	9
410.91	25	11	5
421.0	1	0	0
428.0	1	0	0
Total	119	58	20

Table 3–A–3 Average Length of Stay (ALOS) and Numbers of Patients with Length of Stay (LOS) Two Days or Less, DRGs 121, 122, and 123

	DRG 121	DRG 122	DRG 123
ALOS	5.6 days	3.6 days	3.5 days
LOS ≤ 2 days	26	18	10

CHAPTER 4

Measures of Central Tendency and Variability

KEY TERMS	Population	Measures of variation
	Population parameter	Range
	Sample	Standard deviation
	Sample statistic	Variance
	Measures of central tendency	Polarization
	Mean	Uniformity
	Trimmed mean	Individuality
	Winsorized mean	Class interval
	Weighted mean	Real limits
	Median	Apparent limits
	Mode	

LEARNING OBJECTIVES

At the conclusion of this chapter, you should be able to:

1. Define key terms.
2. Calculate measures of central tendency—mean, median, and mode—for grouped and ungrouped frequency distributions.
3. Calculate measures of variability—range, variance, and standard deviation—for grouped and ungrouped frequency distributions.
4. Use statistical software to calculate measures of central tendency and variation for ungrouped frequency distributions.
5. Explain why measures of central tendency and variation differ in grouped and ungrouped frequency distributions.

Two main types of measures are used to describe frequency distributions: measures of central tendency and measures of variability. **Measures of central tendency** measure location; measures of central tendency focus on the typical value of a data set. Variation emphasizes differences. **Measures of variation** measure distance and/or dispersion around the typical value of a data set. Generalizations about populations from samples are based on the variation of the variables in the data set.

Descriptive measures may be computed from both populations and samples. A **population** is a group of persons or objects about which a researcher or investigator wishes to draw conclusions. A **sample** is a subset of the population. Measures that result from the compilation of data from populations are called parameters. Measures that result from analysis of data from samples are called statistics. For example, if we were interested in determining the average age of all members of the American Health Information Management Association (AHIMA), all members of the association would make up the population; the average age would be a **population parameter**. But, if we were to draw a sample from the membership list and then calculate the average age, the average would be a **sample statistic**.

MEASURES OF CENTRAL TENDENCY

As previously stated, measures of central tendency summarize the typical value of a variable. When we think of measures of central tendency, we usually think of averages; however, averages or the arithmetic mean may not always be the most appropriate way of summarizing the most typical value of a data set. There are three major measures of central tendency; the selection of the relevant measure of central tendency is related to the scale of measurement used in data collection.

1. The **mode**, symbolized by M_O, is defined as the most frequently occurring observation in a frequency distribution; it is the only measure of central tendency that is appropriate for nominal data.
2. The **median**, symbolized by M_D, is the midpoint of a frequency distribution; it is appropriate for both ordinal and metric data.
3. The **mean**, symbolized by $\overline{X}$ (pronounced "x-bar"), is the arithmetic average; it is appropriate for metric data.

Mode

The mode is the simplest measure of central tendency. With the mode, we are indicating the most frequently occurring observation for metric data and/or the most frequently occurring category for nominal data.

The mode is an important measure of central tendency for nominal-level data because an average cannot be taken from data that are placed in categories. Averages work only when a variable has a unit of measurement. The mode is an important measure of central tendency in the sense that it shows what the typical category on a variable is. For example, if we group the membership of AHIMA by sex, on average, the typical health information management (HIM) professional is female. We can say this because approximately 92% of the membership of AHIMA is female.

Another interpretation of the mode is that if the goal is to be as accurate as possible, the mode provides the best "guess" as to the category an observation may take on a variable. That is, no other guess for a random case will be correct as often as the mode. Continuing with our example, if one were to guess the sex of a typical HIM professional, the best "guess" would be that the sex of the practitioner was female. In making this guess, one would be correct approximately 92% of the time.

The mode offers several advantages: it is easy to obtain and to interpret, it is not sensitive to extreme values, and it is easy to communicate and explain to others. However, there are inherent disadvantages in using the mode. First, the mode may not be descriptive of the data because the most common category may not occur very often, especially when there are a large number of categories. Second, the mode may not be unique. That is, two categories or metric measures may be equally likely and more common than any other category or metric measure; when this occurs, we have a bimodal or multimodal distribution. If each category occurs with equal frequency, there is no mode. Third, the mode does not provide information about the entire frequency distribution—it only tells us the most frequently occurring value or category in the frequency distribution.

Also, the mode may be overly affected by sampling variation in cases where there is a bimodal distribution. If several samples are taken from the same population, the mode may fluctuate widely from sample to sample. For nominal-level data, the mode is also sensitive to how categories are combined. The classification scheme should be at the same level of generality for all categories rather than having broad categories for some and more specific categories for others. The mode can be manipulated by making the level of generality of different categories unequal. When reading a statistical analysis that reports the mode, we should always examine the categories to make sure that the modal categories were not manipulated by use of categories at different levels of generality. For example, compare the following hypothetical data on hospital admissions:

Hospital Admissions by Race—A		Hospital Admissions by Race—B	
White	60%	White	60%
African American	15%	African American	15%
Hispanic	12%	Other	25%
Asian	8%		
Other	5%		

In example A, hospital admissions by race are distributed in a way that might be expected in an urban population. However, in example B, a biased view of admissions is presented by lumping two of the categories, Hispanic and Asian, into the "other" category. In this example, the individual presenting the data may be interested in emphasizing the low percentage in the African American category. Combining two racial categories into the other category creates a biased view of the racial makeup of hospital admissions.

For interval or ratio level data, the mode can be graphically represented in a frequency polygon. Figure 4–1 displays the frequency of the ages of a group of 20 nursing home residents, which are presented below:

76 76 78 78 78 78 78 80 80 80
82 82 82 84 84 86 88 88 90 90

The modal age is 78 (n = 5).

Figure 4–1 Frequency Polygon for Age of 20 Nursing Home Residents

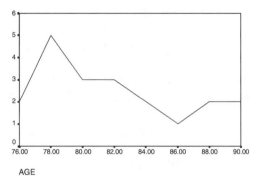

For nominal data, the mode may be depicted in a bar chart (Figure 4–2).

Figure 4–2 Bar Graph for Hospital Admissions by Race

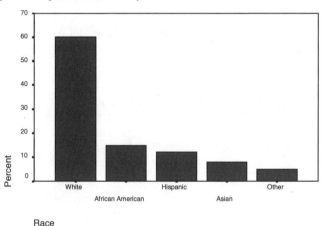

Median

When categories of a variable are ordered, the measure of central tendency should take order into account. The median does so by finding the value of the variable that corresponds to the middle case. It is a positional measure that indicates the point at which 50% of the cases fall above and 50% of the cases fall below.

If there is an odd number of observations in the frequency distribution, the median is the middle number. In the following frequency distribution, the median is 5—there are four cases above and four cases below the value 5.

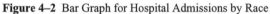

1   2   3   4   5   6   7   8   9

If there is an even number of observations, the median is the midpoint between the two middle observations. It is found by averaging the two middle scores $[(x + y)/2]$. In the following frequency distribution, the median is 5.5 $[(5 + 6)/2]$.

1   2   3   4   5   6   7   8   9   10

If the two middle observations take on the same value, the mode is that value. When determining the mode, it does not matter if there are duplicate observations in the frequency distribution. Consider the following frequency distribution:

1   2   2   3   4   4   4   5   6   7

In this distribution there are 10 observations, so the median falls between cases between the fifth and sixth observation. Therefore, the median is 4 $[(4 + 4)/2 = 4]$.

The median is an important measure for data that fall on the ordinal scale of measurement. This is due to the limitations of other measures for ordered data. The mode can be used for ordinal data, but it does not take "order" into account, which is the characteristic that makes the measure more than just a nominal classification. The mode can also be unrepresentative for an ordinal measure. It is also not meaningful to take an average of ordered variables because the distance between the intervals is not necessarily equal. This concept is illustrated in Table 4–1, hospital ranking by severity of illness. Hospitals with adjacent ranks differ by as little as .001 (1.826–1.825) on their severity of illness scores or by as much as .127 (1.753–1.626).

Table 4–1 Hospital Ranking by Severity of Illness

Hospital Ranking	Severity of Illness	Distance between Severity of Illness Scores
1	2.152	—
2	2.027	.125 (2.152 – 2.027)
3	1.965	.062
4	1.876	.089
5	1.826	.050
6	1.825	.001
7	1.753	.072
8	1.626	.127
9	1.594	.032

Averages are often calculated on ordered variables, but the results may be misleading. Therefore, when choosing a measure of central tendency, you should consider not only the scale of measurement upon which the variable falls but also the purpose of the measure.

There are several advantages of using the median. First, it is relatively easy to obtain; second, it is based on the whole distribution rather than just a small portion of the distribution, as is the case with the mode. Third, the median is not influenced by extreme values or unusual outliers, so it is considered a resistant statistic. The median has another advantage in that it can be computed when a distribution is open ended at the extremes. For example, consider the median length of stay for a group of five patients who were admitted to the hospital on the same day. If two patients are discharged on day 2 and one patient is discharged on day 4, the median length of stay is four days. The median can be determined without waiting to see how long the remaining two patients stay in the hospital. While we can determine the median in this example, we cannot determine either the mode or the mean until the two remaining patients are discharged.

Mean

The most effective way of summarizing the center of metric data is to average the values on the variable. The mode and median can be computed on metric data but they do not take full advantage of the numeric data inherent in the data in the frequency distribution. The formula for calculating the mean is

$$\overline{X} = \sum_{i=1}^{n} X_i / N$$

where $\sum$ is summation, X_i is each successive observation in the frequency distribution (from the first observation, $i = 1$, to the last observation, n), and N is the total number of observations in the distribution.

To calculate the average daily census for the data in Table 4–2, we substitute into the above formula as follows:

$$\overline{X} = \sum_{i=1}^{n} X_i / N$$
$$= (167 + 185 + 173 + 182 + 179 + 173 + 170) / 7$$
$$= 1,229/7$$
$$= 175.6$$

Table 4–2 Daily Census, Critical Care Hospital, Week of July 1, 19xx

Day of Week	Daily Census
Sunday	167
Monday	185
Tuesday	173
Wednesday	182
Thursday	179
Friday	173
Saturday	170
Average daily census	175.6

The properties of the mean are presented in Exhibit 4–1.

Exhibit 4–1 Properties of the Arithmetic Mean

1. The total sum of the deviations around the mean is zero.
2. The total sum of the negative deviations from the mean is always equal to the sum of the positive deviations from the mean—therefore, the mean is the balance point for the distribution.
3. The sum of the squared deviations around the mean is smaller than the sum of the squared deviations around any other value.
4. The mean is more stable over repeated measures than any other measure of center.
5. Other important statistics, namely, standard deviation and standard error of the mean, are based on deviations from the mean.

There are two disadvantages associated with the mean. First, the mean can take on a fractional value even when the variable itself can take on only integer values. Consider the example in Table 4–2, which gives the daily inpatient census for one week. The average daily census results in a fractional number even though we do not have fractional patients. However, fractional values are considered more as a problem of interpretation than as a nonmeaningful result. For the data in Table 4–2, we could interpret the average daily census as "On average, the number of inpatients per day was between 175 and 176."

A second disadvantage is that the mean is sensitive to extreme measures. That is, the mean is strongly influenced by outliers; therefore, it is considered a nonresistant measure. For example, if in Table 4–2, the daily census for Sunday was 225 instead of 167, the average daily census would increase to 183.9.

Weighted Mean

Often in the health care setting, we are involved in analyzing several data sets that contain the same information but for different time intervals. That is, we have several samples with separate means for each, and each sample may be of a different size. Review the data presented in Table 4–3.

What is the overall mean for the three months? One might be tempted to sum the means and divide by 3, which would result in an "average of the means." This would be inappropriate because it would not take into account the difference in the sample sizes for each month. We need to calculate the **weighted mean**, which takes into account the difference in the size of each sample. We calculate the weighted mean by

$$\text{Weighted } \overline{X} = \sum N_i \overline{X}_i / N$$

where $\sum$ is summation, N_i is the number of observations in each frequency distribution, N is the total number of observations in combined frequency distributions, and $\overline{X}_i$ is the mean of each distribution.

Table 4–3 Calculation of Arithmetic and Weighted Means for Average Length of Stay (ALOS)

Month	Discharges (n)	Discharge Days	ALOS
Jan.	947	4,228	4.46
Feb.	763	3,965	5.20
Mar.	574	1,842	3.21

Average of Means: (4.46 + 5.20 + 3.21) / 3 = 4.29
Weighted Mean: [4.46(947)] + [5.20(763)] + [3.21 (574)] / 2,284 = 4.39

To calculate the weighted mean for the data in Table 4–3, we have

$$\text{Weighted } \overline{X} = \sum N_i \overline{X}_i \ / \ N$$
$$= [4.46(947)] +$$
$$[5.20(763)] + [3.21(574)] \ / \ 2,284$$
$$= 4.39$$

Compare the calculations in Table 4–3. The weighted mean takes into account the difference in the number of discharges for each month and is therefore more precise.

The mean can also be calculated for dichotomous data. We have already discussed the mode as the appropriate measure of central tendency for categorical data. Sometimes, however, when we have only two categories, it is more relevant to express the mean as the proportion of cases that fall into a certain category. When we are dealing with dichotomous data, we must first code the data; by convention, the variable of interest is coded as "1." For example, if the number of females in a class in mathematics is the variable of interest, "sex" is coded as follows: 1 = female; 0 = male. The proportion of cases with a score of 1 is denoted as p. p is a mean with an intuitive interpretation—the proportion of cases that fall in the category scored "1." Review the data presented in Table 4–4. In this context, the mean is related to the category of interest, not necessarily the most typical category. The interpretation is that the proportion of women in the math class is .15.

Table 4–4 Proportion of Females in Math Class

Sex	Code	f	p
Female	1	30	.15 (p)
Male	0	170	.85 (1 − p)
Total	—	200	1.00

Mean = $p = f_1/n$ = 30/200 = .15

As we have already discussed, one of the disadvantages of using the mean is that it is sensitive to extreme measures. To eliminate the effects of extreme measures, the outliers may be "trimmed" from the frequency distribution before the mean is calculated. An example of **trimmed mean** occurs in some competitive sports where the top and bottom scores are discarded before the mean score is computed.

Another method for improving the calculated mean's resistance to extreme measures is to "winsorize" the mean. In winsorizing, the most extreme values are changed to equal the next less extreme values rather than being dropped totally from the data set, as in trimming. For example, the 5% trimmed mean drops the highest 5% of the observations and lowest 5% of the observations before the mean is computed. The 5% **winsorized mean** with 20 observations changes the highest value (highest 5%) to the second highest value and changes the lowest value (lowest 5%) to the second lowest. Exhibit 4–2 compares these methods.

In Exhibit 4–2, we can see that the arithmetic mean is 1,257.7, which is vastly different from the trimmed mean, 1,217.5, and the winsorized mean, 1,216.6. The latter two adjusted

Exhibit 4–2 Calculations for Arithmetic Mean, Trimmed Mean, Winsorized Mean

Data Set:

660	1,070	1,220	1,430
740	1,100	1,250	1,475
800	1,100	1,250	1,550
820	1,140	1,250	1,600
880	1,150	1,300	1,700
930	1,150	1,300	1,850
1,000	1,200	1,400	2,900

Before calculations are made, arrange the data in order from lowest to highest.

Arithmetic Mean: Sum the observations and divide by the total number of observations:
$660 + 740 + \ldots + 2,900 = 35,215/28 = 1,257.7$

Trimmed Mean: Eliminate the lowest number, which is 660.
Eliminate the highest number, which is 2,900.
Subtract these values from the previous sum: $35,215 - (660 + 2,900) = 31,655$
Divide by the remaining number of observations: $31,655/26 = 1,217.5$

Winsorized Mean: Identify the lowest 5%, 660 and 740, which are each replaced by 800.
Identify the highest 5%, 1,850 and 2,900, which are each replaced by 1,700.
$35,215 - 660 - 740 - 1850 - 2900 = 29,065$
$29,065 + 800 + 800 + 1,700 + 1,700 = 34,065$
Divide by the total number of observations:
$34,065/28 = 1,216.6$

Median: 1,220

Summary:

Arithmetic Mean	1,257.7
Trimmed Mean	1,217.5
Winsorized Mean	1,216.6

means are actually similar to the median, 1,220. Which measure of central tendency best represents the distribution? This is where judgment is important. The statistical analyst must "eyeball" the raw data to make this decision. It appears that the highest score, 2,900, is strongly influencing the arithmetic mean. Therefore, the trimmed mean, the winsorized mean, and/or the median better represent this data set. The data analyst should select the measure of central tendency that best describes the typical value in the frequency distribution. The analyst should include an explanation of why an alternative to the more traditional measure of central tendency, the mean, was used to describe the frequency distribution.

We can use SPSS or other statistical software to calculate the mean, median, and mode. The SPSS output is displayed in Exhibit 4–3. From the "Analyze" menu, choose "Descriptive Statistics," then "Frequencies." In the dialog box, select Statistics," and click "Mean, Median, and Mode." SPSS summarizes our data set in a frequency table.

Exhibit 4–3 SPSS Output for Measures of Central Tendency

Statistics	
Data Set	
N	
Valid	*28*
Missing	*0*
Mean	*1257.6786*
Median	*1210.0000*
Mode	*1250.00*

To obtain the mean, median, and mode using SPSS:
- From the menus, choose:
  Analyze
  →Descriptive Statistics
  →Frequencies
- In the Frequencies dialog box, click Statistics.
  →Select Mean, Median, Mode

MEASURES OF VARIABILITY

Measures of central tendency are not the only statistics used to summarize a frequency distribution. We also want to consider the spread of the distribution, which tells us how widely the observations are spread out around the measure of central tendency. The most commonly used measures of spread are the variance and the standard deviation. The scales of measurement appropriate for the use of the variance and standard deviation are the interval and ratio scales.

Measures of spread increase in value with greater variation on the variable. Measures of spread equal zero when there is no variation. Maximum spread for metric and ordinal variables occurs when cases are evenly split between two extreme groups. This is called **polarization**. Maximum dispersion for nominal variables is defined as when there is an even distribution of cases across the categories regardless of the number of categories, which is called **uniformity**. When each category of a nominal variable occurs just once, it is called **individuality**.

Range

The simplest measure of spread is the **range**. It is simply the difference between the smallest and largest values in a frequency distribution:

$$\text{Range} = X_{\max} - X_{\min}$$

The range is easy to calculate but is affected by extreme measures. Therefore, it is a non-resistant measure of spread. The range varies widely from sample to sample. Only the two most extreme scores affect its value, so it is not sensitive to other values in the distribution. Also, the range is dependent upon sample size: in general, the larger the sample size, the greater the range.

Two frequency distributions may have the same range, but the observations may have variabilities that greatly differ. For example, consider the following two frequency distributions:

Distribution 1
1   2   3   4   5   6   7   8   9   10

Distribution 2
1   1.5   3   3.5   3.7   7   8   8.26   10   10

The range for both distributions is 9 $(10 - 1 = 9)$. But if we compare the two distributions, we see that there is more variation in distribution 2 than in distribution 1. This is confirmed when the variance for each distribution is calculated—the variances for distributions 1 and 2 are 3.03 and 3.44, respectively.

Variance and Standard Deviation

The **variance** (s^2) is the average of the squared deviations from the mean. The variance of a frequency distribution will be larger when the observations within the distribution are widely spread. The variance (and, as we shall see, the **standard deviation**) is maximized when the data are polarized. The formula for calculating the variance is:

$$s^2 = \sum_{i=1}^{n}(X_i - \overline{X})^2 / N - 1$$

The squared deviations of the mean are calculated by subtracting the mean of a frequency distribution from each value in the distribution, $X - \overline{X}$. The difference between the two values is then squared, $(X - \overline{X})^2$. The squared differences are summed and divided by $N - 1$.

The term $N-1$ is a concept referred to as the number of degrees of freedom. If the mean of a frequency distribution is known, then only $N-1$ observations are free to vary. Stated another way, if we know the mean, and $N-1$ scores, we can determine the nth score. The effect of dividing by $N-1$ increases the value of s^2 slightly and is considered to be a less biased estimate of the population variance. However, when N is large, the effect of using $N-1$ instead of N is negligible. We will encounter this concept again in later chapters.

As an example, we will calculate the variance for the census data that appear in Table 4–2. The average daily census is 175.6. To calculate the variance, we set up the problem as follows:

Day	Census	Census – Mean $X - \bar{X}$	(Census – Mean)^2 $(X - \bar{X})^2$
Sunday	167	−8.6	73.96
Monday	185	9.4	88.36
Tuesday	173	−2.6	6.76
Wednesday	182	6.4	40.96
Thursday	179	3.4	11.56
Friday	173	−2.6	6.76
Saturday	170	−5.6	31.36
Total	1,229	≈ 0*	259.72

*Approximate due to rounding.

Note that the property of the mean that is described in Exhibit 4–1, the sum of the deviations from the mean is equal to 0, is displayed in the above calculations. (In the above example, the sum is approximately equal to 0.0 because the mean is rounded.) Substituting into the formula, we calculate the variance as

$$s^2 = \sum_{i=1}^{n}(X_i - \bar{X})^2 / N - 1$$
$$= 259.72 / 6$$
$$= 43.28$$

The variance is equal to 43.28, but what does this mean? The interpretation of the variance is not easy at the descriptive level because the original units of measure are squared to arrive at the variance. However, if we take the square root of the variance, we return to the original units of measurement. The square root of variance is the standard deviation (s).

$$s = \sqrt{\sum_{i=1}^{n}(X_i - \bar{X})^2 / N - 1}$$

Continuing with the census example, the standard deviation is calculated as

$$s = \sqrt{\sum_{i=1}^{n}(X_i - \overline{X})^2 / N - 1}$$
$$= \sqrt{43.28}$$
$$= 6.58$$

The standard deviation is the most widely used measure of variation used in descriptive statistics. The standard deviation measures variability in the same units of measurement as the sample (i.e., height, age, length of stay, etc.). Since the standard deviation is easier to interpret, it is the preferred measure of dispersion for a frequency distribution. The standard deviation is interpreted in relation to the normal distribution, which we will discuss in Chapter 5.

As we already noted, the variance is of little use in descriptive statistics, but it is important in procedures related to statistical inference. The standard deviation, which is the square root of the variance, is defined in terms of deviations from the mean. It is an important measure at the descriptive level. Procedures for calculating the mean, variance, and standard deviation of a frequency distribution are outlined in Exhibit 4–4.

Exhibit 4-4 Calculation of Mean, Variance, and Standard Deviation for Ages of Nursing Home Residents

Patient No.	Age	$(X - \bar{X})$	$(X - \bar{X})^2$	Patient No.	Age	$(X - \bar{X})$	$(X - \bar{X})^2$
1	76	−6	36	11	82	0	0
2	76	−6	36	12	82	0	0
3	78	−4	16	13	82	0	0
4	78	−4	16	14	84	+2	4
5	78	−4	16	15	84	+2	4
6	78	−4	16	16	86	+4	16
7	80	−2	4	17	88	+6	36
8	80	−2	4	18	88	+6	36
9	80	−2	4	19	90	+8	64
10	80	−2	4	20	90	+8	64
				Σ	1,640	0	376

Using a random sample of 20 nursing home residents, calculate the average age of nursing home residents.

Mean:

1. Sum the observations (s): 1,640
2. Divide by the number of observations (N): 20
   1640/20 = 82

Interpretation: The average age or typical age of any nursing home resident is 82.

Variance:

1. Subtract the mean from each observation: $(X - \bar{X})$
2. Square each deviation from the mean: $(X - \bar{X})^2$
3. Sum the squared deviations from the mean: $\sum (X - \bar{X})^2$
4. Divide the sum of the squared deviations from the mean by $N - 1$ (19).

$$s^2 = \sum (X - \bar{X})^2 / N - 1$$
$$= \ 376/19$$
$$= \ 19.8$$

Standard Deviation: Square root of the variance

$$s = \sqrt{\Sigma (X - \bar{X})^2 / N - 1}$$
$$= 4.45$$

Interpretation: Approximately 68% of the nursing home residents are between the ages of 77.55 ($\bar{X} - 1s$) and 86.45 ($\bar{X} + 1s$).

CALCULATING MEASURES OF CENTRAL TENDENCY AND VARIABILITY USING SPSS

Thus far, we have reviewed the formulas for calculating the mean, range, variance, and standard deviation. Exhibit 4–5 displays the SPSS output for the measures of central tendency and variation for the nursing home data presented in Exhibit 4–4. To calculate these measures using SPSS, select "Descriptive Statistics" from the analyze menu, then select "Frequencies." In the dialog box, select "Options." You can now "click" the measures of central tendency and variation that you are interested in. A frequency table is prepared as part of the output. This allows you to verify the actual observations that were entered on the data sheet. Each age, as well as the number of times it was entered on the data sheet, appears in columns 2 and 3 respectively.

Note that for the statistics table, there is a note indicating that the distribution contains multiple modes with the smallest value displayed in the report. Thus, the mode may not be a

Exhibit 4–5 SPSS Output for Nursing Home Data

Statistics

Age

N

Valid	20
Missing	0
Mean	82.0000
Median	81.0000
Mode	78.0[a]
Std. Deviation	4.4485
Variance	19.7895
Range	14.00

[a] Multiple modes exist. The smallest value is shown.

AGE

		Frequency	Percent	Valid Percent	Cumulative Percent
	76.00	2	10.0	10.0	10.0
	78.00	4	20.0	20.0	30.0
	80.00	4	20.0	20.0	50.0
	82.00	3	15.0	15.0	65.0
Valid	84.00	2	10.0	10.0	75.0
	86.00	1	5.0	5.0	80.0
	88.00	2	10.0	10.0	90.0
	90.00	2	10.0	10.0	100.0
	Total	20	100.0	100.0	

fair representation of the distribution. The frequency table tells us that there are two modes, 78 and 80.

In reviewing the data, you can see that the results are similar to the results that were calculated with the assistance of a hand-held calculator. Notice that the results indicate the number of observations that were included in the calculation. This should always be reviewed to verify that the correct number of observations was entered on the SPSS data sheet. Computer packages also provide more precision in our results. SPSS carried out the calculations to more than four decimal places.

DICHOTOMOUS DATA

Just as we could compute the mean for dichotomous data, we can also determine the variance and standard deviation for dichotomous data:

variance: $s^2 = p(1 - p)$

standard deviation: $s = \sqrt{p(1 - p)}$

where p is equal to the variable of interest. In our coding scheme, for the variable "sex," the category of interest, "female," is coded 1, and the "male" category is coded 0. Calculations of the variance and standard deviation for the variable "sex" are presented in Exhibit 4–6.

Exhibit 4–6 Computation of Variance and Standard Deviation for Dichotomous Data

Sex	Code	f	p
Female	1	30	.15
Male	0	170	.85
Total		200	1.00

Mean: $p = f_1/n = 30/200 = .15$
Variance: $s^2 = p(1-p) = 15(1 - .15) = .1275$
Standard Deviation: $s = \sqrt{p(1-p)} = .357$

GROUPED FREQUENCY DISTRIBUTIONS

Since it is inconvenient to work with large data sets, sometimes data are grouped into class intervals for analysis. Table 4–5 presents an example of an ungrouped frequency distribution. There are 58 patients with varying lengths of stay (LOSs). In this format, the data are difficult to interpret, so we will group the LOSs into **class intervals**. Intervals are ways of classifying and/or summarizing raw data into categories.

Table 4–5 Patient Length of Stay (LOS)

LOS (X)	Frequency (f)	fX
1	0	0
2	2	4
3	6	18
4	6	24
5	6	30
6	11	66
7	6	42
8	8	64
9	5	45
10	3	30
11	1	11
12	2	24
13	1	13
14	1	14
Total	58	385

Grouping Data

The first step in grouping data is to determine the number of class intervals (categories) to use. There is no fixed rule as to how many intervals are appropriate; some recommend 5 to 15 class intervals, while others recommend 10 to 20. All agree, however, that there should not be more than 20. As an example, we will group the LOS frequency distribution that appears in Table 4–5.

To construct the grouped frequency distribution, we will arbitrarily select five as the number of class intervals for grouping the LOS data. Next, we need to determine the width of each of these intervals. This is accomplished by dividing the range of the distribution by the number of class intervals: $(14 - 2)/5 = 2.4$. The nearest odd integer value is used to select the width of the class interval; thus, the width will be 3. To construct the class interval, determine what the highest and lowest class intervals should be. These class intervals will contain the highest and lowest values in the frequency distribution. In the LOS data in Table 4–5, the number 14 is the highest observation and the number 2 is the lowest observation; thus, the highest and lowest class intervals must contain these values. The class interval containing the highest value should be placed at the top of the grouped frequency distribution, and the lowest class interval should be placed at the bottom of the grouped frequency distribution. Intervals should be continuous throughout distribution: that is, there should not be any gaps in values in the distribution. Using the ungrouped data, tally the frequencies that occur in each interval. The LOS data in Table 4–5 are presented as a grouped frequency distribution in Table 4–6.

Table 4–6 Grouped Frequency Distribution, LOS Data

Class Interval Apparent Limits	Class Interval Real Limits	Tally	f	M
13–15	12.5–15.5	//	2	14
10–12	9.5–12.5	### /	6	11
7–9	6.5–9.5	### ### ### ////	19	8
4–6	3.5–6.5	### ### ### ### ///	23	5
1–3	0.5–3.5	### ///	8	2
			58	

Table 4–6 groups the LOS data into five class intervals, each having a width of 3. Also, notice that there are two columns—one indicating the **apparent limits** of the class interval and the other indicating the **real limits** of the class interval. The real limits depict the continuous nature of the distribution. The interval width is the difference between the upper and lower real limits of the class interval—for example, $3.5 - 0.5 = 3$. The highest value, 14, is contained in the class interval "13–15," and the lowest value, 2, is contained in the class interval "1–3." Keep in mind that the distribution should not contain any gaps; even if there are no values that fall within a given interval, it should be included in the distribution. The midpoint (M) of the intervals is obtained by adding the apparent limits of the class intervals and dividing by 2—for example, $(1 + 3)/2 = 2$; $(4 + 6)/2 = 5$. The midpoint will be used in calculating the mean, median, and mode of the grouped distribution.

As an alternative to the above procedure for constructing class intervals, we can use the "Sturges" rule as a guide:

$$k = 1 = 3.3\log_{10}(n)$$

where $\log_{10}$ is the usual base 10 logarithm, k is the number of class intervals, and n is the number of data items to be grouped into class intervals.

Using the LOS data from Table 4–5, the number of class intervals (k) required for the grouped frequency distribution would be calculated as follows:

$k = 1 + 3.3\log_{10}(n)$
$\log_{10}(58) = 1.7635$
$k = 1 + 3.3(1.7635)$
$\quad = 6.82$

Since our result is a fraction, we will round to the nearest whole number. Thus, seven class intervals are needed for grouping the frequency distribution in Table 4–5.

After the number of class intervals has been determined, the next step is to determine the width of the intervals:

$$\text{width} = \text{max} - \text{min (range)}/k$$

where max is the largest value in data set, min is the smallest value in data set, and k is the number of class intervals.

$$\text{width} = (14 - 2)/7 = 12/7 = 1.7 = 2$$

The results appear in Table 4–7. The data in Table 4–7 are usually summarized as presented in Table 4–8. The proportion of the total in each class interval is called the relative

Table 4–7 Class Intervals for Length-of-Stay Data

Apparent Limits	Real Limits	Tally	f	M
13–14	12.5–14.5	//	2	13.5
11–12	10.5–12.5	///	3	11.5
9–10	8.5–10.5	### ///	8	9.5
7–8	6.5–8.5	### ### ////	14	7.5
5–6	4.5–6.5	### ### ### //	17	5.5
3–4	2.5–4.5	### ### //	12	3.5
1–2	0.5–2.5	//	2	1.5
			58	

Table 4–8 Grouped Frequency Distribution of Length-of-Stay Data

Class Interval	f	Cum f	Rel f	Cum %
13–14	2	58 (56 + 2)	.034 (2/58)	100.0 (96.5 + 3.4)
11–12	3	56 (53 + 3)	.052	96.5 (13.8 + 5.2)
9–10	8	53 (45 + 8)	.138	91.3 (77.5 + 13.8)
7–8	14	45 (31 + 14)	.241	77.5 (29.3 + 24.1)
5–6	17	31 (14 + 17)	.293	53.4 (24.1 + 29.3)
3–4	12	14 (2 + 12)	.207	24.1 (3.4 + 20.7)
1–2	2	2	.034	3.4

frequency (rel f) and is obtained by dividing the frequency (f) or number of observations in a given interval by the total number of observations (N). The cumulative frequency (cum f) is obtained by summing the observations in each interval with the number of observations (frequencies) in the next interval, beginning with the lowest class interval and proceeding upward. The first class interval (1–2) contains two observations; thus, the cumulative frequency is 2. The next class interval contains 12 observations; thus, the cumulative frequency is 14 (2 + 12). Proceed in this manner until the last class interval is reached. Exhibit 4–7 outlines the steps for constructing a grouped frequency distribution.

Exhibit 4–7 Steps in Constructing a Grouped Frequency Distribution

1. Determine the number of class intervals needed by the Sturges rule. It is suggested that the number of intervals be limited to 20.
2. Determine the width of the class intervals by dividing the range of the frequency distribution by the number of class intervals obtained in step 1. Intervals should be set up so that one score cannot belong to more than one class interval.
3. Determine the point at which the lowest class interval should begin.
4. Record the limits of all class intervals, placing the interval containing the highest score value at the top. Intervals should be continuous and of the same width. Do not leave out class intervals in which no observations occur; to do so would create a misleading impression.
5. Using the tally system, place a tally for each observation in the corresponding class intervals.
6. Summarize the tallies for each class interval in a frequency (f) column.
7. Record the total (f) at the bottom of the frequency column.

There are several disadvantages associated with grouped frequency distributions. First, precision in the resulting statistical calculations is lost. When values are grouped into an interval, the values may be spread evenly throughout the interval, or the values may be concentrated at either end of the interval. When data are grouped, the assumption is that the observations are spread evenly across the class intervals. Second, as we have seen, different groupings can result from the same frequency distribution. Grouping a set of values does not result in a unique set of grouped scores. That is, if the same frequency distribution were grouped into slightly different class intervals, the sample statistics would not be exactly the same.

Calculating the Mean from a Grouped Frequency Distribution

The first step in calculating the mean from a grouped frequency distribution is to determine the midpoint of each interval. Table 4–9 presents the grouped LOS with the corre-

Table 4–9 Grouped LOS Data for Calculating the Mean

Class Interval	Midpoint (X)	f	fX
13–14	13.5	2	27
11–12	11.5	3	34.5
9–10	9.5	8	76
7–8	7.5	14	105
5–6	5.5	17	93.5
3–4	3.5	12	42
1–2	1.5	2	3
		$\Sigma = 58$	$\Sigma = 381$

$$\bar{X} = \Sigma fX / N$$
$$= 381 / 58$$
$$= 6.57$$

sponding midpoint (X) for each interval. The midpoint represents all observations that fall into that interval. For example, the observations 13 and 14 (from Table 4–5) fall into the class interval "13–14"; the midpoint, 13.5, represents both of these observations. The mean is obtained by multiplying the midpoint (X) of each class interval by its corresponding frequency (f); these observations are summed and then divided by the total number of observations (N):

$$\bar{X} = \sum fX / N$$

where X is the midpoint of each interval.

Therefore, for the grouped LOS data, the mean is

$$\bar{X} = 381 / 58 = 6.57$$

The mean for the grouped data, 6.57 (Table 4–9), does not equal the mean for the ungrouped data, 6.64 (385/58). This discrepancy illustrates the loss of precision that occurs when grouping frequency distributions.

Calculating the Median from Grouped Data

Recall that the median is the point in a distribution that 50% of the observations fall above and 50% of the observations fall below. To determine the median in a grouped distribution, we first need to determine which observation meets this definition. For the LOS data in Table 4–9, the median would be the 29th value, as calculated below:

$$50\% \text{ of } N = .5 \times 58 = 29$$

Thus, the 29th value will be the median for the grouped distribution. Inspection of the data in Table 4–8 shows that the 29th observation falls in the interval "5–6." How is this determined? Begin counting the frequencies (f) in the lowest class interval, 1 to 2, until the interval containing the 29th observation is located ($2 + 12 + 17 = 31$). The interval 5 to 6 contains the 15th, 16th, 17th, 18th, 19th, and so on up to the 31st observation. Thus the 29th observation occurs in this interval. The cumulative frequency column provides this information for us. The median is obtained by

$$\text{Mdn} = L + w(1/2n - c)/f_{\text{mdn}}$$

where L is the real lower limit of the class interval containing the median, W is the width of the interval, c is the total number of values falling below the interval containing the median (cumulative frequency), and f_{mdn} is the frequency of the values in the interval containing the median value.

Substituting into our formula, since $L = 4.5$, $w = 2$, $c = 14$, and $f_{\text{mdn}} = 17$, we have

$$4.5 + \{2[\tfrac{1}{2}(58) - 14]\}/17$$
$$= 4.5 + [2(15)]/17$$
$$= 4.5 + 30/17$$
$$= 4.5 + 1.76$$
$$= 6.26$$

The median for the grouped frequency distribution is 6.26 days; the median for the ungrouped distribution is 6 days.

Calculating the Mode from Grouped Data

There are several ways to determine the mode from grouped data. The simplest is to take the midpoint of the most frequently occurring class interval. For the LOS data in Table 4–9, the mode is 5.5 because 17 observations fall in this interval. This is referred to as the crude mode.

The second way to determine the mode from a grouped distribution adjusts the modal value in relation to the relative frequencies in the class intervals adjacent to the class interval containing the modal value. It pulls the modal value toward the adjacent class interval that has greater frequency. This mode is referred to as the refined mode and is calculated as follows:

$$\text{Refined mode} = L + w(f_{mo} - f_b) / (f_{mo} - f_b) + (f_{mo} - f_a),$$

where L is the real lower limits of the class interval containing the modal value, w is the width of the class interval, f_{mo} is the number of values (f) in the class interval containing the mode, f_b is the number of values (f) in the adjacent class interval below the class interval containing the mode, and f_a is the number of values (f) in the adjacent class interval above the class interval containing the mode.

For the grouped LOS data in Table 4–10, $L = 4.5$, $w = 2$, $f_{mo} = 17$, $f_b = 12$, and $f_a = 14$, so the refined mode is calculated as follows:

$$
\begin{aligned}
\text{Refined mode} &= L + w(f_{mo} - f_b)/(f_{mo} - f_b) + (f_{mo} - f_a) \\
&= 4.5 + [2\,(17 - 12)] / (17 - 12) + (17 - 14) \\
&= 4.5 + 2\,[5/(5 + 3)] \\
&= 4.5 + 10/8 \\
&= 4.5 + 1.25 \\
&= 5.75
\end{aligned}
$$

Table 4–10 Grouped Length-of-Stay Data for Calculating the Mean

Class Interval	Midpoint (X)	f	FX	f(X²)
13–14	13.5	2	27	364.5
11–12	11.5	3	34.5	396.75
9–10	9.5	8	76	722.0
7–8	7.5	14	105	787.5
5–6	5.5	17	93.5	514.25
3–4	3.5	12	42	147.0
1–2	1.5	2	3	4.5
		$\Sigma=58$	$\Sigma=381$	$\Sigma=2{,}936.5$

Thus, the refined mode is 5.75, and the crude mode is 5.5.

You can see from the calculations for the refined mode that the number of observations in the class interval that is immediately above ($f_a = 14$), the interval containing the mode is pulling the modal value in that direction. Compare the refined mode to the mode in the ungrouped frequency distribution for the LOS data in Table 4–5, where the mode is 6. The length of stay—six days—occurred 11 times.

Calculating the Variance and Standard Deviation from Grouped Data

To compute the variance and standard deviation from grouped data, we will use what is called the raw score formula. The data from Table 4–9 are reproduced in Table 4–10, but we need to add another column—$f(X^2)$—which is the midpoint (X) squared multiplied by the frequency (f).

The raw score formula for calculating the variance is

$$s^2 = \sum x^2 / (N-1)$$

and the standard deviation is

$$s = \sqrt{\sum x^2 / (N-1)}$$

where the $\sum x^2$ is

$$\sum x^2 = \sum f(X^2) - \left[\sum (X)^2 / N \right]$$

To calculate the variance and standard deviation, we have

$$\sum x^2 = \sum f(X^2) - \left[\sum (X)^2 / N \right]$$
$$= 2{,}936.5 - (381^2 / 58)$$
$$= 2{,}936.5 - 2{,}502.78$$
$$= 433.7$$

$$s^2 = \sum x^2 / (N-1)$$
$$= 433.7 / 57$$
$$= 7.61$$

and

$$s = \sqrt{\sum x^2 / N - 1}$$
$$= \sqrt{7.61}$$
$$= 2.76$$

The variance and standard deviation for our LOS data are 7.61 and 2.76, respectively.

Measures of central tendency and variation for the ungrouped and grouped frequency distributions are compared in Table 4–11. Note that the grouped distribution results in greater variation than the ungrouped distribution because only the midpoint of each interval is con-

Table 4–11 Measures of Central Tendency and Variation, Ungrouped Data versus Grouped Data

	Ungrouped Distribution	Grouped Distribution
Mean	6.64	6.57
Median	6	6.26
Mode	6	5.75
Variance	2.76	7.61
SD	1.66	2.76

sidered in the calculations rather than the entire data set.

CONCLUSION

The mean, median, and mode are measures of central tendency that are commonly used to describe frequency distributions. Measures of central tendency describe the "most typical" value or observation in a frequency distribution. The measure used to describe the distribution should be based on both the scale of measurement and determination of which measure best describes the most typical observation in the frequency distribution.

Measures of spread are the variance, the standard deviation, and the range. The range tells us the distance between the lowest value in a distribution and the highest value, so in general, it does not provide much information about the frequency distribution. The standard deviation is the most common descriptive statistic used to describe the spread of a frequency distribution for metric variables.

ADDITIONAL RESOURCES

Duncan, R.C., et al. 1977. *Introductory biostatistics for the health sciences.* Albany, NY: Delmar Publishers.

Edwards, A.L. 1966. *Statistical methods for the behavioral sciences.* New York: Holt, Rinehart & Winston.

Jekel, J., et al. 1996. *Epidemiology, biostatistics and preventive medicine.* Philadelphia: W.B. Saunders.

Minium, E.W. 1978. *Statistical reasoning in psychology and*

education. New York: John Wiley & Sons.

Phillips, D.S. 1978. *Basic statistics for health science students.* San Francisco: W.H. Freeman & Co.

Stockburger, D.W. 1998. Introductory statistics: Concepts, models and applications. Available on the Internet at http://www.psychstat.smsu.edu/introbook/sbk13m.html

U.S. Department of Health and Human Services, Public Health Service. 1992. *Principles of epidemiology: An introduction to applied epidemiology and biostatistics.* Atlanta, GA: USDHHS.

Weisberg, H.F. 1992. *Central tendency and variability.* Newbury Park, CA: Sage Publications.

Appendix 4–A

Exercises for Solving Problems

KNOWLEDGE QUESTIONS

1. Define the key terms listed at the beginning of this chapter.

2. What is the difference between a population parameter and a sample statistic?

3. Compare and contrast the following measures of central tendency: mean, median, and mode.

4. Define polarization, individuality, and uniformity in relation to variability in a frequency distribution.

5. Why do measures of central tendency and variation of ungrouped frequency distributions differ from those of grouped frequency distributions?

MULTIPLE CHOICE

1. There are 40 students in section I of a medical terminology class and 20 students in section II. The mean score on a midterm exam for section I is 60, and the mean score for section II is 70. What is the mean score for the two classes combined?
   a. 63.3
   b. 65
   c. 67
   d. not enough information provided to answer question

2. For the two scores 8 and 12, $\sum (X - \overline{X})^2$ is:
   a. 2
   b. 4
   c. 8
   d. 12

3. In a frequency distribution, the lowest score is 25 and the highest score is 50; the mean is 37.5. The range is:
   a. 11
   b. 12.5
   c. 24
   d. 25

4. In grouping a set of scores from a frequency distribution, the width of the class intervals should:
   a. be equal
   b. be at least one
   c. vary according to the frequency within the interval
   d. be no more than 10

5. The first class interval in the grouped frequency distribution is 5–10. The width of the interval is:
   a. 5
   b. 5.5
   c. 6
   d. 6.5

6. The midpoint of the class interval 5–10 is:
   a. 7
   b. 7.5
   c. 8
   d. 8.5

7. The width of a class interval is 3. The midpoint is 9. The apparent lower limit of the interval is:
   a. 7
   b. 7.5
   c. 8
   d. 8.5

8. The "real limits" of the class interval 1–3 are:
   a. 0.5–3.5
   b. 1–3
   c. 0–4
   d. 1.5–2.5

The following table displays a cumulative frequency distribution of the length of stay of patients discharged from Community Behavior Health Care during the week of April 1. Use the table below to answer questions 9 through 14.

Class Interval for Length of Stay	f	Cum. f	Cum. %
20–24	4	20	100
15–19	8	16	80
10–14	6	8	40
5–9	0	2	10
0–4	2	2	10

9. Six patients had lengths of stay that fall:
   a. below 14.5 days
   b. at 12 days
   c. above 9.5 days
   d. between 9.5 days and 14.5 days

10. Twelve patients had lengths of stay that were greater than:
    a. 14.5 days
    b. 15 days
    c. 17 days
    d. 19.5 days

11. Sixteen patients had lengths of stay below:
    a. 20 days
    b. 19.5 days
    c. 17 days
    d. 14.5 days

12. The cumulative frequency value of "8" means that 8 cases fall below:
    a. 14.5 days
    b. 14 days
    c. 12 days
    d. 10 days

13. Forty percent of the patients discharged had lengths of stay that fell below:
    a. 14.5 days
    b. 14 days
    c. 12 days
    d. 10 days

14. Eighty percent of the patients discharged had lengths of stay that fell below:
    a. 19.5 days
    b. 19 days
    c. 17 days
    d. 14.5 days

15. Which of the following is *not* a measure of spread?
    a. mode
    b. range
    c. standard deviation
    d. variance

16. Review the following two frequency distributions:
    1:   200 210 190 220 195
    2:   210 170 180 235 240

    The standard deviation for distribution 1 is:
    a. the same as that for set 2
    b. less than that for set 2
    c. greater than that for set 2
    d. not enough information provided

17. The standard deviation of a frequency distribution is 5. The variance is:
    a. 10
    b. 15
    c. 20
    d. 25
    e. not enough information provided

18. In a frequency distribution, the mean is 32. If each score is divided by 2, the mean of the new distribution is:
    a. 64
    b. 32
    c. 16
    d. not enough information provided

19. In the following frequency distribution, the number 4 is the:
        4   4   5   7
    a. mean
    b. mode
    c. median
    d. range

20. Review the grouped frequency distribution below:

Class Interval	f
40–44	2
35–39	3
30–34	6
25–29	5
20–24	4

After the data were grouped into class intervals, it was determined that a value of 35 was really a value of 39. Correcting this error will change the calculated value of:
a. the mean
b. the median
c. the mode
d. all of the above
e. none of the above

PROBLEMS

1. Review the data in Tables 4–A–1 and 4–A–2 and answer the questions that follow. Use an electronic spreadsheet to assist you in preparing the answers.

Table 4–A–1 Male Deaths Due to Leukemia (ICD-9-CM Codes 200–208.9) in the State of Ohio, 1996

Age Group	Leukemia Deaths in Men	p	Cum. p	M	f(M)
5–14	9				
15–24	14				
25–34	38				
35–44	59				
45–54	123				
55–64	166				
65–74	414				
75–84	391				
85–94	137				
	1,351				

Source: Data from Centers for Disease Control and Prevention, CDC Wonder Data Base, http://wonder.cdc.gov.

Table 4–A–2 Female Deaths Due to Leukemia (ICD-9-CM Codes 200–208.9) in the State of Ohio, 1996

Age Group	Leukemia Deaths in Women	p	Cum. p	M	f(M)
5–14	11				
15–24	9				
25–34	14				
35–44	44				
45–54	62				
55–64	134				
65–74	338				
75–84	435				
85–94	213				
	1,260				

Source: Data from Centers for Disease Control and Prevention, CDC Wonder Data Base, http://wonder.cdc.gov.

a. What is the mean age of death for men? For women?

b. What are the crude modes and median ages of death for men? For women?

c. What are the refined mode and the refined median for men? For women?

d. Compare and contrast the crude and refined results for each group. Explain any disparities that may exist.

e. In analyzing the results of your data for men and women, what conclusions can you draw?

2. Use the data of the ages of 100 nursing home residents that appear in Exhibit 4–A–1 to solve the following:

a. Use statistical software to calculate the mean, median, mode, variance, and standard deviation for the ungrouped frequency distribution and to prepare a frequency table.

b. Group ages into class intervals. Prepare a table that displays the frequencies for each class interval, the cumulative frequency, the relative proportion, and the cumulative percent.

c. Compute the mean, median, mode, variance, and standard deviation for the grouped data.

d. Compare the results of the grouped and ungrouped frequency distributions.

Exhibit 4–A–1 Ages of 100 Nursing Home Residents

65	68	71	73	75	76	78	80	81	85
65	68	71	74	75	76	78	80	82	86
65	69	72	74	75	76	78	80	82	86
66	69	72	74	75	77	78	80	82	87
66	69	72	74	75	77	78	80	82	88
66	70	72	74	75	77	78	80	83	89
67	70	72	75	75	77	79	80	83	90
67	70	73	75	75	77	79	81	83	90
67	71	73	75	76	77	79	81	84	90
67	71	73	75	76	78	79	81	84	91

3. The lengths of stay for a group of patients discharged with a principal diagnosis of barbiturate poisoning are presented in Exhibit 4–A–2.

Exhibit 4–A–2 Patient Length of Stay for Barbiturate Poisoning, 20xx

1	2	3	5	6	10	13	16
1	2	3	5	6	10	13	17
1	2	3	5	6	10	13	17
1	2	4	5	6	10	14	17
1	2	4	5	8	11	14	18
1	2	4	5	8	11	14	19
1	2	4	5	8	11	14	19
1	2	4	6	8	11	15	20
2	3	4	6	8	12	15	20
2	3	5	6	9	12	16	20

a. Use statistical software to calculate the mean, median, mode, variance, and standard deviation for the ungrouped frequency distribution and to prepare a frequency table.
b. Group ages into class intervals. Prepare a table that displays the frequencies for each class interval, the cumulative frequency, the relative proportion, and the cumulative percent.
c. Compute the mean, median, mode, variance, and standard deviation for the grouped data.
d. Compare the results of the grouped and ungrouped frequency distributions.

CLASS ACTIVITY

An important aspect of the health information manager's job is to be able to collect and analyze data. But data are not always useful in their raw form—they must be turned into information. This activity is designed to provide you with the experience in preparing a written report based on the analysis of the collected data. For this activity, you will:

a. set up an SPSS (or other microcomputer statistical package) data sheet
b. define and label variables for the data sheet
c. summarize data
d. prepare charts and graphs

Instructions

1. Complete the survey that follows these instructions.
2. Turn the survey in to the instructor. Copies of each student's responses will be distributed to the class.

3. Set up the SPSS (or other) data sheet. Define the variables for the data input sheet. Categorical variables have been coded on the data sheet. An example of how to enter the variable information on the data sheet appears in Figure 4–A–1.

Figure 4–A–1 Example of How To Enter Variable Information for Class Activity on SPSS Data Sheet. *Source:* SPSS 9.0 for Windows, Copyright SPSS Inc. 1998, Chicago, Illinois, USA.

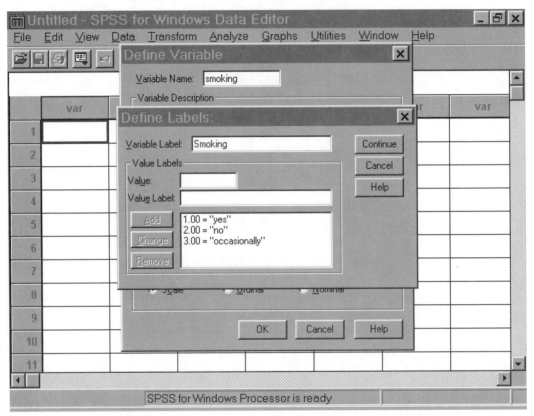

4. Input the data from each completed survey onto the data sheet.
5. Answer the questions below.
6. Prepare a two- to three-page written report describing the characteristics of the HIM class, based on your analysis of the data. Include statistical tables/charts/graphs to support your findings.

Survey Questions

1. What percentage of students live on campus? Off campus?

2. What percentage of the class is female? Male?

3. What is the average height of the class? What is the average height of the men in the class? What is the average height of the women in the class?

4. What are the average heights of the mothers and the fathers?

5. What proportion of the class is right handed? What percentage of the mothers are right handed? How many fathers are right handed?

6. Prepare a bar graph that displays the actual frequency distribution of the hair color of your classmates. What is the modal hair color? Prepare a pie chart that displays hair color by percentage.

7. Prepare a table displaying the frequency distribution of the eye color of your classmates.

8. What proportion of the class went to a public high school?

9. What is the average amount of time that the class spends studying for HIM classes? Prepare a histogram that displays the frequency distribution of time spent studying.

10. What is the average amount of money spent on haircuts for the class? What is the average amount for men? For women?

11. What is the average amount of CDs owned by the class? How many CDs do the men own? The women?

12. What is the average amount of time spent exercising by the class per week? What is the average amount of time for men? For women?

13. What is the average number of hours per week spent watching television? What is the average amount of time for men? For women?

HIM CLASS SURVEY

1. Where do you live?
   ☐ campus housing   (1)
   ☐ off-campus housing   (2)

2. Sex
   ☐ male   (1)
   ☐ female   (2)

3. What is your height in inches? ____

4. What is your father's height in inches?____

5. What is your mother's height in inches? ____

6. What is your shoe size (length not width)? _____

7. Do you smoke?
   ☐ yes   (1)
   ☐ no   (2)
   ☐ occasionally   (3)

8. Are you:
   ☐ left handed   (1)
   ☐ right handed   (2)

9. Is your father:
   ☐ left handed   (1)
   ☐ right handed   (2)

10. Is your mother:
    ☐ left handed   (1)
    ☐ right handed   (2)

11. What is your hair color?
    ☐ black   (1)
    ☐ brown   (2)
    ☐ blond   (3)
    ☐ red   (4)
    ☐ other   (5)

12. What is your eye color?
    ☐ black   (1)
    ☐ brown   (2)
    ☐ blue   (3)
    ☐ green   (4)
    ☐ gray   (5)
    ☐ hazel   (6)
    ☐ other   (7)

13. What type of high school did you attend?
    ☐ public high school   (1)
    ☐ private high school   (2)

14. On average, how many hours per week do you spend studying for HIM classes? ___

15. How much did you spend, to the nearest dollar, on your last haircut, including tip? ____

16. How many CDs do you own? ____

17. On average, how many hours per week do you spend exercising? ____

18. On average, how many hours per week do you spend watching television? ____

CHAPTER 5

The Normal Distribution and Statistical Inference

KEY TERMS	Normal distribution	Sampling methods
	Symmetrical	Simple random sampling
	Asymptotic curve	Stratified random sampling
	Skewness	Systematic sampling
	Kurtosis	Cluster sampling
	Standard normal distribution	Null hypothesis
	z values	Alternative hypothesis
	Standard normal deviate	Type I error
	Central limit theorem	Type II error
	Point estimate	Level of significance
	Standard error of the mean	p value
	Confidence interval	

LEARNING OBJECTIVES

At the conclusion of this chapter, you should be able to:

1. Define key terms.
2. Describe the characteristics of the normal distribution and the standard normal distribution.
3. Compare and contrast the normal distribution and the standard normal distribution.
4. Compare the standard deviation and the standard normal deviate.
5. Convert normal distributions to standard normal distributions using computer statistical software.
6. Explain the central limit theorem.
7. Calculate the standard error of the mean and confidence intervals for samples.
8. Explain how sample size and variation affect the standard error of the mean.
9. Explain the following sampling techniques: simple random sampling, stratified random sampling, systematic sampling, and cluster sampling.

10. Explain the differences between the null and alternative hypotheses.
11. Explain the factors that affect type I and type II errors.
12. Differentiate between the alpha level and the *p* value.
13. Identify the factors that influence sample size.
14. Calculate sample size for given situations.

Much of statistical inference is based on the **normal distribution**, also called the Gaussian distribution for Johann Karl Gauss, the person who best described it. The normal distribution is not a single distribution but an infinite number of possible distributions. This is important in statistical inference because the population mean can take on any positive or negative value, and the population standard deviation can take on any positive or negative value. Thus, the normal distribution is the most widely used theoretical distribution; many naturally occurring phenomena, such as blood pressure, height, and weight, approximate the normal distribution.

CHARACTERISTICS OF THE NORMAL DISTRIBUTION

There are several characteristics of the normal distribution with which you should be familiar. First, the curve is bell shaped and **symmetrical** about the mean (the population mean is symbolized by μ, pronounced "mu"). Second, because the distribution is symmetrical, approximately 50% of the observations lie above the mean and 50% of the observations lie below the mean. The total area under the curve is equal to 1.00. Third, in a normal distribution, the mean, median, and mode are equal. The values of the normal distribution range from minus infinity ($-\infty$) to plus infinity ($+\infty$).

As we move out from the center of the normal curve bilaterally, the height of the curve descends gradually at first, then faster, and finally more slowly as it approaches the horizontal axis. Each tail of the curve approaches the x axis but never touches the x axis, no matter how far from center we go. This type of curve is called an **asymptotic curve** because it is considered asymptotic to the horizontal axis.

Figure 5–1 displays the normal distribution and how the values in the distribution are arranged around the population mean, μ. Approximately 68% of the values lie within 1 standard deviation from the mean ($\mu \pm 1 \delta$); 95% of the observations lie within 1.96 standard deviations from the mean ($\mu \pm 1.96 \delta$); and 99% of the observations lie within 2.58 standard deviations of the mean ($\mu \pm 2.58 \delta$). These characteristics of the normal curve are important when making inferences about population parameters from sample statistics. The symbols used to distinguish between population parameters and sample statistics appear in Table 5–1.

In a normal distribution, we know that the population μ can take on any value and that the population μ is the midpoint of the distribution. Compare Figures 5–1 and 5–2. Even though the means for each distribution—6 and 15, respectively—are different, the shapes of the distributions are the same. Any change in μ without a corresponding change in δ does not change the shape of the distribution. However, changes in the value δ do change the shape of the distribution but do not affect the midpoint. Basically, changes in δ affect the dispersion of the values in the distribution. Dispersion can affect the **skewness** of the distribution.

Figure 5–1 Histogram of Normal Distribution 1

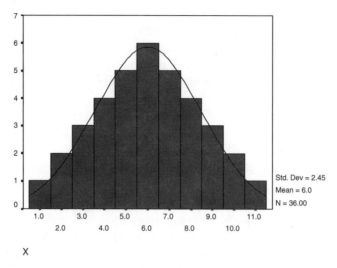

Table 5–1 Statistical Symbols

	Population Parameter	Sample Statistic
Mean	μ	$\overline{X}$
Variance	δ^2	s^2
Standard deviation	δ	s

Figure 5–2 Histogram of Normal Distribution 2

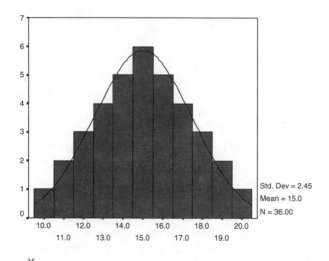

A frequency distribution that is asymmetrical is skewed, and in this case the mean, median, and mode will take on different values. Skewness is the horizontal stretching of a frequency distribution to one side or the other, so that one tail is longer than the other. The longer tail has more observations. Because the mean is sensitive to extreme values, the mean moves in the direction of the long tail when a distribution is skewed. When the direction of the long tail is off to the right, the distribution is said to be positively skewed or skewed to the right. Conversely, when a distribution's long tail is off to the left, the distribution is said to be negatively skewed or skewed to the left. We can determine if a distribution is skewed through SPSS by checking these items in the dialog box after requesting "Frequencies" or "Descriptives" from the "Analyze" menu. An obtained skewness value greater than 1 is an indication that the distribution differs significantly from normal. Another way to assess the skewness of a distribution is to compare the mean and median. If the mean and median approximate one another, the distribution is probably not significantly skewed.

Kurtosis is the vertical stretching of the frequency distribution. If the distribution appears to be more peaked or more flattened than the normal distribution, it is considered to be kurtotic. For a normal distribution, the value of the kurtosis statistic is zero. A positive kurtosis indicates that the frequency distribution has longer tails than the normal distribution and that the observations are clustered toward the center (peakedness). If the kurtosis statistic is negative, the frequency distribution has tails shorter than the normal distribution, and there is less clustering of the observations (flattened).

THE STANDARD NORMAL DISTRIBUTION (z DISTRIBUTION)

Since there are an infinite number of normal distributions, which may have any mean and any standard deviation, the observations in the distribution must be standardized when we want to make comparisons between distributions. When we standardize a frequency distribution, such as one for the variable "age," we are transforming the units of measurement (age) to a unit-free form—that is, the age units become z **values**. The z distribution is referred to as the **standard normal distribution**; it has a mean of 0 and a standard deviation equal to 1. The z value, also called the **standard normal deviate**, is the number of standard deviation units that the observed value lies away from the mean, μ. Transforming our raw observations to z values makes it possible to make comparisons between distributions.

In the standardized normal distribution, the area between the z values of ± 1.0 is 68%, the area between the z values of ± 1.96 is 95%, and the area between +3 and –3 is 99.7%. Any normal distribution may be transformed into a standardized normal distribution through the formulas in Exhibit 5–1. The transformation of a set of observations to z values is a linear transformation that does not change the shape of the distribution. This is illustrated in Figure 5–3, where the normal distribution in Figure 5–1 is transformed into a standard normal distribution with a mean equal to 0 and a standard deviation equal to 1.

For a "real-life" example, we will now compare a normal distribution with a standardized normal distribution to explain some of these concepts. In Exhibit 4–A–1 in Chapter 4, a frequency distribution of the age of 100 nursing home residents is displayed. Using these same data, we will construct a histogram of the frequency distribution for age using SPSS.

Exhibit 5–1 Formulas for Transforming Observed Scores into *z* Scores

z *Value in a Population*	z *Value in a Sample*
$z = (X - \mu) / \delta$	$z = (X - \bar{X}) / s$
Where X is the value of the observation, μ is the mean of the population distribution, and δ is the standard deviation of the population distribution	Where X is the value of the observation, $\bar{X}$ is the mean of the sample distribution, and s is the standard deviation of the sample distribution

Figure 5–3 Standard Normal Distribution

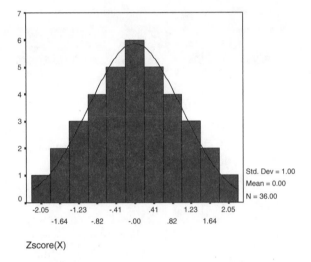

Zscore(X)

Std. Dev = 1.00
Mean = 0.00
N = 36.00

We will also request descriptive statistics and statistics on skewness and kurtosis to evaluate the "normality" of the distribution. The histogram appears in Figure 5–4.

The descriptive statistics in Exhibit 5–2 indicate that the mean, median, and mode are similar; 76.36, 76.0, and 75, respectively. We will interpret the distribution as "normal" because of the similarity between the three measures of central tendency. The skewness statistic is .261, indicating that the distribution does not depart significantly from normal. However, the distribution is somewhat flat, as indicated by the kurtosis statistic, −.281.

Figure 5–4 SPSS Output for Histogram on Ages of 100 Nursing Home Residents

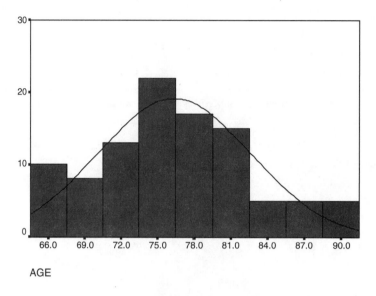

AGE

Exhibit 5–2 SPSS Output of Descriptive Statistics, Ages of Nursing Home Residents

AGE		
N	Valid	100
	Missing	0
Mean		76.3600
Median		76.0000
Mode		75.00
Std. Deviation		6.2386
Variance		38.9196
Skewness		.261
Std. Error of Skewness		.241
Kurtosis		−.281
Std. Error of Kurtosis		.478

We will now convert our "normal" distribution to a standardized normal distribution. The histogram and descriptive statistics appear in Figure 5–5 and Exhibit 5–2. We can convert the scores to standard scores by checking the "Save standardized values as variables" option in the "descriptives" dialog box, as shown in Exhibit 5–3. The SPSS program will create and save a new variable on the data sheet. The mean of the new standardized distribution is 0, and the standard deviation is 1. The skewness statistics and kurtosis statistic remain the same, indicating that the shape of the distribution did not change when the distribution was standardized (Exhibit 5–4).

Figure 5–5 SPSS Output for Histogram on Ages of 100 Nursing Home Residents, Standardized Distribution

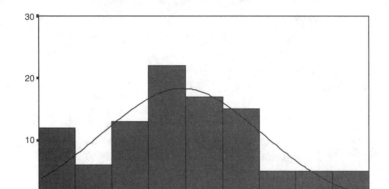

Zscore(AGE)

Exhibit 5–3 SPSS Screen for Requesting Standardized Variables. *Source:* SPSS 9.0 for Windows, Copyright SPSS Inc. 1998, Chicago, Illinois, USA.

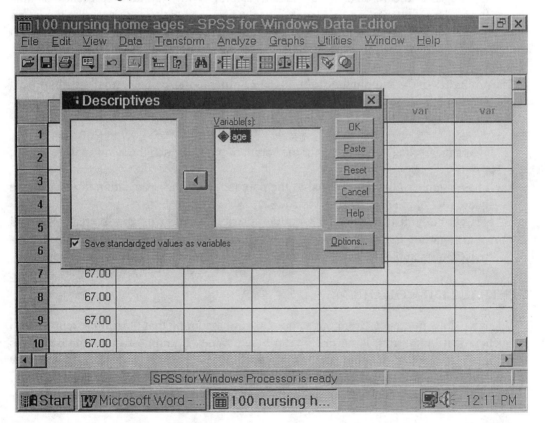

Exhibit 5–4 SPSS Output for Standardized Descriptive Statistics on Ages of 100 Nursing Home Residents

Z score (AGE)		
N	Valid	100
	Missing	0
Mean		–2.2E–15
Median		–5.8E–02
Mode		–.21800
Std. Deviation		1.0000000
Variance		1.0000000
Skewness		.261
Std. Error of Skewness		.241
Kurtosis		–.281
Std. Error of Kurtosis		.478

STATISTICAL INFERENCE

In analyzing health care data, we are usually dealing with data that represent a sample drawn from a larger population. We want to use the sample statistics to describe the larger population. A single sample statistic such as the mean is actually a point estimate. A point estimate is a single numerical value computed from the sample that is assumed to best represent the actual population parameter.

The properties of the sampling distribution are similar to those of a normal distribution. If the population is normally distributed with a mean μ, and a standard deviation δ, the sampling distribution of $\bar{X}$ has the following properties:

1. It has a mean equal to the mean for the population from which the samples were drawn, $\mu_{\bar{x}} = \mu$.
2. It has a standard deviation equal to the population standard deviation divided by the square root of the sample size, $\delta_{\bar{x}} = \delta \sqrt{n}$.
3. It is normally distributed. The sampling distribution of $\bar{X}$ is approximately normal when sampling is from a non-normal population distribution. As the sample size increases, the sample's approximation to normality improves (central limit theorem).

CENTRAL LIMIT THEOREM

When we draw inferences from our sample, we are assuming that the sample represents a frequency distribution that is normally distributed. When a graph of our sample appears normal, we assume that the population from which the sample was drawn is also normally distributed. This is true regardless of the size of the sample drawn from the same population. However, many populations are not normally distributed. Regardless of the type of population distribution, the sampling distribution, if sufficiently large, is approximately normal. The **central limit theorem** summarizes the relationship between the shapes of the population distribution and the sampling distribution of the mean, $\overline{X}$:

> If repeated random samples of size N are drawn from a population, and if a mean is calculated for each sample, the distribution of the sample means approaches the normal distribution as N becomes large. The mean of the sampling distribution will approach the population mean, μ. This is true even if the population distribution is not normal.

The central limit theorem assures us that regardless of the shape of the population distribution, the sampling distribution of $\overline{X}$ approaches normality as the sample size increases. This is true even when data in individual samples are skewed. In reality, the samples do not have to be very large for the sampling distribution of $\overline{X}$ to be approximately normal. In most instances, the approximation to normality is quite rapid as N increases.

These concepts can be illustrated by using the age of nursing home residents' data. Recall that the population mean is 76.4 and the population standard deviation is 6.2. A simple random sample of 30 nursing home residents was drawn from the population. A frequency distribution for the sample is displayed in Table 5–2, and a histogram is displayed in Figure 5–6. The sample mean is 77.7 (Exhibit 5–5), and the sample standard deviation is 5.9. The

Table 5–2 Frequency Distribution of Random Sample of Ages of Nursing Home Residents

Age	Frequency	%	Valid %	Cumulative %
66.00	1	3.3	3.3	3.3
67.00	1	3.3	3.3	6.7
69.00	1	3.3	3.3	10.0
70.00	1	3.3	3.3	13.3
71.00	1	3.3	3.3	16.7
72.00	1	3.3	3.3	20.0
74.00	4	13.3	13.3	33.3
75.00	1	3.3	3.3	36.7
76.00	2	6.7	6.7	43.3
78.00	2	6.7	6.7	50.0
79.00	2	6.7	6.7	56.7
80.00	3	10.0	10.0	66.7
81.00	2	6.7	6.7	73.3
82.00	2	6.7	6.7	80.0
83.00	2	6.7	6.7	86.7
85.00	1	3.3	3.3	90.0
86.00	1	3.3	3.3	93.3
87.00	1	3.3	3.3	96.7
90.00	1	3.3	3.3	100.0
Total	30	100.0	100.0	

Figure 5-6 Histogram of Ages of 30 Nursing Home Residents

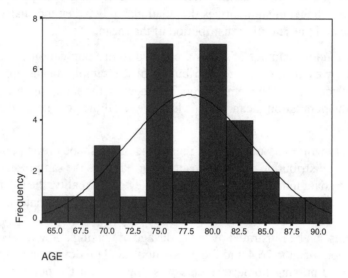

AGE

Exhibit 5–5 Descriptive Statistics on Ages of 30 Nursing Home Residents

AGE		
N	Valid	30
	Missing	0
Mean		77.7333
Median		78.5000
Mode		74.00
Std. Deviation		5.9477
Variance		35.3747
Skewness		−.100
Std. Error for Skewness		.427
Kurtosis		−.436
Std. Error for Kurtosis		.833

sample distribution does not significantly depart from normality, as indicated by the skewness statistic of –0.1. However, the distribution is flatter than the population distribution, as indicated by the kurtosis statistic of –0.436. The difference between the population parameters and the sample statistics is sampling error.

STANDARD ERROR OF THE MEAN

When inferences are made about normally distributed data, conclusions are based on the relationships of the standard deviation and mean to the normal curve. The mean of the sample may or may not be the same as the population mean. The difference between the sample mean and the population parameter μ is sampling error. For example, if we draw three different samples from a population, we will get three different means. In addition, if we take many samples from the same population, we will have as many different means, and these means will be normally distributed. The mean of the means will be close to the true population mean.

To determine how close the sample mean is to the population mean, we find the standard deviation of the distribution of means. The standard deviation of the distribution of means is called the **standard error of the mean** or standard error. The smaller the standard error, the closer the sample mean is likely to be to the population mean. However, we do not need to draw a lot of samples to calculate the standard error; it can be calculated from a single sample:

$$\text{Standard error of the mean (SE)} = s / \sqrt{N}$$

The standard error is influenced by the standard deviation and the sample size. The greater the dispersion around the mean, the less certain we are about the actual population mean, and the greater the standard error of the mean. The larger the sample size, the more confidence we have in the mean and the smaller the standard error of the mean. The smaller the standard error, the more reliable the statistic.

The effects of sample size and standard deviation on the standard error are illustrated in the following examples. In a hypothetical frequency distribution on the average age of college graduates, the mean is 22.5 and the standard deviation is 3.5. With a sample size of 100, the standard error of the mean is .35; if we increase the sample size to 200, and the mean and standard deviation remain the same, the standard error of the mean decreases to .25. If the sample size remains at 100 but the standard deviation increases to 5.5, the standard error of the mean increases to .55. These data are summarized in Table 5–3.

Table 5–3 Statistical Comparisons by Sample Size

	Sample 1	*Sample 2*	*Sample 3*
N	100	200	100
Mean	22.5	22.5	22.5
SD	3.5	3.5	5.5
SE	.35	.25	.55

The data in Exhibit 5–6 further illustrate these principles. Three simple random samples were drawn from a population in which the mean is 109.2 and the standard deviation is 30.2.

Exhibit 5–6 Sample Means and Population Mean

Population Data:	68	72	76	85	87	90	93	94	94
	95	97	98	103	105	105	107	114	117
	118	119	123	124	127	151	159	217	

Sample 1	Sample 2	Sample 3	
76	72	72	103
85	85	76	105
87	93	85	105
93	95	87	107
98	97	90	117
103	98	93	118
105	103	94	119
105	105	95	124
117	107	97	151
118	114	98	217
119	117		
123	118		
127	119		
151	124		
217	127		

$\overline{X}_1 = 114.9$ $\overline{X}_2 = 104.9$ $\overline{X}_3 = 107.7$

$s_1 = 34.1$ $s_2 = 15.3$ $s_3 = 31.4$

$s_{\overline{x}1} = 8.8$ $s_{\overline{x}2} = 4.0$ $s_{\overline{x}3} = 7.0$

The sample size in samples 1 and 2 is 15. In sample 1, the mean is 5.7 units above the population mean, and in sample 2 the mean is 4.3 units below the population mean. The mean's sensitivity to extreme scores is demonstrated in sample 1 because the sample mean is pulled in the direction of the outlier (217). The standard deviation for sample 1 ($s = 34.1$) is greater than that for sample 2 ($s = 15.3$), indicating more variation and a greater standard error for sample 1 over sample 2—8.8 versus 4.0, respectively.

However, when we increase the sample size to 20, the observed mean is closer to the population mean, even when the outlier was drawn as part of the sample. However, the outlier increases the variation in the sample, resulting in a standard error of 7.0—a standard error less than that for sample 1 but greater than that for sample 2. Sample 3 is further demonstration that the sample size and standard deviation influence the standard error.

CONFIDENCE INTERVALS

The sample mean, $\overline{X}$, is a **point estimate** of the population mean, μ. With the additional information of the standard error of the mean, $s_{\overline{x}}$, and our knowledge of the normal curve, we can estimate the limits within which the true population mean probably lies. This is called a **confidence interval** on μ and gives a range of values that might reasonably contain the true population mean. The confidence interval is represented as

$$a \le \mu \le b$$

Using the data from sample 1 in Exhibit 5–6, we can add and subtract the standard error of the mean from the sample mean:

$$\text{Point estimate} \pm \text{error} = \overline{X}_1 \pm s_{\overline{x}1} = 114.9 \pm 8.8$$

or

$$106.1 \le \mu \le 123.7$$

The results indicate that the true population mean falls within ± 1 standard error on each side of the sample mean. This is interpreted as meaning that if we draw a number of samples from the population, 68% of these sample means will fall between 106.0 and 123.7. From this we can infer that we are 68% confident that the population mean lies within these limits.

But when developing confidence intervals, we generally want to be more confident about the sample statistic. Generally, the confidence intervals are set at 95%. As noted earlier in this chapter, 95% of the area under the standard normal curve lies between +1.96 and −1.96 standard deviations of the mean. The 95% confidence interval (CI_{95}) may be constructed as follows:

$$\text{CI}_{95} = \overline{X} \pm 1.96(s_{\overline{x}})$$

Substituting into our formula the CI_{95} for sample 1 in Exhibit 5–6 yields

$$\text{CI}_{95} = 114.9 \pm 1.96(8.8) = 114.9 \pm 17.2$$

Thus, we can say that we are 95% confidant that our true population mean lies between 97.7 and 132.1. This confidence interval is expressed as:

$$97.7 \le \mu \le 132.1$$

As you can see from the population data in Exhibit 5–6, the true population mean, 109.2, lies within this band. Note that by increasing the confidence interval from 68% to 95% we have increased the range within which the true mean may fall. Increasing the size of the confidence interval increases our confidence that the true population mean lies within that interval.

Correspondingly, we can compute the CI_{95} for samples 2 and 3:

Sample 2:

$CI_{95} = 104.9 \pm 1.96(4.0) = 104.9 \pm 7.8$

$97.1 \leq \mu \leq 112.7$

Sample 3:

$CI_{95} = 107.8 \pm 1.96(7.0) = 107.8 \pm 13.7$

$94.1 \leq \mu \leq 121.5$

Sample 1 has the greatest variation, as indicated by the standard deviation; thus, it also has the greatest standard error and the widest confidence band.

The general formula for calculating the confidence interval is

$$CI_\mu = \bar{X} \pm \alpha(s_{\bar{x}})$$

where α is the confidence coefficient. For the normal distribution, the 95% confidence interval, the confidence coefficient is equal to 1.96; for a confidence interval of 99%, the confidence coefficient is equal to 2.58 (± 2.58 standard deviations from the mean).

SAMPLING METHODS

Before we can make inference about a population, we must select a sample. Samples should be as representative of the underlying population as possible. If the sample is representative, inferences made from the sample about the population will be correct. There are two general sampling techniques: probability and nonprobability sampling. In probability sampling, each member of a population has a known probability of being selected for the sample. Nonprobability samples are those in which members of a sample are deliberately selected for a specified purpose. One example is the selection of patients admitted to the emergency department in January to study the effects of a new anticoagulant. In nonprobability sampling, generalization of results to a population is extremely limited. Nonprobability sampling is often used in conducting clinical trials.

We will limit our discussion to several methods of probability sampling: **simple random sampling**, **stratified random sampling**, **systematic sampling**, and **cluster sampling**. In simple random sampling, each member of a population has an equal chance of being selected for inclusion in the sample. The selection of one member of the population has no influence on the selection of another. The drawing of numbers in state lotteries is an example of a simple random sample.

Occasionally we are interested in studying different strata within a population. A stratum is a variable by which the population can be subdivided. Common examples in health care include dividing the human population by age or sex, or categorizing acute care facilities by size. Basically, we group the population into subcategories. In stratified random sampling, we want to draw a sample so that each stratum within the population is proportionately represented in the sample. Before drawing the sample, we must divide the population into the strata we are interested in studying and then randomly draw the appropriate sample from each stratum. If we are studying a problem where sex is an important variable, we will want a stratified sample that is composed of 50% men and 50% women.

In systematic sampling, we select every *k*th member of a population from a list—such as selecting the records of every 5th patient discharged for clinical pertinence review. If we want to select a sample of 10 from a population of 100, we will select every 10th name from the discharge list. Caution must be exercised with systematic sampling if the list is ordered in any way. For example, if a list of university students is listed by class rank, the resulting sample may not be representative of the population. In systematic sampling, every member of the population does not have an equal chance of being selected for the sample. Selection for inclusion in the sample is dependent upon the first member selected for inclusion in the sample.

In cluster sampling, the sampling units are groups rather than individuals. For example, if we want to survey physicians in the state of Ohio, we can define the population as physicians practicing in acute care facilities in the state of Ohio. The units to be sampled are hospitals—clusters; then, from each hospital included in the sample, a sample of physicians is surveyed. This is two-stage sampling. We first randomly select hospitals and then randomly select physicians that practice at the hospitals.

HYPOTHESIS TESTING AND STATISTICAL SIGNIFICANCE

With statistical inference, we are interested in making generalizations about a particular population from a sample drawn from that population. When we generalize, we are describing the population from our sample statistics. Often, however, we are interested in determining whether two population means are different with respect to a given variable, such as age, length of stay (LOS), and/or total charges. To determine whether two means are different, we must first develop a hypothesis and perform a statistical test to determine if the observed differences between the means are statistically significant—or, stated another way, whether the observed difference between the group means is greater than what would be expected by chance alone.

To understand the concept of statistical significance, consider the following example. Let's say that the researcher is interested in determining whether physician A's practice profile is superior to physician B's, as indicated by the LOSs of their respective patients. The researcher will evaluate the differences between practice profiles of these two physicians on the basis of the patients' average length of stay (ALOS) for physicians A and B. In addition, the researcher will want to know if the "observed" difference between the two mean LOSs is due to something other than measurement error. The observed differences in the patients' mean LOSs could be due to the following reasons:

1. The practice profile of physician A is actually superior to the practice profile of B.
2. Some confounding factor that was not controlled in any way, such as the age or type of patient, may account for the difference.
3. Random variation could account for the difference.

Only after the second and third reasons have been ruled out can we say that the practice profile of physician A is superior to the practice profile of physician B. To rule out reason 2, we have to design a study that does not permit any extraneous factors that may bias the comparison. To rule out reason 3, we test for statistical significance.

But before we select a statistical test for comparing the two means, we must develop a hypothesis for statistical testing. For tests involving the comparison of two or more groups, the null hypothesis states that there is no difference between the population means from which the two samples were drawn. The **null hypothesis** is consistent with the idea that the observed difference between the means of two or more groups is due to random variation in the data. The null hypothesis is expressed as

$$H_0: \mu_A = \mu_B$$

The interpretation is that the population mean for group A is equal to the population mean for group B.

After we have developed the null hypothesis, we must state the alternative hypothesis. The **alternative hypothesis** states what our theory is or what we expect to happen as a result of the statistical test. The alternative hypothesis may take one of several forms:

1. $H_A: \mu_A \neq \mu_B$
2. $H_A: \mu_A < \mu_B$
3. $H_A: \mu_A > \mu_B$

In the first example, we are stating that we expect that the two population means will not be equal. We are interested only in whether the observed differences between the two population means are significant. In the latter two examples, we are stating a direction in which we expect the population means to differ. In the second example, we are stating that we expect the mean for population A to be significantly less than the mean for population B. And in the third example, we are stating that we expect the mean for population A to be greater than the mean for population B.

For our comparison of the practice profiles of the two physicians, our alternative hypothesis will take the form of the second example. This could indicate that physician A was superior to Physician B in regard to LOS.

LEVEL OF SIGNIFICANCE

To determine if physician A is more effective than physician B, we select an appropriate test of statistical significance and establish an appropriate alpha level, such as $\alpha = 0.05$ or 0.01. The alpha level is the maximum probability of rejecting the null hypothesis when it is true. This is referred to as a **type I error**. If alpha is set at 0.05, we run a 5% risk of error when we reject the null hypothesis—that is, when we state that the means of the two groups are different. A **type II error** occurs when we accept the null hypothesis when it is false.

The null hypothesis is rejected only if the sample results are so different from the hypothesis that the probability of such a difference occurring by chance alone is very low or insignificant. The lower the significance level—for example, $\alpha = 0.01$—the more the sample data must depart from the null hypothesis to be statistically significant. An alpha set at 0.01 is considered to be more strict than an alpha set at 0.05.

When we reject the null hypothesis, we actually support what we believe to be true. Rejecting the null hypothesis supports our theory. Failure to reject the null hypothesis does not mean that the null hypothesis is true; it only means that we did not prove that the observed difference between the means of the two groups was statistically significant beyond a reasonable doubt.

The **level of significance** refers to the probability of making a type I error. For type I error, the level of significance is designated by α (alpha). The level of significance is usually set at .01 or .05. For small sample sizes, alpha is usually set at .05; for large sample sizes, alpha is usually set at .01. If the significance for α is set at .05 and the null hypothesis is rejected, the probability of a type I error is 5%. In the long run, with the drawing of multiple samples from the same population, the rejection of a true null hypothesis will occur 5% of the time. Conversely, the sample data will justify accepting the true null hypothesis 95% of the time.

The probability of committing a type II error is designated by β (beta). Type II errors occur only when we incorrectly fail to reject the null hypothesis. Because the level of significance is set to reduce the probability of type I error, the probability of a type II error is increased. However, the probability of making a type II error decreases as the sample size increases. Table 5–4 shows the probabilities of type I and type II errors.

Table 5–4 Probabilities of Type I and Type II Errors

Action	Null Hypothesis	
	H_0 Is True	H_0 Is False
Reject H_0	Type I error α	Correct $1 - \beta$
Accept H_0	Correct $1 - \alpha$	Type II error β

THE *p* VALUE

The level of significance is determined before conducting the statistical test of significance, or *a priori*. The **p value** is obtained from the statistical test of significance and indicates the probability that the observed difference between the means could have been obtained by chance alone, given random variation and a single test of the null hypothesis. If the obtained *p* value is .03, the correct interpretation is that the probability of obtaining the test statistic at least as extreme as the one calculated is 3%. That is, only 3% of all possible samples will produce a test statistic as extreme as the calculated test statistic if the null hypothesis is true. If the *p* value obtained from the statistical test is less than or equal to the preset alpha level, the result is considered sufficiently rare so that the null hypothesis is rejected.

Exhibit 5–7 provides an example of a statistical test for the difference between two population means, using Excel. In the example, the z test for the difference between two population means was conducted to determine if the ALOS varied by sex for a particular diagnosis-related group (DRG). In the example, the LOSs for males and females discharged from DRG XXX were compared. The mean LOS for males is 4.26 days, and the mean LOS for women is 4.95 days. Prior to conducting the z test, the null and alternative hypotheses were stated and the alpha level was set:

$$H_0: \mu_1 = \mu_2$$
$$H_A: \mu_1 \neq \mu_2$$
$$\alpha = .05$$

The null hypothesis states that there is no difference between the ALOS for patients by sex for DRG XXX; the alternative hypothesis states that there is a difference between the ALOS of the patients by sex for DRG XXX.

Exhibit 5–7 z Test for the Difference between Two Population Means, Excel Output

	Male	Female
Mean	4.2612	4.9470
Known Variance	9.6000	9.0000
Observations	134.0000	151.0000
Hypothesized Mean Difference	0	
z	−3.2733	
P(Z<=z) one-tail	0.0005	
z Critical one-tail	1.6449	
P(Z<=z) two-tail	0.0011	
z Critical two-tail	1.9600	

The Excel output provides the calculated z statistic and its corresponding p values, which indicate whether the means of the two groups are significantly different from each other. (Exhibit 5–8 provides an explanation of each row in the Excel output.) In Exhibit 5–7, the calculated value of z is −3.27. In comparing the LOSs for the two groups, the procedure automatically transformed the LOSs for the two groups to z scores. Excel provides two other z values: 1.96 and 1.64. These values are interpreted as ±1.96 and ±1.64. These are the critical values of z for both one- and two-tailed tests when alpha is set at .05. Recall that in the standard normal distribution, 95% of the observations fall between +1.96 and −1.96 standard deviations of the mean. This means that 5% of the observations fall outside ±1.96 standard

Exhibit 5–8 Explanation of Excel Output, z Test for the Difference Between Two Population Means

> **Mean:** The arithmetic means for each group, male and female
> **Known Variance:** The population variance for each group must be provided in order to conduct the z test. This will be discussed in Chapter 6.
> **Observations:** The size of the sample for each group.
> **Hypothesized Mean Difference:** When conducting the z test, the investigator may specify the difference between the two means that he/she believes to be important. No difference was specified for this example.
> **Z:** The **calculated** value of z (–3.2733) as a result of conducting the statistical test.
> **P(Z<=z) one-tail:** The *p* value. The probability that the **critical** value of z (1.64) is less than or equal to the **calculated** value of z (–3.2733) for a one-tailed test.
> **z critical one-tail:** The **critical** value of z (1.64) for a one-tailed test when α = .05. It should be interpreted as ±1.64 depending on the direction of the test.
> **P(Z<=z) two-tail:** The *p* value. The probability that the **critical** value of Z (1.96) is less than or equal to the **calculated** value of z (–3.2733) for a two-tailed test.
> **z Critical two-tail:** The **critical** value of z (1.96) for a two-tailed test when α = .05.

deviations. The remaining 5% of the observations are divided between the two tails of the standard normal distribution—2.5% in the left tail and 2.5% in the right tail. The critical *z* value for a one-tailed test is ±1.64. In a one-tailed test, we are interested in whether one population mean is greater or less than the other population mean. When alpha equals .05, this is interpreted as 95% of observations falling above or below 1.64, depending on the direction of the test. The remaining 5% of the observations are located in either the right tail or the left tail of the standard normal distribution. The calculated value of *z*, –3.27, must equal or exceed the critical value of *z* if we are to reject the null hypothesis.

The Excel output provides two *p* values, one for a one-tailed test and one for a nondirectional test or two-tailed test. Our alternative hypothesis states that we are interested in whether the mean LOSs for males and females for DRG XXX are significantly different. We will use the *p* value for the two-tailed test. The *p* value is .0011, which is less than the preset alpha level of .05. The interpretation of the *p* value is that the probability of obtaining a *z* statistic as extreme as –3.27, given the corresponding sample size, is 0.11%, or less than 1.0%. Since the *p* value is less than the previously stated alpha level, we reject the null hypothesis and conclude that the mean LOSs for males and females are significantly different from each other.

We will discuss one-tailed and two-tailed tests in more detail in Chapter 6.

Remember that the *p* value is not the level of significance; the level of significance, or alpha level, is set prior to conducting the statistical test. The *p* value is obtained as a result of the statistical test. The *p* value is the probability of obtaining the resultant test statistic when all possible samples are drawn. The *p* value is a statistic that indicates how rare the particular sample is, whereas the level of significance is an independent criterion for evaluating the sample result and is in no way dependent upon that particular result.

SAMPLE SIZE AND INTERPRETATION OF STATISTICAL SIGNIFICANCE

When our statistical analysis results in a nonsignificant difference, we should evaluate the sample size. When the sample size is small, sampling error is likely to be large, and this often leads to a nonsignificant test result even when the observed difference is caused by a real effect. There is no way to determine whether a nonsignificant difference is the result of the small sample size or whether the null hypothesis is correct. It is for this reason that when our statistical test is not significant, we should almost always regard it as inconclusive rather than as an indication of no effect.

On the other hand, very large samples are very likely to result in statistical significance. With large samples, the alpha level is set at 0.01, which requires very strong evidence to reject the null hypothesis. Even with an alpha as strict as 0.01, one must judge the practical implications of the findings. Yes, the test may result in statistical significance, but does this difference have any practical application? When working with data, one cannot solely rely on the results of statistical tests; the knowledge and judgment of the researcher play a vital role in the interpretation of statistical procedures. We will discuss sample size in relation to type I and type II error in greater detail in a later chapter.

Calculating Sample Size

Procedures for calculating the sample size necessarily vary depending on the type of statistical test to be used and the type of research study to be conducted. In general, the size of the sample (n) is based on

1. the size of the population from which the sample is to be drawn
2. the desired alpha level, which controls for type I error
3. the choice on the bounds on the error of the estimate—how close the sample estimate is to be to the true population value

Sample size procedures may control for type I error or for both type I and type II errors. The procedures that we will discuss control only for type I error.

Sample sizes will be large when the underlying population is large, when variation within the population is great, when the designated alpha level is strict ($\alpha = .01$), and when the interval on the error of the sample estimate is narrow. Various procedures for calculating sample size are presented in Exhibits 5–9 through 5–14.

USING COMPUTER SOFTWARE TO SOLVE PROBLEMS

Many computer programs are available that can assist you in solving statistical problems. The advantage of using an electronic spreadsheet or a dedicated statistical package is that the data can be entered directly, and databases can be designed to help evaluate these problems on a more timely basis. If you will recall from Chapter 3, the more timely the data, the more valuable they are in the decision-making process. The health information manager should

Exhibit 5–9 Sample Size Calculation To Estimate Proportion or Rate When Population *N* Is Known

Problem 1: Calculation of size of a simple random sample to estimate a proportion or rate when the size of the total population is known.

$$\text{Sample size} = n/[n(B^2) + 1]$$

where *B* is the bound on the error of the estimate.

Example: There are 600 students in the School of Allied Medical Professions at XYZ University. We want to know what proportion of the student body is male within ±0.5% of the true population proportion. If we want the population proportion to be within ½ of 1.0% of the true population proportion, the bound on the error of the estimate is 1.0% (.5% × 2).

$$\begin{aligned}
\text{Sample size} &= n/[n(B^2) + 1] \\
&= 600/[600(.01^2) + 1] \\
&= 600/1.06 \\
&= 566.04, \text{ or } 566 \text{ cases}
\end{aligned}$$

Why do we need a sample size of 566 cases, which would constitute 94.3% of the population? Because we based our calculations on a very narrow bound on the estimate—±0.5%. We are not willing to tolerate much error when making inferences regarding the true population proportion from the sample mean. If we increase the bounds on the estimate to ±2.5%, we have:

$$\begin{aligned}
\text{Sample size} &= n/[n(B^2) + 1] \\
&= 600/[600(.05^2) + 1] \\
&= 600/2.5 \\
&= 240 \text{ cases}
\end{aligned}$$

Increasing the interval around our sample estimate decreases the sample size required by 58%.

Exhibit 5–10 Sample Size Calculation To Estimate Proportion or Rate When Population *N* Is Unknown

Problem 2: Calculation of size of a simple random sample to estimate a proportion or rate when the size of the total population is unknown.

$$\text{Sample size} = [(1.96^2)(pq)]/B^2$$

where *p* is the estimated proportion or rate, *q* is 1 – estimated proportion or rate, and *B* is the bound on error of estimate (1.96 varies depending on the desired confidence level sought in estimating proportion or rate).

Example: We want to conduct a study of members of the American Health Information Management Association (AHIMA). We know that in AHIMA 10% of the population is male. What is the size of the sample needed if we want to be sure we have enough men in our sample within ±1.0% of the true population proportion?

$$\begin{aligned}
\text{Sample size} &= [(1.96^2)(pq)]/B^2 \\
&= \{(1.96^2)[(.1)(.9)]\}/.02^2 \\
&= [3.8416(.09)]/.0004 \\
&= 864.36, \text{ or } 864
\end{aligned}$$

Again, we ask why we need such a large sample size. We need it primarily because we placed such a narrow bound on our estimate. If we increase the bound on the estimate to ±2.5%, the resultant sample size reduces to 138.

$$\begin{aligned}
\text{Sample size} &= [(1.96^2)(pq)]/B^2 \\
&= \{(1.96^2)[(.1)(.9)]\}/.05^2 \\
&= [3.8416(.09)]/.0025 \\
&= 138.3, \text{ or } 138 \text{ cases}
\end{aligned}$$

Increasing the interval around our sample estimate decreases the sample size required by 84%.

become proficient not only in data collection but also in the analysis of the data so that the data are useful to health care providers, planners, and researchers. Examples have been limited to the use of SPSS, but electronic spreadsheets such as Excel may also be used.

Selection of statistical computer software is a matter of choice. An example of using Excel for descriptive statistics is presented in Exhibit 5–15. The output displayed is provided auto-

Exhibit 5–11 Sample Size Calculation To Estimate Mean When Population N Is Known

Problem 3: Calculation of size of a simple random sample to estimate the mean when the size of the total population is known.

$$\text{Sample size} = \frac{n(\text{SD})^2}{n-1[B^2/1.96^2] + (\text{SD})^2}$$

where SD = standard deviation, which can be estimated by dividing the range by 4 ($R/4$).

Example: We want to select a sample to study the mean number of days in the surgical intensive care unit (SICU) for patients having coronary artery bypass graft (CABG) surgery. Last year, 400 patients were discharged; for these patients, the number of SICU days ranged from 2 to 9. We want to estimate the mean number of days within ±.25 days of the true population mean.

$$\text{SD} = R/4 = 9 - 2 = 7/4 = 1.75$$

$$\begin{aligned}
\text{Sample size} &= \frac{n(\text{SD})^2}{n - 1[B^2/1.96^2] + (\text{SD})^2} \\
&= \frac{400(1.75)^2}{399[(.5^2)/1.96^2] + 1.75^2} \\
&= 1{,}225/\{[399(.065)] + 3.0625\} \\
&= 1{,}225/28.9975 \\
&= 42.25, \text{ or } 42 \text{ cases}
\end{aligned}$$

Exhibit 5–12 Sample Size Calculation To Estimate Mean When Population N Is Unknown

Problem 4: Calculation of size of a simple random sample to estimate the mean when the size of the total population is unknown.

$$\text{Sample size} = [1.96^2(\text{SD})^2]/B^2$$

where SD is the standard deviation, which can be estimated by dividing the range by 4 ($R/4$).

Example: We want to select a sample to study the mean number of surgical intensive care unit (SICU) days for patients having coronary artery bypass graft (CABG) surgery. The CABG benchmarking literature indicates that the number of SICU days ranges from 2 days to 11 days. We want to estimate the mean number of days within ±.25 days of the true population mean.

$$\text{SD} = R/4 = 11 - 2 = 9/4 = 2.25$$

$$\begin{aligned}
\text{Sample size} &= [1.96^2(\text{SD})^2]/B^2 \\
&= [1.96^2(2.25)^2]/.5^2 \\
&= 19.4481/.25 \\
&= 77.79, \text{ or } 78 \text{ cases}
\end{aligned}$$

matically by Excel when one is using the "Descriptive Statistics" option. Dedicated statistical packages, such as SPSS, are often easier to use in that less manipulation of the data is required. Also, dedicated statistical packages can offer the user more choices in the types of statistical tests that are available, and most include both parametric and nonparametric procedures. Excel does not include options for nonparametric procedures.

CONCLUSION

The normal and standard normal distributions are theoretical distributions used for testing statistical problems in health care, since many naturally occurring phenomena follow the normal distribution. The normal distribution is actually a family of distributions in which the population mean can take on any value. The normal distribution is a symmetrical, bell-shaped distribution where 50% of the observations fall above the mean and 50% of the obser-

Exhibit 5–13 Stratified Sample Size Calculation To Estimate Mean When Population N Is Known and n in Each Stratum Is Known

---

Problem 5: Calculation of size of stratified random sample to estimate the mean when the size of the total population is known and the n in each stratum is known.

$$\text{Sample size} = q/\{[(N)(B^2/1.96^2)] + (q/n)\}$$

where $q = \Sigma[(n)(SD)]^2$ for each stratum, n is the population size of each stratum, N is the total population size, SD is the standard deviation, and B is the bound on error of estimate.

Example: We want to select a stratified random sample to study the mean drug charges for congestive heart failure (CHF) patients treated during the previous year. The population consists of 370 patients stratified by three physicians. We want the mean charge estimate to be within ± $25 of the true population mean. Information related to physicians A, B, and C appears below:

	Phys. A	Phys. B	Phys. C
No. of patients	120	160	90
p of total patients	.324	.433	.243
Range of drug charges	$1,000	$900	$852
SD ($R/4$)	$250	$225	$213

$$
\begin{aligned}
\text{Sample size} &= q/\{[(N)(B^2/1.96^2)] + (q/n)\}\\
&= [120(250)]^2 + [160(225)]^2 + [90(213)]^2/\\
&\quad 370(50^2/1.96^2) + (2{,}563{,}488{,}900/370)\\
&= 358 \text{ total cases needed (rounded)}
\end{aligned}
$$

For each stratum:

Physician A = 358 × .324 = 116 cases
Physician B = 358 × .433 = 155 cases
Physician C = 358 × .243 = 87 cases

---

vations fall below the mean. In the normal distribution, the mean, median, and mode are equal.

To make comparisons between distributions, the normal distribution may be standardized. The standard normal distribution has many of the same properties as the normal distribution except that in the standard normal distribution, the mean is equal to 0, and the standard deviation is 1. There is only one standard normal distribution. In the standard normal distribution, 68% of the observations fall between +1.0 and −1.0 standard deviations of the mean, and 95% of the observations fall between +1.96 and −1.96 standard deviations of the mean.

The standard normal distribution is important in statistical inference. The standard normal distribution can be used to make comparisons between populations. In statistical testing, we are interested in whether one population is the same as or differs from another population on a variable of interest.

When making comparisons between populations, we must first draw a sample from the population. Probability sampling is the preferred sampling technique. Types of probability

Exhibit 5–14 Sample Size Calculation To Estimate Difference between Two Means

Problem 6: Calculation of size of a simple random sample to estimate the difference between two means at the 95% confidence level.

Sample size = $\{1.96^2[(SD_1)^2 + (SD_2)^2]\}/B^2$

where SD_1 = standard deviation of group 1, SD_2 = standard deviation of group 2, and B^2 = size of the difference to be detected.

Example: We want to select a sample to determine if the difference between the mean average length of stay (ALOS) between two physicians is at least ±.25 days. The standard deviation for ALOS for the patients of physician A is 1.98; for physician B, it is 1.52.

$$\begin{aligned}
\text{Sample size} &= \{1.96^2[(SD_1)^2 + (SD_2)^2]\}/B^2 \\
&= \{1.96^2[(1.98^2 + 1.52^2)]\}/.5^2 \\
&= \{3.8416(3.9204 + 2.3104)\}/.25 \\
&= 23.94/.25 \\
&= 95.74, \text{ or } 96 \text{ cases per group}
\end{aligned}$$

Exhibit 5–15 Excel Output for Descriptive Statistics on Age

Age	
Mean	77.733
Standard Error	1.085
Median	78.5
Mode	74
Standard Deviation	5.947
Sample Variance	35.374
Kurtosis	–0.435
Skewness	–0.099
Range	24
Minimum	66
Maximum	90
Sum	2,332
Count	30
Confidence Level (95.0%)	2.220

sampling include simple random sampling, stratified random sampling, systematic sampling, and cluster sampling. It is important to take care when drawing samples so that we have some level of confidence when making inferences from the sample to the underlying population. In general, the larger the sample size, the more confidence we have in our results.

With statistical inference, we are interested in making generalizations about our population parameters from sample statistics. For example, if we are interested in comparing two population means for significant differences, we must set up a hypothesis. For statistical testing we set up two hypotheses—the null and alternative hypotheses. The null hypothesis states that there is no difference between the population parameters of interest; the alternative hypothesis states that there is a statistically significant difference in the population parameters of interest.

After formulating our hypotheses, we must set an alpha level for rejection of the null hypothesis. For large samples, alpha is usually set at .01 because it is easy to achieve statistical significance with large samples. Conversely, for small samples, alpha is usually set at .05 because it is more difficult to achieve statistical significance with smaller samples. The alpha level also indicates the probability of making a type I error. In a type I error, we reject the null hypothesis when it is true. A type II error is made when we fail to reject a null hypothesis that is false.

ADDITIONAL RESOURCES

Clark, J.J., and M. Clark. 1983. *A statistics primer for managers*. New York: Free Press.

Duncan, R.C., et al. 1983. *Introductory biostatistics for the health sciences*. Albany, NY: Delmar Publishers.

Jekel, J., et al. 1996. *Epidemiology, biostatistics, and preventive medicine*. Philadelphia: W.B. Saunders.

Phillips, D.S. 1978. *Basic statistics for health science students*. San Francisco: W.H. Freeman & Co.

Schott, S. 1990. *Statistics for health professionals*. Philadelphia: W.B. Saunders.

Stockburger, D.W. 1998. Introductory statistics: Concepts, models and applications. The normal curve. http://www.psychstat.umsu.edu/introbook/sbk13m.html

U.S. Department of Health and Human Services, Public Health Service. 1992. *Principles of epidemiology: An introduction to applied epidemiology and biostatistics*. Atlanta, GA: USDHHS.

Appendix 5–A

Exercises for Solving Problems

KNOWLEDGE QUESTIONS

1. Define the key terms listed at the beginning of this chapter.

2. Compare the normal distribution with the standard normal distribution.

3. What is the difference between the standard deviation and the standard normal deviate?

4. You have been analyzing discharges by sex from DRG 462, Rehabilitation, for Critical Care Hospital. Specifically, you are interested in determining if there is a difference in average age by sex. Review the data in Table 5–A–1, and answer the questions that follow.

Table 5–A–1 Mean Age of Patients, by Sex, DRG 462, Rehabilitation, in 1997 at XYZ Hospital

	Male	Female	Total
N	178	364	542
Mean	73.39	76.70	75.61
Standard deviation	15.27	12.4	13.49
Standard error	1.14	0.65	0.58
Lower bound 95% CI	71.13	75.43	74.48
Upper bound 95% CI	75.65	77.98	76.75
Minimum age	18	32	18
Maximum age	97	98	98

a. State the null and alternative hypotheses; state the a priori alpha level.
b. What is the average age for the entire group? For men? For women?
c. Why is the standard error larger for the male group than for the female group?
d. Why is the standard error for the total group smaller than either of the standard errors for the male or female groups?

e. What is the 95% confidence interval for men? For women? For the entire group?

f. What is your interpretation of the 95% confidence interval?

5. You have been analyzing hospital discharges from DRG 15, Transient Ischemic Attack and Precerebral Occlusions. The average length of stay (ALOS) for patients discharged from DRG 15 is 2.2 days. The national length of stay for DRG 15 is 4.1 days. You are interested in determining whether the hospital's length of stay for DRG 15 is significantly different from the national ALOS.

a. State the null and alternative hypotheses.

b. Set the alpha level.

6. You are interested in studying patient average length of stay (ALOS) for three physicians. You want to determine if there is a significant difference between the ALOSs of the three physicians.

a. State the null and alternative hypotheses.

b. Set the alpha level.

7. Explain the differences between the alpha level and the *p* value.

8. What are type I and type II errors? What factors contribute to making either a type I or type II error?

9. The mean length of stay for patients discharged from DRG 005, Extracranial Vascular Procedures, is 3.33. The standard deviation for the group is 3.18, and the number of patients discharged is 21. Calculate the 95% confidence interval for the mean length of stay.

MULTIPLE CHOICE

1. In a normal distribution, 68% of the observations fall within:
   a. $\pm 1\ \sigma$ of the mean
   b. $\pm 2\ \sigma$ of the mean
   c. $\pm 3\ \sigma$ of the mean
   d. $\pm 1\frac{1}{2}\ \sigma$ of the mean

2. In a normal distribution, 32% of the scores fall outside:
   a. $\pm 1\ \sigma$ of the mean
   b. $\pm 2\ \sigma$ of the mean
   c. $\pm 3\ \sigma$ of the mean
   d. $\pm 1\frac{1}{2}\ \sigma$ of the mean

3. The normal distribution is:
   a. continuous
   b. a family of distributions
   c. symmetrical about the mean
   d. all of the above

4. Which of the following is *not* a characteristic of the normal curve?
   a. It is unimodal.
   b. It is a discrete distribution.
   c. It is asymptotic to the x axis.
   d. The mean may take on any value.

5. The lengths of stay for DRG 123 were standardized so that comparison could be made across hospitals. What percentage of the lengths of stay would have a z value greater than or equal to 1.00?
   a. 32%
   b. 16%
   c. 8%
   d. 4%

6. In a standard normal distribution, what percentage of the lengths of stay for DRG 123 would fall above $z = -1.96$?
   a. 99%
   b. 97.5%
   c. 95%
   d. 68%

7. If a distribution has a long tail to the right, it is:
   a. bimodal
   b. abnormal
   c. positively skewed
   d. negatively skewed

8. In a standard normal distribution, the mean:
   a. is 0.00
   b. is -1.00
   c. is +1.00
   d. may take on any value

9. A normal distribution has a mean of 20 and a standard deviation of 5. Ninety-five percent of the scores fall between:
   a. 15 and 25
   b. 10 and 30
   c. 5 and 35
   d. Not enough information provided

10. The standard deviation of a distribution is 24; the sample size is 9. The standard error of the mean is:
   a. 3
   b. 8
   c. 75
   d. 225
   e. not enough information provided

11. A condition that is fundamental to statistical inference is:
    a. random sampling
    b. that the population is normally distributed
    c. that the mean of the population is known
    d. all of the above

12. The null hypothesis is a statement that is:
    a. probably true
    b. considered to be false until proven true
    c. evaluated statistically as either true or false
    d. all of the above

13. When $\alpha = .05$, the null hypothesis will be:
    a. rejected 5% of the time
    b. rejected 5% of the time when it is true
    c. accepted 5% of the time
    d. accepted 5% of the time when it is false

14. A type I error occurs when:
    a. we reject the null hypothesis when it is true
    b. we reject the null hypothesis when it is false
    c. we accept the null hypothesis when it is true
    d. we accept the null hypothesis when it is false

15. A type II error occurs when we:
    a. use a two-tailed test when a one-tailed test is more appropriate
    b. use a one-tailed test when a two-tailed test is more appropriate
    c. reject the null hypothesis when it is true
    d. accept the null hypothesis when it is false

16. If we change the alpha level for a statistical test from .05 to .01, we are:
    a. increasing the risk of making a type I error
    b. decreasing the risk of making a type I error
    c. decreasing the risk of making a type II error
    d. increasing the probability of finding statistical significance

17. In general, large sample sizes:
    a. reduce the risk of type I error
    b. reduce the risk of type II error
    c. make it easier to detect significant differences
    d. all of the above

18. The p value is the:
    a. power of a statistical test
    b. probability that the null hypothesis is true
    c. probability of making a type II error
    d. probability of getting a result as extreme as the one observed if the null hypothesis is true

19. We have drawn a simple random sample of 100 patients who were discharged from Critical Care Hospital in January. Of all the patients discharged during January, 55% were women and 45% were men. To match the population, our sample should contain:
   a. 45 men and 55 women
   b. 50 men and 50 women
   c. 55 men and 45 women
   d. The ratio of men to women in the sample size is not important.

20. You are assisting a physician who is conducting a study on the number of cancer cases at Critical Care Hospital. You jointly decide to take a 5% random sample of the estimated 20,000 charts. This is an example of:
   a. cluster sampling
   b. simple random sampling
   c. stratified random sampling
   d. two-stage random sampling

21. The physician now decides to draw his 5% sample of cancer cases by selecting every 20th chart by medical record number. This is an example of:
   a. random cluster sampling
   b. two-stage random sampling
   c. systematic random sampling
   d. stratified random sampling

22. You decide to study coding quality by randomly selecting hospitals in your state. From each of the hospitals selected, you review coded charts of randomly selected coders. This is an example of:
   a. cluster sampling
   b. simple random sampling
   c. stratified random sampling
   d. two-stage random sampling

PROBLEMS

1. Review the data on length of stay that appear in Table 5–A–2 to answer the questions below.
   a. Using a microcomputer statistical package, calculate the average length of stay for the entire group, for men, and for women.
   b. You are interested in determining if there is a difference in the average length of stay by sex. State the null and alternative hypotheses; state the *a priori* alpha level.
   c. Calculate the standard error of the mean length of stay for the entire group, for men, and for women.
   d. Calculate the 95% confidence interval for length of stay for the entire group, for men, and for women.

Table 5–A–2 Critical Care Hospital, Length of Stay of Patients by Sex, DRG 127, Heart Failure, 1997

Sex

LOS Days	Male	Female	Total
1.00	12	10	22
2.00	25	24	49
3.00	31	17	48
4.00	28	28	56
5.00	11	23	34
6.00	6	15	21
7.00	6	12	18
8.00	5	9	14
9.00	3	2	5
10.00	3	4	7
11.00	1	2	3
12.00	1	1	2
13.00	1	2	3
14.00	1		1
15.00		2	2
18.00		1	1
25.00	1		1
Total	135	152	287

CHAPTER 6

Hypothesis Testing of the Difference between Two Population Means

KEY TERMS   Hypothesis testing
    One-tailed test
    Two-tailed test
Critical region
Noncritical region
z test
    z test for comparing two independent population means
    z test for comparing two population proportions
Effect
Degrees of freedom (df)
t test
    t statistic
    one-sample t test
    t test for comparison of two independent sample means
    paired t test

LEARNING OBJECTIVES   At the conclusion of this chapter, you should be able to:

1. Define key terms.
2. Calculate one- and two-tailed tests of significance for one and two independent samples using z.
3. Use z for comparing two population proportions.
4. Compare and contrast the normal distribution and t distribution.
5. Calculate one- and two-tailed tests of significance for one and two independent samples using t.
6. Conduct a paired-sample t test.
7. Use statistical software to calculate the various t tests.

In our discussion of **hypothesis testing** of the difference between population means, we will be dealing with examples where population parameters are both known and unknown. If population parameters are known and we have sufficiently large samples ($N \geq 30$), the standard normal distribution is used as the basis for statistical decision making in the form of a z test. If we are comparing means when population parameters are unknown, and if our samples are smaller, Student's t test is used as the basis for statistical decision making. Our discussion will first focus on the use of the z test and the standard normal distribution and then consider the t test and the t distribution for comparing sample means to population means, comparing the means of two populations, and comparing pre- and posttest scores of matched pairs.

THE STANDARD NORMAL DISTRIBUTION AND THE z TEST FOR COMPARING POPULATION MEANS

Before we conduct a statistical test such as the z test, we must develop a hypothesis for the test. We select a statistical test based on our research questions, which are developed into statistical hypotheses. A statistical hypothesis may involve comparing a sample mean to a population mean or comparing two or more sample means drawn from two populations. The hypothesis may be either one tailed (directional) or two tailed (nondirectional). In a **one-tailed test**, we are seeking to determine if our sample mean, $\overline{X}$, is significantly greater or less than the population parameter μ. If we are interested in determining whether our sample $\overline{X}$ is significantly greater than the population parameter μ, we look for a critical z value in the positive tail of the distribution. Conversely, if we are interested in determining whether our sample $\overline{X}$ is significantly less than the population parameter μ, we look for a critical z value in the negative tail of the distribution. In a one-tailed test with an alpha of .05, we look for statistical significance in either the upper or lower tail of the distribution.

In a nondirectional or **two-tailed test**, we are interested only in determining whether the sample mean, $\overline{X}$, and the population parameter μ are significantly different from each other; the direction of the inequality is not an issue. In this case, both tails of the z distribution are used in the statistical decision making. A two-tailed test divides alpha in half, placing .025 in each tail. That is, when alpha is set at .05, we look for statistical significance in either the positive or negative tails of the standard normal distribution.

The null and alternative hypotheses may take the following forms:

$$H_0\ \mu_1 = 5.5 \text{ or } H_0\text{: } \mu_1 = \mu_2$$
$$H_A\text{: } \mu_1 \neq 5.5 \text{ or } H_A\text{: } \mu_1 \neq \mu_2 \text{ (two-tailed tests)}$$
$$H_A\text{: } \mu_1 < 5.5 \text{ or } H_A\text{: } \mu_1 < \mu_2 \text{ (one-tailed tests)}$$
$$H_A\text{: } \mu_1 > 5.5 \text{ or } H_A\text{: } \mu_1 > \mu_2 \text{ (one-tailed tests)}$$

We will illustrate a one-tailed test using the z test. From our discussion in Chapter 5, we know from the central limit theorem that we can expect that 95% of the sampling means will fall between +1.96 and −1.96 standard deviations of the true mean and that 99% of the sampling means will fall between +2.58 and −2.58 standard deviations of the true mean. For a two-tailed test, these standard deviations correspond to the significance levels of .05 and .01

respectively. In a one-tailed test, $z = \pm 1.64$ when $\alpha = .05$, and $z = \pm 2.33$ when $\alpha = .01$. A one-tailed test is considered more "robust" than a two-tailed test because statistical significance is easier to achieve. In a one-tailed test when $\alpha = .05$, ± 1.65 is required to achieve statistical significance; in a two-tailed test, ± 1.96 is required for statistical significance. The space between the critical values of z is called the **noncritical region**; the space outside or equal to the critical values of z is called the region of rejection. The critical values for the standard normal distribution are displayed in Table 6–1.

Table 6–1 Critical Values for Standard Normal Distributions

	Alpha	Critical Value z
Two-tailed test	.05	±1.96
	.01	±2.58
One-tailed test	.05	±1.65
	.01	±2.33

A one-tailed test is considered more "robust" than a two-tailed test because it is easier to achieve statistical significance. When conducting a statistical test, we "calculate" the value of z and compare it to the critical value of z. On a one-tailed test when $\alpha = .05$, a z of ± 1.65 is required to achieve statistical significance, so our calculated value of z must fall outside ± 1.65 in order to be statistically significant. In a two-tailed test, a z of ± 1.96 is required for statistical significance, so our calculated value of z must fall outside ± 1.96 in order to be statistically significant. In a two-tailed test, the space between ± 1.96 when $\alpha = .05$ is called the noncritical region or the area where we do not reject the null hypothesis. Thus, if the calculated value of z falls between ± 1.96, we fail to reject the null hypothesis. On the other hand, the space outside or beyond ± 1.96 when $\alpha = .05$ is called the **critical region**. If the calculated value of z is greater than or equal to $+1.96$ or less than or equal to -1.96, we reject the null hypothesis.

When we are conducting either a one-tailed or a two-tailed z test, the population parameters μ and σ are known. In our first example, we will conduct a two-tailed test in which we are interested in whether the hospital's average length of stay (ALOS) for patients discharged from DRG 089, Simple Pneumonia and Pleurisy, Age > 17, with CC, is different from the national ALOS. The 1997 national mean length of stay (LOS) (μ) for DRG 089 is 6.3 days, and the hypothetical standard deviation is 2.44 (σ). (We are using a hypothetical standard deviation because the actual population parameter is not available.) At Critical Care Hospital in 1997, 104 patients were discharged from DRG 089 with an ALOS of 5.49 days and a standard deviation equal to 3.44. In determining whether the observed difference in the ALOSs is statistically significant, we need to first state the null and alternative hypotheses and alpha level:

$$H_0: \mu_1 = \mu_2$$
$$H_A: \mu_1 \neq \mu_2$$
$$\alpha = .05$$

The null hypothesis states that the hospital's ALOS is equal to the national ALOS for DRG 89. The alternative hypothesis states that the hospital ALOS for DRG 89 is significantly different from the national ALOS. Since the alternative hypothesis is one of inequality, we are conducting a two-tailed test. The calculated value of z must fall outside or equal the critical value of z, ± 1.96. The z value is calculated as follows:

$$z = \frac{\bar{X} - \mu}{\sigma / \sqrt{n}}$$

$$= \frac{5.49 - 6.30}{2.44 / \sqrt{104}}$$

$$= \frac{-.81}{2.44 / 10.19}$$

$$= -3.39$$

The results would be reported as

$$Z_{calc} = -3.39$$
$$Z_{crit} = -1.96$$

Since our calculated value is negative, we refer to the negative tail of the distribution. The calculated value of z, -3.39, falls outside the critical value of z, -1.96, when $\alpha = .05$. We therefore reject the null and conclude that the ALOS at Critical Care Hospital is significantly different from the national ALOS for DRG 089.

In our second example, we will conduct a one-tailed test. The quality improvement team at Critical Care Hospital is interested in determining if the administration of a new antibiotic has had any effect in reducing the ALOS for patients discharged from DRG 089, Simple Pneumonia and Pleurisy, Age > 17, with CC. (An **effect** is a change in one variable—in this case, the ALOS—that may be associated with another variable—in this case, the antibiotic.) In 1997, the ALOS for the 104 patients discharged from DRG 089 at Critical Care Hospital was 5.49 days, and the standard deviation was 3.44. Specifically, we want to know if the antibiotic resulted in significant reduction of the ALOS.

We will first construct our null and alternative hypotheses. In the null hypothesis, we are assuming that the antibiotic will have no effect. If we reject the null hypothesis on the basis of our statistical test, we are saying that the probability of getting such a mean value by random chance is too small for us to believe that the null hypothesis is true. If we fail to reject the null hypothesis, we are stating that the probability associated with the observed mean is large, that such samples are common, and that there is not enough evidence that the antibiotic was effective in reducing the ALOS.

The null and alternative hypotheses are

$$H_0: \mu_1 = 5.49$$
$$H_A: \mu_1 < 5.49$$
$$\alpha = .05$$

The null hypothesis states that the hospital ALOS is equal to 5.49, the hospital's ALOS for DRG 89 in 1997. The alternative hypothesis states that the hospital ALOS is significantly less than the national ALOS, 5.49 days.

In this one-tailed test, we are interested in determining if the ALOS for DRG 89 is significantly less than the ALOS prior to administration of the new antibiotic. So we will look for statistical significance in the negative end of the tail. For a one-tailed test in which alpha is set at .05, the critical value of z is -1.64, so the calculated value of z must be less than or equal to -1.64 in order for the results to be statistically significant.

Now that we have stated the null and alternative hypotheses, we need to determine the sample size necessary to provide us with results in which we can be confident. Using the formula in the previous chapter in Exhibit 5–11, we will calculate the sample size, with a bound on the estimate equal to .25. The bound on the estimate indicates that we want to be within ±.25 of our true population mean. The sample size is calculated as follows:

$$\frac{N(sd^2)}{[N-1(B^2/1.96^2)]+sd^2}$$
$$=\frac{104(3.44^2)}{[103(.5^2/1.96^2)]+3.44^2}$$
$$=66.39=66$$

The sample size for our study is 66; the size of the standard deviation indicates that there is quite a bit of variation in the LOS for the 1997 discharges. Thus, for the amount of precision required in the study, a comparatively large sample is required. The sample was randomly drawn from all discharges from DRG 89. The descriptive statistics relating to our sample appear in Exhibit 6–1. The sample mean for the 66 patients who make up the sample who were treated after implementation of the antibiotic is 4.71.

Exhibit 6–1 Descriptive Statistics for Sample from DRG 089 (SPSS Output)

		LOS	Valid N (listwise)
N	Statistic	66	66
Minimum	Statistic	1.00	
Maximum	Statistic	11.00	
Mean	Statistic	4.7121	
Std. Deviation	Statistic	2.6181	
Skewness	Statistic	.601	
	Std. Error	.295	
Kurtosis	Statistic	.608	
	Std. Error	.582	

We calculate z as follows:

$$z = \frac{\bar{X} - \mu}{\sigma / \sqrt{n}}$$

$$= \frac{4.7121 - 5.49}{2.44 / \sqrt{66}}$$

$$= -.7779 / [(2.44) / (8.12)]$$

$$= -2.59$$

Our calculated value of z is –2.59. Our critical value of z for a one-tailed test is –1.64 when alpha equals .05. Since our calculated value is less than or equal to the critical value of z, we reject the null and conclude that the new antibiotic may have had an effect on reducing LOS for patients discharged from DRG 089. Note that this example is used for illustrative purposes only. Other factors may be at work that account for the reduction in the ALOS.

We can find the critical value of z by referring to a statistical table. Appendix B contains a table for the z scores in the standard normal distribution (Table B–1). The table contains three columns:

z	Cum p	Tail p
0.00	0.5000	0.5000
0.01	0.5040	0.4960
.	.	.
.	.	.
3.90	1.000	0.0000

The first column contains the values of z from 0.00 to 3.90; these should be read as both positive and negative, since the normal distribution is symmetrical. As you recall, the z score, 0.00, is the mean or center of the distribution. The second column is the cumulative probability of z from the lower end to the distribution to the location of z in the standard normal distribution. The third column is the tail probability, or the area beyond the location of z in the remaining portion of the distribution. For each value of z, the sum of these two probabilities is equal to 1.00.

To locate the exact probability of a calculated value of z, such as –3.39, locate 3.39 in the z column. The third column indicates that the exact p value for a one-tailed test is .0003. This is the portion of the standard normal distribution that is in one tail of the distribution beyond the z value ±3.39. If we are conducting a two-tailed test, we must double the p value to .0006.

THE z TEST FOR COMPARING TWO POPULATION PROPORTIONS

Often in quality improvement activities or various types of medical research, we are interested in comparing population proportions rather than population means. For example we may be interested in comparing the proportion of patients in medical and surgical intensive care who acquire nosocomial infections or comparing the proportion of patients who survive five years after experiencing two different surgical procedures. We can use a variation of z for comparing two population means or comparing two population proportions. The z test for comparing two population proportions may be either directional or nondirectional. Just as when we compare two population means using z, we assume that the two samples are selected independently and randomly from their respective populations and that the samples are normally distributed.

The null and alternative hypotheses may take the following forms:

$$H_0: p_1 = p_2$$
$$H_A: p_1 \neq p_2 \text{ (two-tailed tests)}$$
$$H_A: p_1 < p_2 \text{ or } p_1 > p_2 \text{ (one-tailed tests)}$$

The formula for calculating z for comparing two proportions is

$$z = \frac{(p_1 - p_2) - \left[1/2\left(1/n_1 + 1/n_2\right)\right]}{\sqrt{pq\left[\left(1/n_1\right) + \left(1/n_2\right)\right]}}$$

where p is the proportion of p_1 and p_2 when considered together as one sample and q is $(1 - p)$.

Consider the hypothetical example where we are comparing five-year survival rates following surgery for breast cancer. In group 1, 100 patients were followed after undergoing lumpectomy. In group 2, 100 patients were followed after undergoing mastectomy of the affected breast. In group 1, 80% of the patients were still alive after five years; in group 2, 85% were still alive after five years. The research question is whether there is a significant difference in the five-year survival rates between the two groups. The null and alternative hypotheses for a nondirectional test are

$$H_0: p_1 = p_2$$
$$H_A: p_1 \neq p_2$$
$$\alpha = .05$$

The null hypothesis states that the proportion of patients who survived in group 1 is equal to the proportion who survived in group 2. The alternative hypothesis states that the proportions of patients who survived in each group are not equal. The test we will conduct is a nondirectional test for the difference between two population proportions. In order for the test to be statistically significant, the calculated value of z must fall outside or equal the critical value of z, ± 1.96.

For a nondirectional test for an alpha of .05, the critical value of z is ±1.96, and z is calculated as

$$z = \frac{(p_1 - p_2) - [1/2(1/n_1 + 1/n_2)]}{\sqrt{pq[(1/n_1) + (1/n_2)]}}$$

$$= \frac{(.8 - .85) - [1/2(1/100 + 1/100)]}{\sqrt{(.825)(.175)(1/100 + 1/100)}}$$

$$= \frac{(-.05) - [1/2(.01 + .01)]}{\sqrt{.144(.01 + .01)}}$$

$$= -0.06 / .054$$

$$= -1.12$$

Since our calculated value of z, -1.12, does not fall outside or equal the critical value of z, -1.96, we fail to reject the null and conclude that the five-year survival rates following these two different surgical procedures are not significantly different. In other words, the type of surgical procedure had no effect on the five-year survival rate for breast cancer.

In the above example, the z calculations were performed with the assistance of a hand-held calculator. Neither SPSS, version 9.0.0, nor Excel provides a procedure for conducting a z test for the difference between two population proportions.

THE t TEST

Thus far in this text, we have discussed only the normal and standard normal distributions. There are other distributions from which statistical inferences can be made, one of which is the t distribution, sometimes referred to as Student's t. Student's t is named for William Gosset, who published under the pseudonym of Student. He was the first to describe this family of distributions. We conduct a t **test** when the population parameter σ is unknown. The σ is estimated from the sample statistic s. Before conducting the actual t test, we will compare the standard normal distribution with the t distribution.

The t distribution is used for statistical testing when population parameters are unknown and/or when the sample size is small. The definition of *small* varies; some researchers state that a sample size of less than 500 is small, while others consider a sample size of less than 90 small. Others have used the various forms of the t test with sample sizes of less than 30. With very large samples (e.g., $N \geq 1,000$), the t distribution and the normal distribution are approximately the same. In fact, the standard normal curve is a special case of the t distribution when df = ∞.

Both the standard normal and t distributions are symmetrical about a mean of zero. Like the normal distribution, the t distribution is actually a family of distributions based on sample size. This additional parameter is referred to as degrees of freedom (df) and is calculated by subtracting 1 from the sample size (df = $N - 1$). Exhibit 6–2 provides an explanation of **degrees of freedom**. The normal distribution is bell shaped; the shape of the t distribution is related to the number of degrees of freedom. A distribution with a small number of degrees of freedom is flatter; this results in a greater area in the tails of the distribution. Because the t distribution is so spread out, it is more difficult to achieve statistical significance with a small sample size.

Exhibit 6–2 Degrees of Freedom

The term *degrees of freedom* refers to the number of values that are free to vary after certain restrictions have been placed on the data. For example, in any set of interval-level data, we can sum the data to get a total. Assume that for a given frequency distribution, the sum is 100 and there are 10 cases ($N = 10$). If we arbitrarily assign a value of 10 to the first case, 5 to the second case, 15 to the third, 8 to the fourth, 2 to the fifth, 18 to the sixth, 23 to the seventh, 4 to the eighth, and 6 to the ninth, the cumulated sum will be:

$$10 + 5 + 15 + 8 + 2 + 18 + 23 + 4 + 6 = 91$$

The first nine values sum to 91. For all 10 cases to sum to 100, the 10th case must be equal to 9. Nine scores were arbitrarily set before the 10th was determined. Nine scores were free to vary; thus, we have nine degrees of freedom. Degrees of freedom are the number of elements in a set that can be arbitrarily defined before the rest of the elements in the set are determined.

In the t distribution when $\alpha = .05$, the critical value required to achieve statistical significance varies with the size of the sample. With the t distribution for a sample size of 10 (df = 9) and for a two-tailed test, a value outside or equal to ±2.262 must be obtained to achieve statistical significance as compared to ±1.96 in the standard normal distribution. In the t distribution with nine degrees of freedom, 95% of the observations fall between –2.262 and +2.262 standard deviations of the mean. If the size of the sample is increased from 10 to 20 (df = 19), the critical value required to achieve statistical significance decreases to ±2.093. Thus, the critical value needed to achieve statistical significance decreases as the sample size increases. As the sample size increases, the t distribution becomes less broad and flat and approaches the bell shape of the normal curve. With a sample size of 500, the critical value for the t distribution, when alpha is set at 0.05, is ±1.965, similar to the critical value of ±1.96, when alpha is set at 0.05, for the normal distribution. To test a hypothesis using the t distribution, we compare the calculated value of t to the critical value of t that is contained in the t table (Appendix B, Table B–2). Remember that the t distribution is actually a family of distributions where the tabled value of t is dependent upon the number of degrees of freedom in the sample, where df $= N - 1$.

The assumptions for the t test are that the samples are drawn randomly and independently from their respective populations and that they are normally distributed. In addition, it is assumed that the population variances of the two groups are approximately equal.

Two-tailed t Test

In a nondirectional t test, our question is just whether our sample mean is significantly different from the population mean, regardless of direction. In this case, both tails of the t distribution are used in the statistical decision making. A two-tailed t test divides alpha in half, placing half in each tail. That is, when alpha is set at .05, 2.5% of the area under both the upper and lower tails of the curve is considered when deciding whether to accept the null hypothesis.

Given this information about the t test and the t distribution, let us work through the same LOS problem that we used with the one-tailed z test. To restate our question of interest, we are interested in determining whether the hospital's ALOS for DRG 89 is significantly different from the national ALOS for DRG 089. The national ALOS is 6.3 days; our hospital mean LOS is 5.49, and the standard deviation is 3.44. There were 104 discharges from DRG 89. The first step in the process is to state our null and alternate hypotheses and to set the alpha level at which we will reject our null hypothesis:

$$H_0: \mu_1 = \mu_2$$
$$H_A: \mu_1 \neq \mu_2$$
$$\alpha = .05$$

As with the nondirectional z test, the null hypothesis states that the hospital ALOS for DRG 89 is equal to the national ALOS for DRG 89. The alternative hypothesis states that the ALOS for the hospital is significantly different from the national ALOS for DRG 89.

Since we are interested in determining only whether our hospital mean is different from the national mean, the t test is nondirectional, or a two-tailed test. Next, we determine the critical region for rejection of the null hypothesis. For a sample size of 104 (df $= 103$), the tabled t or critical t ($t_{0.05}$) value is approximately ± 1.98; since H_A is nondirectional, the critical region consists of all values of $t \geq 1.984$ or ≤ 1.984.

To locate the critical value of t, we refer to the tabled critical values of the t distribution in Appendix B, Table B–2. The first column lists the degrees of freedom, and the remaining columns identify the critical values of t for *a priori* alpha levels for both one- and two-tailed tests. Since the table does not list all possible degrees of freedom, we select the row for df $= 100$ for our problem. For a two-tailed test with alpha set at .05, the critical value of t is 1.984. Therefore, our region of rejection for the calculated value of t must equal or fall outside ± 1.984.

Using the formula for a **one-sample t test**, we can now calculate t:

$$t = \frac{\overline{X} - \mu}{s / \sqrt{N}}$$

$$t = \frac{5.49 - 6.30}{3.44 / \sqrt{104}}$$

$$= -.81 / (3.44 / 10.19)$$

$$= -2.399$$

The results would be reported as

$$t_{calc} = -2.399$$
$$t_{crit_{.05}} = -1.984$$

Since our t_{calc} is less than or equal to -1.984, we reject the null and conclude that our hospital LOS is significantly different from the national ALOS for DRG 089.

Notice that the formula for t takes the same general form as that for z. The only difference is that in z, the population parameter σ is used in the calculation, whereas in t, the population σ is estimated from the sample statistic s.

To calculate the CI_{95}, we use the same procedures as presented in Chapter 5, except that we use the critical value of t_{05}, which for 103 df is 1.98.

$$CI_{95} = \overline{X} \pm t_\alpha (s / \sqrt{N})$$

$$= 5.49 \pm 1.98(3.44 / \sqrt{104})$$

$$= 5.49 \pm 1.98(3.44 / 10.19)$$

$$= 5.49 \pm 1.98(.34)$$

$$= 5.49 \pm .668$$

$$[4.82, 6.16]$$

Thus, we are 95% confident that the true population mean lies between 4.82 and 6.16.

We can use SPSS to calculate the one-sample t test. When requesting the one-sample t test, the population parameter (i.e., 6.3) to which the sample mean is being compared must be specified. The output for the one-sample t test appears in Exhibit 6–3 and an explanation of the SPSS output appears in Exhibit 6–4.

✓ **To Obtain a One-Sample t Test Using SPSS:**

- From the menus, choose:
  Analyze
     →Compare Means
        →One Sample t Test
- Select one or more variables to be tested against the hypothesized value. Enter a numeric text value against which each sample mean is compared.

Exhibit 6–3 SPSS Output for One-Sample *t* Test

One-Sample Statistics		One-Sample Test			
	LOS				*LOS*
N	104	Test Value = 6.3	t		−2.399
Mean	5.4904		df		103
Std. Deviation	3.4416		Sig. (2-tailed)		.018
Std. Error Mean	.3375		Mean Difference		−.8096
			95% Confidence Interval	Lower	−1.4789
			of the Difference	Upper	−.1403

Exhibit 6–4 Output for One-Sample *t* Test

Test Value	*Population Parameter to Which the Sample Statistic Is Compared*
t	The calculated value of *t*
df	Degrees of freedom; for the one-sample *t* test the degrees of freedom are equal to $(n-1)$
Sig two-tailed	For a two-tailed or nondirectional statistical test, the *p* value for the calculated value of *t*
Mean difference	The actual difference between the two population means; the hospital mean is subtracted from the national mean
95% confidence interval of the difference	The interval that covers the true difference between the two population means

Note that the calculated *t* for our SPSS output is the same as that calculated with the assistance of a hand-held calculator. (When minor differences occur, they are most likely due to rounding.) The significance level or *p* value is .018, which is less than our previously established alpha level of .05. SPSS reports results in terms of significance—what we previously described as the *p* value. The critical value of *t* for the predetermined alpha level is not reported. The 95% confidence interval of the difference between the means is also provided. The 95% confidence interval of the mean is interpreted as meaning that we are 95% confident that the interval [−.1403, −1.4789] covers the true difference in the LOS between the hospital mean and the national mean for DRG 089. It is calculated as

$$CI_{\left(u_1 - u_2\right)} = (\overline{X}_1 - \overline{X}_2) \pm t_a \left[s\sqrt{(1 / n_1) + (1 / n_2)} \right]$$

One-Tailed *t* Test

Using the same information for the one-tailed z test, we will conduct a one-tailed t test. Recall that the quality improvement team is interested in determining if the administration of a new antibiotic resulted in a decrease in the ALOS. As before, the null and alternative hypotheses are

$$H_0: \mu_1 = 5.49$$
$$H_A: \mu_1 < 5.49$$
$$\alpha = .05$$

From the data in Exhibit 6–1, we know that the mean after administration of the antibiotic is 4.7121. Our previous calculations indicate that the required sample size is 66. Because this is a one-tailed test, the critical t value for an alpha of .05 and for 65 degrees of freedom is approximately -1.664. We had to approximate the critical t value because our t table does not include the critical values of t for all possible degrees of freedom. Our table provides the critical values of t for 60 and 80 degrees of freedom. So a conservative estimate of the critical t for 80 df was selected, -1.664. This is not much different from the critical value of t for 60 df, -1.671.

$$t = \frac{\overline{X} - \mu}{s / \sqrt{N}}$$
$$= 4.71 - 5.49 / (2.62 / \sqrt{66})$$
$$= -.78 / (2.62 / 8.124)$$
$$= -2.41$$

Since our t_{calc}, -2.41, is less than or equal to -1.664, we reject the null hypothesis and state that it appears that the new antibiotic may have been effective in reducing the hospital ALOS for DRG 89. The 95% CI for the mean would be calculated as

$$CI_{95} = \overline{X} \pm t_a (s / \sqrt{N})$$
$$= 4.71 \pm 1.671(2.62 / \sqrt{66})$$
$$= 4.71 \pm 1.67(.322)$$
$$= 4.71 \pm .54$$
$$= [4.17, 5.25]$$

We are therefore 95% confident that the interval from 4.17 to 5.25 covers the true LOS for our hospital patients after administration of the antibiotic.

When we use SPSS for the one-tailed t test, the output is the same as that for the two-tailed test, as displayed in Exhibit 6–5. The significance of the ***t* statistic** or p value for a two-sided test is reported. If we are conducting a one-tailed test, we must divide the p value when reporting the results. For a one-tailed t test, the p value becomes .0095 (.019/2), illustrating

Exhibit 6–5 SPSS Output for One–Sample *t* Test

One-Sample Statistics		One-Sample Test		
	LOS			*LOS*
N	66	Test Value = 5.49 t		−2.414
Mean	4.7121	df		65
Std. Deviation	2.6181	Sig. (2-tailed)		.019
Std. Error Mean	.3223	Mean Difference		−.7779
		95% Confidence Interval	Lower	−1.4215
		of the difference	Upper	−.1343

that it is easier to achieve statistical significance with a one-tailed test than with a two-tailed test.

The *t* Test for Comparing Two Independent Sample Means

Sometimes we are interested in comparing means from two independent samples—for example, comparing average charges by DRG or average charges by physician. In these examples, we would draw independent random samples from their respective populations. The null hypothesis would state that there was no difference in the population means for the two groups; the alternative hypothesis would be that there was a difference between the two population means:

$$H_0: \mu_1 = \mu_2$$
$$H_A: \mu_1 \neq \mu_2$$
$$\alpha = .05$$

The formula for the *t* test for comparison of **two independent sample means** is

$$t = \frac{\overline{X}_1 - \overline{X}_2}{s_p \sqrt{(1/n_1) + (1/n_2)}}$$

where s_p is called the pooled standard deviation. The pooled standard deviation is an average of the sample variances – n_1 and n_2. The pooled standard deviation is found by

$$s_p = \sqrt{(n_1 - 1)s_1^2 + (n_2 - 1)s_2^2 / (n_1 + n_2 - 2)}$$

Degrees of freedom for the *t* test for two independent samples are equal to $n_1 + n_2 - 2$. Exhibit 6–6 outlines the steps for solving the two-sample *t* test. The null hypothesis states that the mean charges for Dr. Sparenocost and Dr. Spendtheleast are equal; the alternative hypothesis states that the mean charges for Drs. Sparenocost and Spendtheleast are significantly different. We are conducting a one-tailed, nondirectional *t* test. The SPSS output for a two-sample *t* test appears in Exhibit 6–7.

Exhibit 6–6 Calculation of t Test for Two Independent Sample Means

At Critical Care Hospital, the average charge for Dr. Sparenocost is \$10,034.70; the average charge for Dr. Spendtheleast is \$6,158.53. The question of interest is whether the average charges for Dr. Sparenocost are significantly different from those for Dr. Spendtheleast.

1. State the null hypothesis and the alternative hypothesis, and set the alpha level.

$H_0: \mu_1 = \mu_2$
$H_1: \mu_1 \neq \mu_2$
$\alpha = .05$

2. Determine the region of rejection for a one-tailed two-sample t test where df $= n_1 + n_2 - 2 = 37$ $t_{crit0.05} = \pm 2.02$.

3. Calculate sample statistics:

Dr. Sparenocost	Dr. Spendtheleast
$\overline{X}_1 = \$10,034.70$	$\overline{X}_2 = \$6,158.53$
$s_1 = 4,390.98$	$s_2 = 3,177.50$
$n_1 = 20$	$n_2 = 19$

The pooled standard deviation:

$$s_p = \sqrt{\frac{(n_1 - 1)s_1^2 + (n_2 - 1)s_2^2}{n_1 + n_2 - 2}}$$

$$s_p = \sqrt{\frac{(20 - 1)4,390.98^2 + (19 - 1)3,177.5^2}{20 + 19 - 2}}$$

$$= 3,848.73$$

Calculation of t:

$$t = \frac{\overline{X}_1 - \overline{X}_2}{s_p = \sqrt{(1/n_1) + (1/n_2)}}$$

$$t = \frac{10,034.70 - 6,158.53}{3,848.73\sqrt{1/20 + 1/19}}$$

$$= 3,876.1737 / 1,232.98$$

$$= 3.144$$

4. Conclusion: $t_{calc} = 3.144$; $t_{calc} \geq t_{crit0.05}$ (df $= 37$) $= 2.021$. We reject the null hypothesis and conclude that it appears that the average charges for Dr. Sparenocost are significantly different from the average charges for Dr. Spendtheleast.

Exhibit 6–7 SPSS Output for Two-Sample *t* Test

Group Statistics

	TOTCHG	
	24	25
N	20	19
Mean	10034.7000	6158.5263
Std. Deviation	4390.9747	3177.4976
Std. Error Mean	981.8518	728.9679

Independent Samples Test

			TOTCHG	
			Equal Variances Assumed	*Equal Variances Not Assumed*
Levene's Test for	F		.248	
Equality of Variances	Sig.		.622	
t test for Equality of Means	t		3.144	3.170
	df		37	34.617
	Sig. (2-tailed)		.003	.003
	Mean Difference		3876.1737	3876.1737
	Std. Error Difference		1232.9839	1222.8766
	95% Confidence Interval	Lower	1377.9110	1392.6197
	of the Difference	Upper	6374.4364	6359.7276

✓ **To Obtain an Independent Samples *t* Test Using SPSS:**

- From the menus, choose
  Analyze
      →Compare Means
          →Independent Samples *t* Test
- Select one or more quantitative variables. A separate *t* test
  is computed for each variable.
- Select a single grouping variable, and click "Define Groups"
  to specify two codes for the groups you want to compare.

The results indicate that the calculated value of *t*, 3.144, is greater than the critical value of t, +2.021. We therefore reject the null hypothesis and conclude that the mean charges for each doctor are significantly different from each other. Why is it important to know if the charges of different physicians are significantly different from one another? The results could help us determine if one physician is more cost-effective than another in the delivery of health care services. Some possible questions that could be explored after obtaining this result include: Does one physician order more diagnostic tests than the other? Is the ALOS for the patients of one physician less than that for the other physician? If so, why? Answers to these and other questions can help us to educate physicians on the variations in their practice patterns. This may lead to more cost-effective delivery of health care services.

It is important to remember that we should be careful in drawing any definitive conclusions before conducting further investigation. In the example, the mean charges for one physician were significantly different from the mean charges for the other. When significant results are achieved, the data analyst must conduct further investigation to determine if there is an explanation for the difference. Perhaps the patients of one physician are older and sicker than the other physicians' patients. It would also be important to compare charges between all physicians who treat similar patients.

The results of our hand calculations are the same as the SPSS results. We are interested in the results in the column labeled "Equal Variances Assumed." SPSS automatically provides the results of Levene's test, which compares the equality of the variances between the groups. One of the assumptions of the t test is that the variances of the populations from which the two samples are drawn are equal. Since the result of the test is not significant, the variances of the two samples are assumed to be equal.

Excel may also be used for conducting the t test for comparing the means of two independent samples. The Excel output appears in Exhibit 6–8. The interpretation of the output is the same as that outlined in Exhibit 5–8, with the exception of the "pooled variance." The pooled variance is the pooled standard deviation squared that appears in Exhibit 6–6.

Exhibit 6–8 Excel Output for Two-Sample t Test, Assuming Equal Variances

	Phys 24	Phys 25
Mean	10034.700	6182.211
Variance	19280659.063	9973822.509
Observations	20	19
Pooled Variance	14753008.848	
Hypothesized Mean Difference	0	
df	37	
t Stat	3.131	
P(T<=t) one-tail	0.002	
t Critical one-tail	1.687	
P(T<=t) two-tail	0.003	
t Critical two-tail	2.026	

Paired *t* Test

In a **paired *t* test**, we are comparing the means of two samples that have been drawn from a single population. In a paired *t* test, the pair may be composed of two individuals who are matched on a set of characteristics such as height and weight, or the individual may be self-paired—serving as his or her own control. In this test, we are trying to determine if there is a difference in the means between the individuals who make up the pair or in the difference between "before" and "after" observations when one individual is serving as his or her control. The null and alternative hypotheses for the paired *t* test are

$$H_0: \overline{D} = 0$$
$$H_{A_1}: \overline{D} \neq 0$$

for a two-tailed test or

$$H_{A_1}: \overline{D} > 0$$
$$H_{A_2}: \overline{D} < 0$$

for a one-tailed test.
In the paired *t* test, *t* is calculated as

$$t = \overline{d} / (s_{\overline{d}})$$

where $\overline{d} = \sum D / N$, $s_{\overline{d}} = \sqrt{\sum d^2 / N(N-1)}$,

and $\sum d^2 = \sum D^2 - \left(\sum D\right)^2 / N$.

D is the difference in the observations before and after treatment for each individual in the study, or it is the difference in the observations between the experimental and control groups. $\overline{D}$ or $\overline{d}$ is the observed mean difference between the "before" and "after" observations or the mean observed difference between the experimental and control groups.

Let's consider an example where we are interested in improving the attitude of health information management (HIM) students toward statistics. There are 10 students in the statistics class; each student is given an attitude assessment prior to watching a video on the role of the HIM professional as a data analyst in health care. Following the video, the students are given a second attitude assessment. The null and alternative hypotheses are

$$H_0: \overline{D} = 0$$
$$H_{A_1}: \overline{D} < 0$$
$$\alpha = .05$$

The null hypothesis states that the difference between the pre- and postvideo assessment scores equals zero. The alternative hypothesis states that the postvideo assessment scores will be less than zero. The "before" and "after" data appear in Table 6–2.

Table 6–2 Pre- and Post-Attitude Assessment of HIM Students

Student	Before X_1	After X_2	Difference D	D^2
1	25	28	-3	9
2	23	19	4	16
3	30	34	-4	16
4	7	10	-3	9
5	3	6	-3	9
6	22	26	-4	16
7	12	13	-1	1
8	30	47	-17	289
9	5	16	-11	121
10	14	9	-5	25
Total	171	208	-37	511

This is a one-directional t test. Why do we expect the average difference to be less than zero? Because we expect the postvideo attitude assessment score to be greater than the prevideo attitude assessment score. When subtracting the postvideo assessment score from the pre-assessment score, the expected result should be negative. The critical value of t for a one-direction test with nine degrees of freedom, $\alpha = .05$, is -1.833 (Appendix B, Table B–2). For the paired t test, degrees of freedom are equal to $n - 1$ where n is the number of pairs.

Before we can calculate t, we must determine the sum of the squares of the difference score.

$$\sum d^2 = \sum D^2 - \left[\left(\sum D\right)^2 / n\right]$$
$$= 511 - [(-37)^2 / 10]$$
$$= 511 - 136.9$$
$$= 374.10$$

The standard error of the difference is

$$S_{\bar{d}} = \sqrt{\sum d^2 / n(n-1)}$$
$$= \sqrt{374.10 / 10(9)}$$
$$= 2.039$$

and

$$\bar{d} = \sum D / n$$
$$= -37 / 10$$
$$= -3.7$$

t is calculated by

$$t = \bar{d} / (s_{\bar{d}})$$
$$= -3.7 / 2.039$$
$$= -1.815$$

Since the calculated value of t, -1.815, does not fall in the region of rejection for the critical value of t when $\alpha = .05$, -1.833, we fail to reject the null and conclude that there is not enough evidence to indicate that the video improved the attitude of HIM students regarding statistics.

We can use SPSS to calculate the paired t test; the results appear in Exhibit 6–9. Note that the SPSS calculated t matches our "hand-calculated" t. For a two-tailed test, the exact p value for a t_{calc} of -1.815 (df = 9) is .103; for a one-tailed test, the p value is halved to 0.052.

Exhibit 6–9 SPSS Output for Paired-Sample t Test

Paired Samples Statistics		
	Pair 1	
	Prevideo	*Postvideo*
Mean	17.0000	20.80000
N	10	10
Std. Deviation	10.2029	12.9168
Std. Error Mean	3.2265	4.0847

Paired Samples Test

			Pair 1 Prevideo- Postvideo
Paired Differences	Mean		−3.7000
	Std. Deviation		6.4472
	Std. Error Mean		2.0388
	95% Confidence Interval	Lower	−8.3121
	of the Difference	Upper	.9121
t			−1.815
df			9
Sig. (2-tailed)			.103

✓ **To Obtain a Paired-Sample *t* Test Using SPSS:**

- From the menus, choose:
  Analyze
      →Compare means
          →Paired Samples t Test
- Select a pair of variables as follows:
      →Click each of two variables. The first variable
          appears in the "Current Selections" group as
          "variable 1," and the second appears as "variable 2."
      →After you have selected a pair of variables, click
          the arrow button to move the pair into the "Paired
          Variables" list. You may select more pairs of
          variables. To remove a pair of variables from the
          "Paired Variables" list, select a pair in the list and
          click the arrow button.

We may also use Excel to calculate a paired-sample *t* test. The Excel output appears in Exhibit 6–10. The Excel output includes the Pearson *r* correlation coefficient, which is +.87 (see Chapter 8).

Exhibit 6–10 Excel Output for Paired-Sample *t* Test

	Prevideo	*Postvideo*
Mean	17.1	20.8
Variance	104.1	166.844
Observations	10	10
Pearson Correlation	0.870	
Hypothesized Mean Difference	0	
Df	9	
t Stat	−1.81	
P(T<=t) one-tail	0.051	
t Critical one-tail	1.833	
P(T<=t) two-tail	0.102	
t Critical two-tail	2.262	

CONCLUSION

In this chapter, we have reviewed statistical procedures for testing hypotheses of the differences between means. We can use the z distribution for testing hypotheses involving one and two independent samples. To use the z distribution, we must assume that the samples are independent and are normally distributed and the sample size must be greater than 30. The population parameters μ and σ must be known if we are to use z.

When population parameters are not known, we can use the t distribution to test hypotheses of differences between population means. We can use t to compare a sample mean with a population mean or to compare the mean of two samples drawn independently from two populations, and we can use the paired t test for comparing means between matched pairs. In using both t and z, we are restricted to comparing means of two samples.

ADDITIONAL RESOURCES

Besag, F.P., and P.L. Besag. 1985. *Statistics for the helping professions*. Beverly Hills, CA: Sage Publications.

Clark, J.J., and M. Clark. 1983. *A statistics primer for managers*. New York: Free Press.

Duncan, R.C., et al. 1983. *Introductory biostatistics for the health sciences*. Albany, NY: Delmar Publishers.

Hall, H.I. 1998. The z test. *Quality Resource* 16, no. 5: 7.

Jekel, J.F., et al. 1996. *Biostatistics, epidemiology, and preventive medicine*. Philadelphia: W.B. Saunders.

Katz, D.L. 1997. *Biostatistics, epidemiology, and preventive medicine review*. Philadelphia: W.B. Saunders.

Appendix 6–A

Exercises for Solving Problems

KNOWLEDGE QUESTIONS

1. Define the key terms listed at the beginning of this chapter.

2. Compare and contrast the z distribution with the t distribution.

3. Describe situations in which we would use one-tailed tests; describe situations in which we would use two-tailed tests.

4. What assumptions must be met when using z and t for hypothesis testing? Why are these assumptions not always strictly followed?

5. In hypothesis testing, what is meant by the term *effect*?

6. Figure 6–9 displays the results of a paired t test in which we were interested in determining if the attitudes of HIM students toward statistics changed after viewing a video. We failed to reject the null hypothesis in this situation. What are some reasons for our failure to reject the null in this situation?

MULTIPLE CHOICE

1. It is easier for a statistical test to achieve statistical significance when we conduct a:
   a. nondirectional test
   b. one-tailed test
   c. two-tailed test
   d. all of the above

2. If a statistical test is significant at the .01 level, it is:
   a. also significant at the .05 level
   b. not significant at the .05 level
   c. also significant at the .001 level
   d. also significant at the .0001 level

For questions 3 through 6, refer to the problem below:

3. We are conducting a study of the age of nursing home patients in the county. The null and alternative hypotheses are

$$H_0: \mu = 80$$
$$H_A: \mu \neq 80$$

We have used the z test for evaluating our results when the critical values of z are ± 1.96 where $\alpha = .05$, and ± 2.58 where $\alpha = .01$.

In this case, the null hypothesis is:
a. directional
b. nondirectional
c. one-tailed z test
d. two-tailed t test

4. If the calculated z is $+2.30$, we would:
a. accept the H_0 at $\alpha = .05$ but reject the H_0 at $\alpha = .01$
b. accept the H_0 at $\alpha = .05$ and accept the H_0 at $\alpha = .01$
c. reject the H_0 at $\alpha = .05$ but accept the H_0 at $\alpha = .01$
d. reject the H_0 at $\alpha = .05$ and reject the H_0 at $\alpha = .01$

5. If the calculated value of z is $+1.80$, we would:
a. accept the H_0 at $\alpha = .05$ but reject the H_0 at $\alpha = .01$
b. accept the H_0 at $\alpha = .05$ and accept the H_0 at $\alpha = .01$
c. reject the H_0 at $\alpha = .05$ but accept the H_0 at $\alpha = .01$
d. reject the H_0 at $\alpha = .05$ and reject the H_0 at $\alpha = .01$

6. If the calculated value of z is -2.80, we would:
a. accept the H_0 at $\alpha = .05$ but reject the H_0 at $\alpha = .01$
b. accept the H_0 at $\alpha = .05$ and accept the H_0 at $\alpha = .01$
c. reject the H_0 at $\alpha = .05$ but accept the H_0 at $\alpha = .01$
d. reject the H_0 at $\alpha = .05$ and reject the H_0 at $\alpha = .01$

7. Which of the following is *not* needed to transform a score to a z score?
a. mean
b. variance
c. raw score
d. standard deviation

8. You believe that the hospital's average length of stay for DRG XXX is significantly less than the national average for the same DRG. Which of the following statistical tests would be most appropriate for answering this question?
   a. single-sample directional *t* test
   b. single-sample nondirectional *t* test
   c. *t* test for two independent samples
   d. any of the above

9. In the above problem, the sample size is 100. The number of degrees of freedom for evaluating the statistical significance of the test result is:
   a. 99
   b. 98
   c. 97
   d. not enough information provided

PROBLEMS

1. As an HIM DRG analyst, you are interested in comparing the mean length of stay (LOS) for Critical Care Hospital and the national mean for DRG 005, Extracranial Vascular Procedures. The hospital mean LOS is 3.381, and the standard deviation is 3.2012 (Table 6–A–1). The national average LOS for DRG 005 is 3.6 days, and the hypothetical standard deviation is 2.56 (actual standard deviation not available). The summary data for Critical Care Hospital appear in Table 6–A–1 and Exhibit 6–A–1.
   a. State the null and alternative hypotheses and the *a priori* alpha level.
   b. Calculate the difference between the hospital mean and the national mean using z. What are the resultant z statistic and the significance level?
   c. Calculate the difference between the hospital mean and the national mean using t. What are the number of degrees of freedom, the resultant t statistic, and the significance level?
   d. State your conclusions.

Table 6–A–1 Frequency Distribution for Length of Stay DRG 005 in 1997 at Critical Care Hospital (SPSS Output)

		Frequency	Percent	Valid Percent	Cumulative Percent
Valid	1.00	4	19.0	19.0	19.0
	2.00	8	38.1	38.1	57.1
	3.00	3	14.3	14.3	71.4
	4.00	2	9.5	9.5	81.0
	5.00	1	4.8	4.8	85.7
	6.00	1	4.8	4.8	90.5
	8.00	1	4.8	4.8	95.2
	15.00	1	4.8	4.8	100.0
	Total	21	100.0	100.0	

Exhibit 6–A–1 Length of Stay Statistics for DRG 005 in 1997 at Critical Care Hospital (SPSS Output)

N	Valid	21
	Missing	0
Mean		3.3810
Std. Error of Mean		.6986
Median		2.0000
Mode		2.00
Std. Deviation		3.2012

2. For the same DRG 005, you want to determine if there is a difference in the length of stay by payer. The summary data appear in Tables 6–A–2 and 6–A–3.
   a. State the null and alternative hypotheses and the *a priori* alpha level.
   b. Use the *t* test for two independent sample means to determine if the observed difference between the two means is statistically significant. What are the number of degrees of freedom, the resultant *t* statistic, and the significance level?
   c. State your conclusions.

Table 6–A–2 Frequency Distribution of Length of Stay by Payer, DRG 005, at Critical Care Hospital in 1997 (SPSS Output)

LOS* Payer Crosstabulation

Count

		Payer		
		Medicare	Commercial PPO	Total
LOS	1.00	2	2	4
	2.00	2	6	8
	3.00	1	2	3
	4.00	1	1	2
	5.00	1		1
	6.00		1	1
	8.00	1		1
	15.00		1	1
Total		8	13	21

Table 6–A–3 Mean and Standard Deviation for Length of Stay by Payer, DRG 005, at Critical Care Hospital in 1997 (SPSS Output)

Payer	Mean	N	Std. Deviation
Medicare	3.2500	8	2.3755
Commercial PPO	3.4615	13	3.7107
Total	3.3810	21	3.2012

3. You have been monitoring the lengths of stay for two of your physicians who discharge the most patients from DRG 127, Heart Failure. The relevant statistics appear in Tables 6–A–4 and 6–A–5. You specifically want to know if the observed difference in the lengths of stay for physicians 1 and 3 is statistically significant.
   a. State the null and alternative hypotheses and the *a priori* alpha level.
   b. Use the *t* test for two independent sample means to determine if the observed difference between the two means is statistically significant. What are the number of degrees of freedom, the resultant *t* statistic, and the significance level?
   c. State your conclusions.

Table 6–A–4 Frequency Distribution of Length of Stay by Physician, DRG 127, in 1997 at Critical Care Hospital (SPSS Output)

LOS* Physician Crosstabulation

Count

		Physician		
		1.00	3.00	Total
LOS	1.00	1		1
	2.00	1		1
	3.00	4	2	6
	4.00	1	1	2
	5.00	4	1	5
	6.00		2	2
	7.00	2	1	3
	8.00		2	2
	9.00		1	1
	10.00	2		2
	11.00		2	2
	15.00		1	1
Total		15	13	28

Table 6–A–5 Length of Stay by Physician, DRG 127, in 1997 at Critical Care Hospital (SPSS Output)

Report

LOS

Physician	Mean	N	Std. Deviation	Std. Error of Mean
1.00	4.8667	15	2.6690	.6891
3.00	7.3846	13	3.5009	.9710
Total	6.0357	28	3.2828	.6204

CHAPTER 7

Analysis of Variance

LEARNING OBJECTIVES

At the conclusion of this chapter, you should be able to:

1. Define key terms.
2. Use ANOVA to calculate the differences between two or more sample means.
3. Use statistical software to calculate ANOVA procedures.
4. When the ANOVA procedure results in a significant F statistic, use post hoc procedures to determine which means are significantly different.
5. Explain the purpose of post hoc tests.
6. Relate the concept of statistical power to beta error and sample size.

In Chapter 6, we discussed procedures for comparing two population means. But what do we do when we want to compare means when more than two groups are involved? If, for example, we had three populations, A, B, and C, for which we wanted to compare sample means, we could conduct multiple t tests by comparing A and B, A and C, and B and C. But this could become quite tedious: if we had 10 groups for which we wanted to compare means, we would have to make 45 comparisons. Also in making these multiple comparisons, we increase the probability of making a type I error—rejecting the null hypothesis when it is true. The **analysis of variance (ANOVA)** procedure is used when we want to compare the observed differences between two or more means from two or more independent samples.

ANALYSIS OF VARIANCE

As the name implies, ANOVA deals with variances rather than standard deviations and standard errors. In statistical terminology, variation refers to the sum of the squared deviations from the mean and is often referred to as the sum of squares: $\sum(X - \overline{X})^2$ or $\sum x^2$. When divided by the appropriate degrees of freedom, it is referred to as the variance: $\sum(X - \overline{X})^2 / (N - 1)$. The goal of the ANOVA procedure is to explain the total variation in the study. To do this, we must obtain two independent estimates of variance, one based on the variability between groups (**sum of squares between, SSB**) and the other based on the variability within groups (**sum of squares within, SSW**). These combined (SSB + SSW) equal the **total sum of squares (TSS)**.

To conduct the ANOVA procedure, the dependent variable must be continuous and/or be at least at the interval or ratio level of measurement. The samples should be drawn independently and randomly and be normally distributed. However, in cases where large samples are drawn, this assumption may be relaxed because of the central limit theorem. The variances of the group populations should be approximately equal. The independent variable is discrete or categorical.

The F distribution is used to test the difference between the two variance estimates. (ANOVA is often referred to as the F test, which is derived from the name of the individual who developed it, Sir Ronald Fisher.) Like the t distribution, the F distribution is a family of distributions based on the number of degrees of freedom associated with the variance estimates. The F distribution is a positively skewed distribution, so the calculated and critical values of F are positive.

The F ratio is obtained by dividing the mean of the between-group variance estimate (SSB) by the mean of the within-group variance estimate (SSW). If the obtained value of F equals or exceeds the critical value of F, the null hypothesis is rejected, and we conclude that the observed means differ more than what would be expected by chance alone. When conducting the ANOVA procedure, the alternative hypothesis is always one of inequality or nondirectional.

We will limit our discussion to the one-way ANOVA procedure. In the one-way ANOVA, we want to determine the effect of only one factor, or independent variable (IV), on the dependent variable (DV): for example, the effect of sex (IV) on length of stay (LOS) (DV). The one-way ANOVA procedure for analyzing two groups is an extension of the t test for comparing two sample means as $t^2 = F$. In the case of two independent samples, the ANOVA procedure is used more often because it is considered more powerful in complex experimental research designs.

The sum of squares is the basic concept in the ANOVA procedure. We have already learned to calculate the sum of squares in computing the variance. The raw score formula for the sum of squares is

$$\sum x^2 = \sum x^2 - \left(\sum X\right)^2 / N$$

which is equal to $\sum(X - \overline{X})^2$, as previously described in Chapter 4.

The TSS can be broken down into the sum of squares within groups (SSW) and the sum of squares between groups (SSB). Thus, the basic ANOVA model is

$$TSS = SSB + SSW$$

The TSS represents the variation of all the observations around the grand mean. The grand mean is the mean of the samples when they are combined or treated as one. The grand mean is represented by $\overline{\overline{X}}$. The SSB represents the variation of the sample means around the grand mean, and the SSW represents the variation of the independent observations in each sample around their respective means.

We will now conduct a simple ANOVA procedure to determine the significance of the difference between two sample means. In Table 7–1, the length of stay (LOS) for patients discharged from the medical intensive care unit (MICU) and surgical intensive care unit (SICU) are displayed. For this problem, we are interested in determining whether there is a significant difference between the average LOSs (ALOSs) for the SICU (X) and the MICU (Y). As with the t test, the first step is to state the null hypothesis and set the alpha level:

$$H_0: \mu_1 = \mu_2$$
$$H_A: \mu_1 \neq \mu_2$$
$$\alpha = .05$$

The null hypothesis states that there is no significant difference in the ALOSs for patients discharged from the MICU and the SICU. The alternative hypothesis states that the observed difference in the ALOSs for MICU and SICU is significant.

In ANOVA, the alternative hypothesis is always nondirectional since the F distribution is a positive distribution.

Table 7–1 Patient Lengths of Stay (LOSs) in Surgical and Medical Intensive Care Units (SICU and MICU), July 1 through 14, 19xx

Patient LOS SICU (X_1)	X_1^2	Patient LOS MICU (X_2)	X_2^2
21	441	9	81
19	361	10	100
18	324	20	400
13	169	14	196
15	225	18	324
20	400	5	25
22	484	8	64
25	625	11	121
17	289	12	144
10	100	13	169
$\sum X_1 = 180$	$\sum X_1^2 = 3,418$	$\sum X_2 = 120$	$\sum X_2^2 = 1,624$
$\overline{X}_1 = 18$		$\overline{X}_2 = 12$	

$$\overline{\overline{X}} = 15$$

To determine the TSS, which is the sum of the squares for the two groups treated as one.

$$\sum x^2 = \sum X^2 - \left[\left(\sum X \right)^2 / N \right]$$
$$= (3{,}418 + 1{,}624) - [(180 + 120)^2 / 20]$$
$$= 542$$

Next, we find the sum of squares within each group (SSW). For the SSW, each group is considered separately. The sum of squares for the SICU is

$$\sum x^2 = \sum X_1^{\,2} - \left[\left(\sum X_1 \right)^2 / N \right]$$
$$= 3{,}418 - (180)^2 / 10$$
$$= 178$$

The sum of squares for the MICU is

$$\sum x^2 = \sum X_2^{\,2} - \left[\left(\sum X_2 \right)^2 / N \right]$$
$$= 1{,}624 - (120)^2 / 10$$
$$= 184$$

So the total SSW is $178 + 184 = 362$.

Since TSS = SSB + SSW, we could subtract the SSW from the TSS to obtain the SSB. But to serve as a check on our calculations, we will directly calculate the SSB. The SSB is a measure of the variation of the group means about the combined mean. When the group means do not differ from each other, the SSB will be equal to zero. The greater the variation between the group means, the larger the SSB will be. The size of the SSB tells us how large the effect of the independent variable is on the dependent variable. In our example, the independent variable is type of care unit, and the dependent variable is the patient's LOS. The SSB is calculated as follows:

$$SSB = \sum n_i (\overline{X}_i - \overline{\overline{X}})^2$$

where n_i is the number of observations in each group, $\overline{\overline{X}}$ is the overall mean, or grand mean, and $\overline{X}_i$ is the mean for each group.

From Table 7–1, we know that the mean for the SICU is 18 days, the mean for the MICU is 12 days, and the grand mean is 15 days. The calculation for the SSB is

$$SSB = \sum n_i (\overline{X}_i - \overline{\overline{X}})^2$$
$$= 10(18 - 15)^2 + 10(12 - 15)^2$$
$$= 180$$

Thus, in terms of our ANOVA model, we now have

$$TSS = SSB + SSW$$
$$542 = 362 + 180$$

Each of these sums of squares has a specified number of degrees of freedom. Since the TSS refers to the two groups as one, the degrees of freedom is equal to $n-1$. The degrees of freedom for the SSW is equal to $n_i - 1$, where n_i is the number of observations in each group. But since we have more than one group, the number of degrees of freedom for the SSW will be equal to $k(n_i - 1)$, where k is equal to the number of groups. This latter formula applies only when the sample size for each group is the same. The number of degrees of freedom for the SSB is equal to $k - 1$ where k is the number of groups. In summary, the degrees of freedom for the F ratio are:

Source of Variation	Degrees of Freedom
SSB	$k-1$
SSW	$k(n_i - 1)$, only when all sample sizes are equal
TSS	$n-1$

After the sum of squares for each source of variation has been calculated, the data are summarized in an ANOVA table, as in Table 7–2. The components of the table are:

Source of Variation	df	Mean Square	F
SSB	$k - 1$	SSB/df	Means square SSB/means square SSW
SSW	$K(n - 1)$	SSW/df	
TSS	$n - 1$		

Table 7–2 ANOVA Table for Patient Length of Stay in Medical and Surgical Intensive Care Units

Source	SS	df	Mean Square	F
SSB	180	1	180.00	8.95
SSW	362	18	20.11	
TSS	542	19		

F TEST

A new column appears in Table 7–2 that we have not yet discussed—the mean square column. In the *F* test, we are comparing the SSB mean square to the SSW mean square. The mean squares are obtained by dividing the sum of squares for the SSB and SSW by their corresponding degrees of freedom. The SSB mean square is an estimate of the common population variance that is independent of the variation in the group means; that is, how much the group means differ from the overall mean. This is the effect on each observation from belonging to that particular group and is due to the effect of the treatment. If the group means tend to cluster around the grand mean, there is no treatment effect.

The SSW mean square is an estimate of the population variance that is independent of the variance within groups; that is, how much the observations within each group are spread out around the group mean. Variation within groups is considered error; this is because if each subject within a group is treated the same, the expected outcome for each member of the group should be similar. That is, the differences in observations within a group cannot be due to differential treatment. Wide variation within a group would indicate that there was no relationship between the independent variable (care unit) and the expected outcome, so any effect could not be attributed to the independent variable. When we reject the null, we are stating that the between-group variation is greater than the within-group variation. To obtain the value of *F*, the SSB mean square is divided by the SSW mean square:

$$F = \frac{\text{Mean square between groups}}{\text{Mean square within groups}}$$

If the population means are equal, indicating no effect, *F* will equal 1. If they differ, the mean square$_{SSB}$ will be greater than the mean square$_{SSW}$, and *F* will be greater than 1.

Recall that the *F* distribution is based on the degrees of freedom associated with the between-group variance estimate and the within-group variance estimate. In our example, there are two groups, so the degrees of freedom for SSB are equal to $k - 1$ or $2 - 1 = 1$. The within-group degrees of freedom are equal to $k(n_i - 1)$ or $2(10 - 1) = 18$.

To determine whether the *F* value is significant at our preset alpha level (0.05), we refer to the *F* table (Appendix B, Table B–3). In the *F* table, the degrees of freedom for the numerator are represented in the columns, and the degrees of freedom for the denominator are represented in the rows. To locate the critical value of *F*, we find the cell where the column and row for the designated degrees of freedom intersect. For 1 and 18 degrees of freedom, the critical value of *F* at .05 is 4.41. Since our calculated *F* ratio, 8.95, is larger than the critical value of 4.41, we reject the null hypothesis and conclude that it appears that the observed difference in the ALOSs for the MICU and the SICU is significant.

When the value of *F* is significant, we conclude that the groups under study differ significantly from each other; that is, the groups show more variation than what can be attributed to random sampling from populations with a common population mean. The greater the effect, the larger the obtained *F* ratio.

From the information contained in the ANOVA table, we can compute a correlation ratio, eta^2:

$$\text{eta}^2 = \text{SSB/TSS}$$
$$= 180/542$$
$$= .33$$

In our example, the correlation ratio is .33, or 33%. The correlation ratio explains how much variation in the dependent variable is explained by the independent variable. So we would state that 33% of the variation in length of stay is explained by the type of care unit.

To calculate this simple ANOVA procedure using SPSS, select "Compare Means" from the "Analyze" dropdown menu. Then select "Means." In the "Means" dialog box, type in "LOS" as the dependent variable and "care unit" as the factor. Click "Options" for the desired descriptive statistics and request the ANOVA table and eta^2. The SPSS output appears in Exhibit 7–1.

Exhibit 7–1 SPSS Output for "Compare Means"

Descriptives

Length of Stay

		MICU	SICU	Total
N		10	10	20
Mean		12.0000	18.0000	15.0000
Std. Deviation		4.5216	4.4472	5.3410
Std. Error		1.4298	1.4063	1.1943
95% Confidence	Lower			
Interval for Mean	Bound	8.7655	14.8186	12.5003
	Upper			
	Bound	15.2345	21.1814	17.4997
Minimum		5.00	10.00	5.00
Maximum		20.00	25.00	25.00

ANOVA

Length of Stay

	Sum of Squares	df	Mean Square	F	Sig.
Between Groups	180.000	1	180.000	8.950	.008
Within Groups	362.000	18	20.111		
Total	542.000	19			

Measures of Association

	Eta	Eta Squared
Length of Stay * Care Unit	.576	.332

In the dialog box, click "Options" to select a wide range of descriptive statistics. In the report section of Exhibit 7–1, the mean, standard deviation, variance, minimum and maximum values (range), and 95% confidence intervals are reported. The ANOVA table that appears in Exhibit 7–1 contains the information that we previously discussed except that the exact p value, .008, is provided. Eta and eta^2 are the same as what we calculated previously.

✓ **To Obtain a One-Way Analysis of Variance Using SPSS:**

- From the menus, choose:
  →Analyze
  →Compare means
  →Select one or more dependent variables
  →Select a single independent factor variable
  →Click "Options" for descriptive statistics and
   ANOVA table

We can also use Excel to conduct the one-way ANOVA procedures; the results appear in Exhibit 7–2. The information provided is similar to the ANOVA output for SPSS. However, Excel also displays the critical value of F, whereas SPSS does not.

Exhibit 7–2 Excel Output for One-Way ANOVA Procedure

Groups	Count	Sum	Average	Variance
SICU	10	180	18	19.778
MICU	10	120	12	20.444

ANOVA

Source of Variation	SS	df	MS	F	P value	F crit
Between Groups	180	1	180	8.950	0.008	4.414
Within Groups	362	18	20.111			
Total	542	19				

ANOVA IN THE THREE-SAMPLE CASE

Determining if there is a difference between two sample means is rather straightforward. But what do we do when we have more than two sample means? How do we know which means are actually different from one another? When we are working with more than two samples, we could have a situation where only two of the three means were different from each other. Follow-up procedures, called post hoc tests, must be conducted to determine which means are significantly different from one another. We will look at two post hoc tests: the **Scheffé test** and Tukey's honest significant difference (HSD) test.

The Scheffé test performs simultaneous joint pairwise comparisons for all possible pairwise combinations of means. The Scheffé test uses the F distribution for testing the significance of the mean differences and is the most conservative method of making post hoc multiple comparisons. The advantage of the Scheffé test is that it can be used when the n's in each group being compared are equal or unequal.

The **Tukey HSD** test uses the Studentized range statistic to make all of the pairwise comparisons between group means.

Let us now review an example where we wish to compare three sample means. Three physicians were compared in regard to the hospital LOS of their respective patients following a minor surgical procedure without complications. A sample of eight medical records were selected for each physician; the LOSs appear in Table 7–3.

Table 7–3 Patient Length of Stay by Physician

			Physician		
A	A²	B	B²	C	C²
4	16	4	16	5	25
5	25	5	25	3	9
5	25	4	16	3	9
4	16	3	9	3	9
6	36	4	16	3	9
6	36	5	25	3	9
4	16	3	9	4	16
5	25	3	9	5	25
$\Sigma A = 39$	$\Sigma A^2 = 195$	$\Sigma B = 31$	$\Sigma B^2 = 125$	$\Sigma C = 29$	$\Sigma C^2 = 111$
$A = 4.875$		$B = 3.875$		$C = 3.625$	

For this problem, we are interested in determining whether there is a significant difference in the ALOS for the patients of these three physicians. The null and alternative hypotheses and alpha level are

$$H_0: \mu_A = \mu_B = \mu_C$$
$$H_A: \mu_A \neq \mu_B \neq \mu_C$$
$$\alpha = .05$$

The null hypothesis states that the ALOSs for the patients of the three physicians are equal. The alternative hypothesis states that the ALOSs of the patients of the three physicians are not equal.

To determine the TSS, we treat the three groups as one group.

$$\sum x^2 = \sum X^2 - \left[\left(\sum X \right)^2 / N \right]$$
$$= (195 - 125 - 111) - [(39 + 31 + 29)^2 / 24]$$
$$= 22.625$$

Next, we find the SSW. For the SSW, each group is considered separately. The sum of SSW for physician A is

$$\sum x^2 = \sum X^2 - \left[\left(\sum X\right)^2 / N\right]$$
$$= 195 - [(39)^2 / 8]$$
$$= 4.875$$

The sum of SSW for physician B is

$$\sum x^2 = \sum X^2 - \left[\left(\sum X\right)^2 / N\right]$$
$$= 125 - [(31)^2 / 8]$$
$$= 4.875$$

The sum of SSW for physician C is

$$\sum x^2 = \sum X^2 - \left[\left(\sum X\right)^2 / N\right]$$
$$= 111 - [(29)^2 / 8]$$
$$= 5.875$$

So the total SSW is $4.875 + 4.875 + 5.875 = 15.625$.

After calculation of the overall mean, 4.125, the SSB is

$$SSB = \sum n_i (\bar{X}_i - \bar{\bar{X}})^2$$
$$= 8(4.875 - 4.125)^2 + 8(3.875 - 4.125)^2 + 8(3.625 - 4.125)^2$$
$$= 4.5 + .5 + 2.0$$
$$= 7.0$$

Thus, in terms of our ANOVA model, we now have

$$TSS = SSB + SSW$$
$$22.625 = 7.0 + 15.625$$

The data are summarized in the ANOVA Table 7–4.

Table 7–4 ANOVA Table for Physicians A, B, and C

Source	SS	df	Mean Square	F
SSB	7.0	2	3.5	4.73
SSW	15.625	21	.74	
SST	22.625	23		

The critical F value for 2 and 21 degrees of freedom when $\alpha = .05$ is 3.47. Since our calculated F is greater than the critical F, we reject the null hypothesis and conclude that it appears that patient LOS does vary by physician. But with three groups of physicians, we do not know if all three means are different from each other or if only two means are different from each other. We must now perform **post hoc procedures** to determine where these differences lie. Calculations for the Tukey and Scheffé post hoc procedures appear in Exhibit 7–3.

Calculating the correlation coefficient eta^2:

$$eta^2 = SSB/TSS$$
$$= 7.415/22.625$$
$$= .32$$

Eta^2 indicates that 32% of the variation in LOS is related to the physician. There could be a multitude of reasons for the patients of a particular physician having a significantly longer LOS, on average, than the other physicians. The physician may treat older patients or sicker patients, or physician A may have practice patterns that are different from those of physicians B and C. Whatever the reason, it should not be ascribed without investigation.

The results of the SPSS ANOVA procedure for the three means are displayed in Exhibit 7–4, and the results of the post hoc procedures appear in Exhibit 7–5. For both the Tukey HSD and the Scheffé, the ALOSs for physicians A and C are significantly different. The SPSS output in Exhibit 7–5 also displays homogeneous subsets by type of post hoc procedure. For both the Tukey HSD and the Scheffé test, the ALOSs for physicians B and C and physicians B and A are not significantly different. The results of the Excel ANOVA procedure are displayed in Exhibit 7–6. Excel does not provide post hoc procedures for analyzing differences for more than two group means.

STATISTICAL POWER

In the previous chapter, we discussed the effect that sample size has on the achievement of statistical significance. We also discussed sample size in relation to type I and type II error. Recall that type I error is the probability of rejecting the null hypothesis when it is true; type II error is the probability of accepting the null hypothesis when it is false. These concepts may be represented as

$$\alpha = \text{Pr (rejecting } H_0 | H_0 \text{ is true)}$$
$$\beta = \text{Pr (accepting } H_0 | H_0 \text{ is false)}$$

Exhibit 7–3 Tukey HSD and Scheffé's Test

Tukey HSD	Scheffé Test
$$\text{HSD} = q(a)\sqrt{\text{MS}_{\text{SSW}} / n}$$ Where MS_{ssw} is the mean square of the SSW, a is the number of means to be compared, n is the number in each group, and q is the df associated with MSssw. In our example, the df associated with MS_{ssw} is 21. From the distribution of the Studentized range statistic (Appendix B, Table B–4) for comparison of three means and 21 degrees of freedom, the critical value of t where $a = .05$ is approximately 3.55. Thus: $$3.55\sqrt{.74 / 8} = 1.08$$ The difference between any two means must be at least 1.08. Therefore: $$\overline{A} = \overline{B}$$ $$\overline{B} = \overline{C}$$ $$\overline{A} \neq \overline{C}$$ The average length of stay for the patients of physician A is significantly different from the average length of stay for patients of physician C.	In the Scheffé test, F must be computed to make the comparison. $$F = (\overline{X}_1 - X_2)^2 / [\text{MS}_{\text{SSW}}(n_1 + n_2)] / n_1 n_2$$ For means A and B, $$F = \frac{(4.875 - 3.875)^2}{.74(8 + 8) / 64}$$ $$= 5.41$$ For means A and C, $$F = \frac{(4.875 - 3.625)^2}{.74(8 + 8) / 64}$$ $$= 8.45$$ For means B and C, $$F = \frac{(3.875 - 3.625)^2}{.74(8 + 8) / 64}$$ $$= 0.34$$ To obtain the critical value of F, we multiply $(k - 1)$ by the critical value for F in the original ANOVA procedure. The number of groups in our analysis is three, so $k - 1 = 2$; and for 2 and 21 degrees of freedom, F_{crit} is 3.47. Therefore, F_{crit} for comparison purposes is 6.47 (2×3.47). For the differences between the two means to be statistically significant, the F's calculated from the above formula must exceed 6.47. In our example, the calculated F exceeds the critical value for F for only one comparison—means A and C. Therefore, $$\overline{A} = \overline{B}$$ $$\overline{B} = \overline{C}$$ $$\overline{A} \neq \overline{C}$$ The average length of stay for the patients of physician A is significantly different from the average length of stay for patients of physician C.

Exhibit 7–4 SPSS Output for Comparing Group Means of More Than Two Groups

Descriptives

Length of Stay

		A	B	C	Total
N		8	8	8	24
Mean		4.8750	3.8750	3.6250	4.1250
Std. Deviation		.8345	.8345	.9161	.9918
Std. Error		.2950	.2950	.3239	.2025
95% Confidence Interval for Mean	Lower Bound	4.1773	3.1773	2.8591	3.7062
	Upper Bound	5.5727	4.5727	4.3909	4.5438
Minimum		4.00	3.00	3.00	3.00
Maximum		6.00	5.00	5.00	6.00

ANOVA

Length of Stay

	Sum of Squares	df	Mean Square	F	Sig.
Between Groups	7.000	2	3.500	4.704	.021
Within Groups	15.625	21	.744		
Total	22.625	23			

Ordinarily, in statistical testing, we control for type I error when we set the alpha level. However, the more strict the alpha level, the more the probability of making a type II error increases. To get around this problem, we often increase the sample size because this reduces type II error. Recall that the standard error of the mean is a function of sample size as demonstrated by

$$SE_{\bar{x}} = \sigma / \sqrt{n}$$
$$SE_{\bar{x}} = \sigma / \sqrt{100} = 1 / 10\sigma$$
$$SE_{\bar{x}} = \sigma / \sqrt{400} = 1 / 20\sigma$$

Therefore, we can say that increasing the sample size decreases sampling error and lowers the probability of committing a type II error.

Another way to avoid making a type II error is to conduct a statistical power analysis. Power analysis helps us decide (1) how large the sample size must be for accurate and reliable statistical judgments and (2) how likely it is that our sample test statistic will detect effects for a given sample size.

We make many compromises when selecting the appropriate sample size. If our resultant decisions are to be accurate, the sample size must be large enough so that sampling error is small. But we do not want to choose sample sizes larger than needed because they are more

Exhibit 7–5 SPSS Output for Post Hoc Procedures Comparing Group Means of More Than Two Groups

Multiple Comparisons

Dependent Variable: Length of Stay

	(I) Physician	(J) Physician	Mean Difference (I–J)	Std. Error	Sig.	95% Confidence Interval Lower Bound	95% Confidence Interval Upper Bound
Tukey HSD	A	B	1.0000	.4313	.075	−8.71E–02	2.0871
		C	1.2500*	.4313	.022	.1629	2.3371
	B	A	−1.0000	.4313	.075	−2.0871	8.710E–02
		C	.2500	.4313	.832	−.8371	1.3371
	C	A	−1.2500*	.4313	.022	−2.3371	−.1629
		B	−.2500	.4313	.832	−1.3371	.8371
Scheffé	A	B	1.0000	.4313	.091	−.1357	2.1357
		C	1.2500*	.4313	.029	.1143	2.3857
	B	A	−1.0000	.4313	.091	−2.1357	.1357
		C	.2500	.4313	.846	−.8857	1.3857
	C	A	−1.2500*	.4313	.029	−2.3857	−.1143
		B	−.2500	.4313	.846	−1.3857	.8857
LSD	A	B	1.0000*	.4313	.031	.1031	1.8969
		C	1.2599*	.4313	.009	.3531	2.1469
	B	A	−1.0000*	.4313	.031	−1.8969	−.1031
		C	.2500	.4313	.568	−.6469	1.1469
	C	A	−1.2500*	.4313	.009	−2.1469	−.3531
		B	−.2500	.4313	.568	−1.1469	.6469

* The mean difference is significant at the .05 level.

Length of Stay

	Physician	N	Subset for alpha = .05 — 1	Subset for alpha = .05 — 2
Tukey HSD[a]	C	8	3.6250	
	B	8	3.8750	3.8750
	A	8		4.8750
	Sig.		.832	.075
Scheffé[a]	C	8	3.6250	
	B	8	3.8750	3.8750
	A	8		4.8750
	Sig.		.846	.091

Means for groups in homogeneous subsets are displayed.

[a] Uses Harmonic Mean Sample Size = 8.000.

Exhibit 7–6 Excel Output for One-Way ANOVA for More Than Two Groups

ANOVA: Single Factor
SUMMARY

Groups	Count	Sum	Average	Variance
A	8	39	4.875	0.696
B	8	31	3.875	0.696
C	8	29	3.625	0.839

ANOVA

Source of Variation	SS	df	MS	F	P value	F crit
Between Groups	7	2	3.5	4.704	0.021	3.467
Within Groups	15.625	21	0.744			
Total	22.625	23				

expensive and time consuming to implement and administer. On the other hand, with small sample sizes, the results may be so imprecise as to be rendered useless.

Power analysis can help us select an appropriate sample size. The power of a statistical test is the ability of the test to reject the null hypothesis given that the null is false. This is represented as

$$\beta = \Pr (\text{rejecting } H_0 | H_0 \text{ is false}) = 1 - \beta$$

In other words, statistical power $(1 - \beta)$ is the probability of obtaining a statistically significant difference when one actually exists. The power of a statistical test is the complement of a type II error.

Calculating statistical power for every possible test is beyond the scope of this text. However, we will review one example in which we calculate sample size controlling for type I error only and a second example in which we control for both type I and type II error.

In most research, a beta error of 20% is set. This is equal to a z_β of 0.84. In most cases where $\alpha = .05$, for a two-tailed test, z_α is 1.96. In our example, we want to use a t test for two independent samples to determine if the mean difference between the LOSs for two special care units, MICU and SICU (Table 7–1), is at least 2 days. The standard deviation for the two groups together, as indicated in Exhibit 7–1, is 5.34. The sample size required, controlling for alpha error only, is

$$N = (z_\alpha)^2 \times 2 \times (s)^2 / \bar{d}^2$$
$$= (1.96)^2 \times 2 \times (5.34)^2 / (2)^2$$
$$= 3.8416 \times 2 \times 28.5156 / 4$$
$$= 219.09 / 4$$
$$= 54.77, \text{ or } 55 \text{ cases}$$

The result, 55 cases, is the sample size required for one sample; however, since we want to compare the ALOS for two samples, we multiply 55 times 2, which equals 110 cases. Or we could state that 55 cases are required in each sample, when we are interested in determining if the difference is at least two days and controlling for alpha error only. When we want to control for both alpha and beta error together, the formula becomes

$$N = (z_\alpha)^2 \times 2 \times (s)^2 / \overline{d}^2$$
$$= (1.96 + .84)^2 \times 2 \times (5.34)^2 / (2)^2$$
$$= (7.84 \times 2 \times 28.5156) / 4$$
$$= 447.125 / 4$$
$$= 111.78, \text{ or } 112 \text{ cases}$$

Notice that when we control for both alpha and beta error together, the size of one sample doubles. This illustrates how larger sample sizes help us control for beta error. If we wanted to detect for even smaller differences between LOSs, such as one day, an even larger sample size would be required. We can readily see this by examining the mean difference expected in the formula above: the denominator would be changed from 4 (2^2) to 1 (1^2). If we are interested in detecting a difference of only one day, 447 cases would be required in each sample (447.125/1).

For other types of statistical problems, the statistical Web site of the University of California at Los Angeles has an on-line calculator for determining the power of a statistical test (www.stat.ucla.edu).

CONCLUSION

When we are interested in comparing means of two or more samples, we use ANOVA procedures. ANOVA also requires that the samples be randomly drawn, normally distributed, and independent of each other. When more than two samples are involved, and statistical significance is found, so that the null hypothesis is rejected, we must conduct post hoc procedures to determine which sample means differ. The Tukey HSD and the Scheffé test were conducted to determine which of the three means differed from one another.

Last, we discussed the concept of statistical power. Statistical power helps us control for beta error in conducting our research. One way to control for beta error is to select large samples. Another is to use various formulas to determine the sample size appropriate for the type of statistical test that we use. If we wish to detect small differences between the means of the population under study, larger sample sizes will be required; if we wish to detect difference between sample means that may be somewhat larger, we can generally get by with a smaller sample size. If the sample size is excessively large, we run the risk of detecting a difference smaller than what is important, thereby not only wasting time and resources but making interpretation of the results more problematic.

ADDITIONAL RESOURCES

Besag, F.P., and P.L. Besag. 1985. *Statistics for the helping professions*. Beverly Hills, CA: Sage Publications.

Clark, J.J., and M. Clark. 1983. *A statistics primer for managers*. New York: Free Press.

Duncan, R.C., et al. 1983. *Introductory biostatistics for the health sciences*. Albany, NY: Delmar Publishers.

Hall, H.I. 1998. The *z* test. *Quality Resource* 16, no. 5: 7.

Jekel, J.F., et al. 1996. *Biostatistics, epidemiology, and preventive medicine*. Philadelphia: W.B. Saunders.

Katz, D.L. 1997. *Biostatistics, epidemiology, and preventive medicine review*. Philadelphia: W.B. Saunders.

Kennedy, J.J. 1978. *An introduction to the design and analysis of experiments in education and psychology*. Lanham, MD: University Press of America.

Stockburger, D.W. 1998. Introductory statistics: Concepts, models and applications. ANOVA. www.psychstat. umsu.edu/introbook

Appendix 7–A

Exercises for Solving Problems

KNOWLEDGE QUESTIONS

1. Define the key terms listed at the beginning of this chapter.

2. Explain each component of the ANOVA model. How is the F ratio obtained?

3. To conduct the ANOVA procedure, the dependent variable must fall upon which scale of measurement? The grouping variable or independent variable falls upon which scale of measurement?

4. When conducting ANOVA to compare the means of three groups, under what conditions would we reject the null hypothesis? What conclusion would be drawn?

5. What is the purpose of conducting post hoc procedures?

MULTIPLE CHOICE

1. The CEO of Critical Care Hospital wants to compare average charges for congestive heart failure patients with those of two other acute care facilities in the community. Which of the following statistical tests would be most appropriate for answering the question?
   a. one-sample t test
   b. t test for two independent samples
   c. one-way ANOVA
   d. any of the above

For questions 2 through 4, refer to the following:

You are using ANOVA to compare the average age of patients discharged from two DRGs. In DRG XXX, there are 16 patients with an average age of 45. In DRG YYY, there are 20 patients with an average age of 50.

2. In the ANOVA table, the number of degrees of freedom for the SSB is:
   a. 3
   b. 2
   c. 1
   d. none of the above

3. The number of degrees of freedom for the SSW is:
   a. 34
   b. 35
   c. 36
   d. none of the above

4. The number of degrees of freedom for the SST is:
   a. 34
   b. 35
   c. 36
   d. none of the above

5. The ANOVA procedure may be used:
   a. with large sample sizes
   b. with small sample sizes
   c. when comparing the means of four groups
   d. all of the above

6. In the ANOVA procedure, we reject the null hypothesis when the calculated value of F is:
   a. zero
   b. greater than the critical value of F
   c. less than or equal to the critical value of F
   d. equal to the critical value of F
   e. b and d
   f. all of the above

7. If we fail to reject the null in the ANOVA procedure:
   a. the treatment had no effect on the subgroups under study
   b. the observed differences between the group means are statistically significant
   c. the observed differences between the group means are not statistically significant
   d. a and c
   e. all of the above

8. In the ANOVA procedure, the variations of the observation around their respective group means is an indication of:
   a. within-group variation
   b. between-group variation
   c. variation among the combined groups
   d. all of the above

9. We have conducted an ANOVA procedure in which we compared three population means. The calculated F equals 4.704, and the critical value of F is 3.467. Under this circumstance, we would:
   a. reject the null hypothesis
   b. conduct post hoc procedures
   c. fail to reject the null hypothesis
   d. a and b

10. You want to use the ANOVA procedure to compare the average length of stay of the patients of two physicians. The ANOVA procedure has the most power when:
    a. the two sample sizes are equal
    b. one sample is twice the size of the second sample
    c. one sample is three times the size of the second sample
    d. sample size has no effect on power

PROBLEMS

1. You have been analyzing hospital discharges from DRG 15, Transient Ischemic Attack and Precerebral Occlusions. You want to know if there is a difference in the average age of men and women discharged from DRG 15. The frequency distribution for discharges by sex appears in Table 7–A–1. You have decided to use the ANOVA procedure to calculate your results.
   a. State the null and alternative hypotheses and the alpha level that you will use.
   b. What is the mean age for men? What is the mean age for women?
   c. What is the calculated value of F? Is it statistically significant?
   d. What is your conclusion?

2. You also want to know if there is a difference in the average length of stay (ALOS) by sex for patients discharged from DRG 15. The frequency distribution for ALOS by sex appears in Table 7–A–2. You have decided to use the ANOVA procedure to calculate your results.
   a. State the null and alternative hypotheses and the alpha level that you will use.
   b. What is the ALOS for men? What is the ALOS for women?
   c. What is the calculated value of F? Is it statistically significant?
   d. What is your conclusion?

Table 7–A–1 Frequency Distribution of Age at Discharge by Sex, DRG 15, in 1997 at Critical Care Hospital (SPSS Output)

AGE * SEX Crosstabulation

Count

AGE		Male	Female	Total
AGE	42.00		1	1
	52.00	1		1
	61.00	2	2	4
	62.00	3	1	4
	65.00	2		2
	67.00	2		2
	68.00	2	1	3
	69.00		2	2
	70.00	3	1	4
	72.00	2		2
	73.00	1	2	3
	74.00	1	2	3
	75.00		1	1
	76.00	1	2	3
	77.00	3	1	4
	78.00	1	2	3
	79.00	1	1	2
	80.00		3	3
	81.00	1	2	3
	82.00		2	2
	84.00	2		2
	85.00		3	3
	86.00	1	1	2
	87.00		1	1
	88.00	2	3	5
	90.00		1	1
	93.00		1	1
	94.00		1	1
Total		31	37	68

Table 7–A–2 Frequency Distribution of ALOS at Discharge by Sex, DRG 15, in 1997 at Critical Care Hospital (SPSS Output)

LOS * SEX Crosstabulation

Count

LOS		Male	Female	Total
LOS	1.00	10	8	18
	2.00	10	15	25
	3.00	5	7	12
	4.00	4	4	8
	5.00		2	2
	8.00		1	1
	9.00	1		1
	12.00	1		1
Total		31	37	68

3. You also want to know if there is a difference in the average age of patients by race for discharges from DRG 15. The frequency distribution for age by race appears in Table 7–A–3. You have decided to use the ANOVA procedure to calculate your results.

   a. State the null and alternative hypotheses and the alpha level that you will use.
   b. What is the average age for whites? What is the average age for nonwhites?
   c. What is the calculated value of F? Is it statistically significant?
   d. What is your conclusion? What factors might explain the difference in average age by race?

Table 7–A–3 Frequency Distribution for Age by Race, DRG 15 (SPSS Output)

AGE * RACE Crosstabulation

Count

		RACE		
		White	Nonwhite	Total
AGE	42.00		1	1
	52.00	1		1
	61.00	3	1	4
	62.00	3	1	4
	65.00	1	1	2
	67.00	1	1	2
	68.00	3		3
	69.00	1	1	2
	70.00	2	2	4
	72.00	2		2
	73.00	2	1	3
	74.00		3	3
	75.00	1		1
	76.00	3		3
	77.00	4		4
	78.00	2	1	3
	79.00	2		2
	80.00	2	1	3
	81.00	2	1	3
	82.00	2		2
	84.00		2	2
	85.00	3		3
	86.00	2		2
	87.00	1		1
	88.00	5		5
	90.00	1		1
	93.00	1		1
	94.00	1		1
Total		51	17	68

CHAPTER 8

Correlation and Linear Regression

LEARNING OBJECTIVES

Upon completion of this chapter, you should be able to:

1. Define key terms.
2. Define the Pearson r product moment correlation coefficient.
3. Construct scatter diagrams for variables X and Y.
4. Construct scatter diagrams using microcomputer statistical software.
5. Interpret the Pearson r.
6. Compare the Pearson r with the coefficient of determination.
7. Explain "line of best fit" in linear regression.
8. Explain "slope" and "intercept" in the regression model.
9. Construct linear regression models using microcomputer statistical software.
10. Conduct hypothesis testing for the Pearson r and linear regression.
11. Interpret regression models for given situations.
12. Differentiate between simple regression and multiple regression.
13. Explain multicollinearity.

Often we are interested in determining relationships between variables such as age and length of stay (LOS), age and survival time, or type of diet and cholesterol levels. To determine the extent to which two variables are related, we can calculate a correlation coefficient.

There are many types of correlation coefficients, but we will limit our discussion to the Pearson r, or, more formally, the **Pearson r correlation coefficient**. The Pearson r is a measure of the linear relationship between two variables; it is used when both variables under study fall on the interval or ratio scale of measurement. There are other measures of association for variables that are either nominal or ordinal; these will be discussed in Chapters 9 and 10.

CHARACTERISTICS OF PEARSON r

To calculate the Pearson r, measures must be taken on two variables, X and Y—for example, height (X) and weight (Y). These measures are taken in pairs for each member of a sample randomly drawn from a population. The values of the calculated Pearson r range from -1.00 to $+1.00$. A correlation coefficient of -1.00 indicates that the two variables have a perfect negative relationship; a correlation coefficient of $+1.00$ indicates that the two variables have a perfect positive relationship; and a correlation coefficient of 0.0 indicates that there is no relationship between the two variables.

A positive relationship between the two variables means that as the measures on one variable increase, so do the measures on the second variable and, conversely, that as the measures on one variable decrease, so do the measures on the second variable. In other words, the measures on each variable move in the same direction. Thus, we can say that there is a direct relationship between the two variables.

A negative relationship means that the observations for the two variables are moving in opposite directions. As measures tend to increase on one variable, they tend to decrease on the second variable. In this situation, we say that there is an inverse relationship between the two variables.

The underlying assumption for the Pearson r is that the relationship between the two variables is linear. Since relationships between variables are not always linear, one should construct a scatter diagram or scatter plot to assess the type of relationship that exists between the two variables. We can construct a **scatter diagram** by plotting one variable, X, on the abscissa (horizontal axis) of a graph and plotting the second variable, Y, on the ordinate (vertical axis). If the points appear to approximate a straight line, then the two variables are linearly related, and it is appropriate to use the Pearson r. Scatter diagrams displaying positive and negative linear relationships appear in Figure 8–1; a scatter diagram indicating no relationship is also displayed.

Figure 8–1 Scatter Diagrams of Linear Relationships

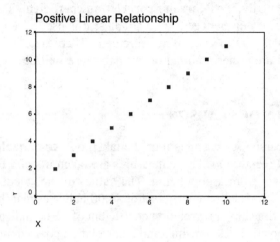

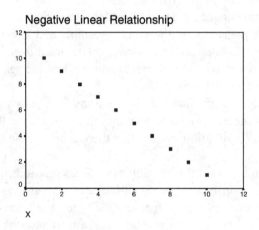

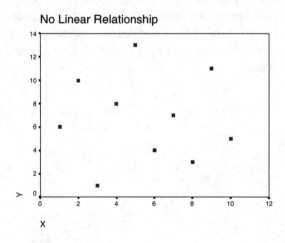

To further illustrate, let's consider a health information management (HIM) example in which we are interested in determining if there is a relationship between age (*X*) and total charges for DRG 336, Transurethral Prostatectomy with CC. The scatter diagram of age (*X*) and total charges (*Y*) appears in Figure 8–2.

Figure 8–2 Scatter Diagram, Age and Total Charges (TOTCHG) for DRG 336

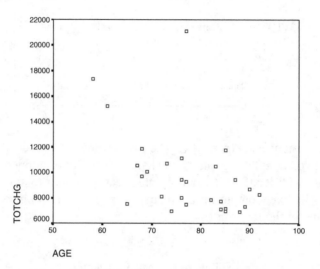

Examination of the scatter diagram indicates that the relationship between the two variables is negative. Imagine a line drawn through the plots from the upper left corner down to the lower right. The diagram indicates that as age increases, total charges decrease. Therefore, the relationship between the two variables is considered negative. The means and standard deviations for age and charges for DRG 336 appear in Exhibit 8–1. The SPSS output for the Pearson *r* verifies that the relationship is negative (Exhibit 8–2). The Pearson *r* is −.471,

Exhibit 8–1 Means and Standard Deviations, Age and Total Charges (TOTCHG), DRG 336 (SPSS Output)

		AGE	TOTCHG
N	Valid	28	28
	Missing	0	0
Mean		77.4286	9803.7500
Median		77.0000	9003.5000
Mode		76.00[a]	6899.00[a]
Std. Deviation		9.1183	3326.6847
Minimum		58.00	6899.00
Maximum		92.00	21093.00

[a] Multiple modes exist. The smallest value is shown.

Exhibit 8–2 SPSS Output for Pearson r, Age and Total Charges (TOTCHG), DRG 336

		AGE	TOTCHG
AGE	Pearson Correlation	1.000	–.471*
	Sig. (2-tailed)		.011
	N	28	28
TOTCHG	Pearson Correlation	–.471*	1.000
	Sig. (2-tailed)	.011	
	N	28	28

*Correlation is significant at the 0.05 level (2-tailed).

which is statistically significant ($p = .011$). The results indicate a moderate negative correlation between our two variables, age and total charges. The SPSS output displays the Pearson r for each variable with itself—for example, the Pearson r for "total charges" with "total charges" is 1.00. The Excel output for the Pearson r appears in Exhibit 8–3. Excel does not provide the p value for the Pearson r.

Exhibit 8–3 Excel Output for Pearson r, Age and Total Charges (TOTCHG), DRG 336

	AGE	TOTCHG
AGE	1	
TOTCHG	–0.47111	1

This relationship seems somewhat paradoxical. Why do total charges tend to decrease with age? Most would expect the opposite to occur. We will consider this situation again later in the chapter.

✓ **To Obtain a Simple Scatter Diagram Using SPSS:**

- From the menus, choose:
  →Graphs
  →Scatter
- Select the icon for "Simple."
- Select "Define."
- Select a variable for the x axis and a variable for the y axis.
  These variables must be numeric but should not be in date format.

CALCULATION OF THE PEARSON *r*

The Pearson *r* is a sample of the true population correlation value, which is denoted by the Greek symbol ρ, and is subject to sampling variation. When calculating the Pearson *r*, we are interested in testing the null hypothesis that ρ = 0; that is, the true population correlation is zero. A value of ρ = 0 indicates that there is no linear relationship between the two variables of interest. A significant *r* indicates that there is a relationship between the two variables of interest. Just as with the *t* and *F* tests, the obtained value of *r* is compared to a critical value of *r* to determine its statistical significance. For the Pearson *r*, we may conduct either a directional or nondirectional test.

The null and alternative hypotheses are

$$H_0: \rho = 0$$
$$H_A: r \neq 0 \text{ (two-tailed alternative)}$$
$$H_A: \rho < 0 \text{ or } \rho > 0 \text{ (one-tailed alternative)}$$

The formula for calculating the Pearson *r* is

$$r = \frac{\sum xy}{\sqrt{\sum x^2 \sum y^2}}$$

Let us now follow the procedure for calculating the Pearson *r* for the two variables, LOS and total charges for DRG 087, Pulmonary Edema and Respiratory Failure. It should be obvious that the longer one stays in the hospital, the greater the charges, so one would expect a positive correlation to result.

We will first construct a scatter diagram to assess the relationship between the two variables. We want to determine whether our assumption of linearity is tenable. The scatter diagram appears in Figure 8–3.

Figure 8–3 Scatter Diagram, Length of Stay (LOS) and Total Charges, DRG 087

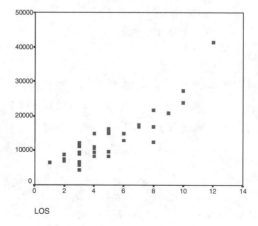

Examination of the scatter diagram indicates a linear relationship between LOS and total charges. As the LOS increases, so do total charges. We would expect the resultant Pearson r to be positive.

The null and alternative hypotheses are

$$H_0: \rho = 0$$
$$H_A: \rho > 0$$
$$\alpha = .05$$

The null hypothesis states that there is no relationship between LOS and total charges. The alternative hypothesis states that there is a positive relationship between LOS and total charges, so we will be conducting a one-tailed test.

We are using a one-tailed test because we expect that the relationship between the two variables will be positive—that is, LOS and total charges will move in the same direction. All cases discharged from DRG 087 are presented in Table 8–1. Microsoft Excel97 was used to prepare the data required for calculating the Pearson r. Before we can calculate the Pearson r, we must first calculate Σx^2, Σy^2, and Σxy^2 (from Table 8–1):

$$\Sigma x^2 = \Sigma X^2 - \left[\Sigma (X)^2 / n \right]$$
$$= 1,125 - [(173)^2 / 34]$$
$$= 1,125 - (29,929 / 34)$$
$$= 1,125 - 880.26$$
$$= 244.74$$

$$\Sigma y^2 = \Sigma Y^2 - \left[\Sigma (Y)^2 / n \right]$$
$$= 7,915,583,426 - [(457,442)^2 / 34]$$
$$= 7,915,583,426 - (209,253,183,364 / 34)$$
$$= 7,915,583,426 - 6,154,505,393.06$$
$$= 1,761,078,032.94$$

$$\Sigma xy^2 = \Sigma XY - \left[\Sigma (X)(Y) / n \right]$$
$$= 2,905,363 - [(173)(457,442) / 34]$$
$$= 2,905,363 - (79,137,466 / 34)$$
$$= 2,905,363 - 2,327,572.53$$
$$= 577,790.47$$

$$r = \frac{\sum xy}{\sqrt{\sum x^2 \sum y^2}}$$

$$= 577,790.47 / \sqrt{(9,244.74)(1,761,078,032.94)}$$

$$= 577,790.47 / \sqrt{431,006,237,781.74}$$

$$= 577,790.47 / 656,510.65$$

$$= .88$$

Table 8–1 Total Charges and Length of Stay (LOS) for Patients Discharged from DRG 087

Patient	LOS X	Total Charges Y	LOS² X²	Total Charges² Y²	LOS × Charges XY
1	3	4,304	9	18,524,416	12,912
2	3	5,867	9	34,421,689	17,601
3	1	6,507	1	42,341,049	6,507
4	3	6,702	9	44,916,804	20,106
5	2	6,971	4	48,594,841	13,942
6	2	7,405	4	54,834,025	14,810
7	4	8,222	16	67,601,284	32,888
8	5	8,285	25	68,641,225	41,425
9	2	8,771	4	76,930,441	17,542
10	3	8,944	9	79,995,136	26,832
11	4	9,389	16	88,153,321	37,556
12	3	9,494	9	90,136,036	28,482
13	5	9,660	25	93,315,600	48,300
14	4	10,566	16	111,640,356	42,264
15	4	10,920	16	119,246,400	43,680
16	3	11,061	9	122,345,721	33,183
17	3	11,133	9	123,943,689	33,399
18	3	11,290	9	127,464,100	33,870
19	3	12,143	9	147,452,449	36,429
20	8	12,462	64	155,301,444	99,696
21	6	12,893	36	166,229,449	77,358
22	6	14,840	36	220,225,600	89,040
23	4	14,917	16	222,516,889	59,668
24	5	15,106	25	228,191,236	75,530
25	5	16,289	25	265,331,521	81,445
26	8	16,892	64	285,339,664	135,136
27	7	16,925	49	286,455,625	118,475
28	8	16,955	64	287,472,025	135,640
29	7	17,375	49	301,890,625	121,625
30	9	20,830	81	433,888,900	187,470
31	8	21,754	64	473,236,516	174,032
32	10	23,915	100	571,927,225	239,150
33	10	27,245	100	742,290,025	272,450
34	12	41,410	144	1,714,788,100	496,920
Total	173	457,442	1,125	7,915,583,426	2,905,363

The calculated Pearson r is +0.88, indicating a strong positive relationship. Referring to Table B–5 in Appendix B, we find that the critical value for r for 32 degrees of freedom, $\alpha =$ .05 (df $= n - 2$, where $n =$ number of pairs), and for a one-tailed test is .287. Since our calculated value for r exceeds the critical value, we reject the null hypothesis and conclude that the relationship between LOS and total charges is statistically significant. The SPSS descriptive statistics and results of Pearson r appear in Exhibit 8–4. The SPSS calculated Pearson r matches the results we obtained by using the hand-held calculator. The Excel output for the Pearson r appears in Exhibit 8–5.

Exhibit 8–4 SPSS Output for Pearson r, DRG 087, Total Charges (TOTCHG) and Length of Stay (LOS)

Descriptive Statistics

	TOTCHG	LOS
Mean	13454.18	5.0882
Std. Deviation	7305.2037	2.7233
N	34	34

Correlations

		TOTCHG	LOS
TOTCHG	Pearson Correlation	1.000	.880*
	Sig. (1-tailed)	.	.000
	N	34	34
LOS	Pearson Correlation	.880*	1.000
	Sig. (1-tailed)	.000	.
	N	34	34

*Correlation is significant at the 0.01 level (1-tailed).

Exhibit 8–5 Excel Output for Pearson r, DRG 087, Total Charges and Length of Stay

	Length of Stay	Total Charges
Length of Stay	1	
Total Charges	0.880	1

✓ **To Obtain Pearson r Using SPSS:**

- From the menus choose:
  Analyze
      →Correlate
          →Bivariate
- Select two or more numeric variables.

It is important to remember that two variables' correlation with one another does not necessarily imply causality. We cannot assume that X causes Y or vice versa. In this example, we cannot state that long LOSs cause high charges. We can only state that there is a strong relationship between the two variables. The two variables have a high correlation because they vary together in some systematic way.

In the previous example, where we were considering the relationship between age and total charges, it would not be logical to conclude that old age causes lower charges. Intuitively, this does not make sense. There must be some other variable at work that results in lower charges for older people.

Just as sample size plays a role in statistical significance when determining the difference between population means, it is also true when calculating the Pearson r. Small values of r may be statistically significant when there are many observations, while large values of r may not be statistically significant when there are a few observations.

From the Pearson r, we can calculate the **coefficient of determination r^2**. The r^2 tells us how much of the variation in Y is accounted for by the X variable. In our LOS (X) and total charges (Y) example, $r^2 = .774$ ($.88^2$). So we conclude that 77.4% of the variation in total charges for DRG 087 is explained by the patient's LOS.

The r^2 is a better measure of assessing the strength of a relationship between the two variables, X and Y, than r. The Pearson r alone can be used to make it seem as if the relationship between the two variables is much greater than it actually is. For example, a Pearson r equal to .50 appears to indicate a fairly strong relationship between two variables, when in fact only 25% ($.50^2$) of the variance is accounted for by the two variables together. We will meet the coefficient of determination again in our discussion of linear regression.

INTRODUCTION TO LINEAR REGRESSION

In the previous section, we learned that two variables may have a linear relationship as designated by the Pearson product moment correlation coefficient. We also learned that correlation does not imply causality. Just because two variables, X and Y, have a high correlation with each other, we cannot assume that X causes Y or vice versa. For example, we would not state that height causes weight.

But we can use this information in other ways. If the relationship between two variables is sufficiently large, we can predict the value of one variable from another. The objective of linear regression is to estimate the value of one variable that corresponds to the value of the other variable. In linear regression, we are trying to construct a mathematical model that explains the relationship between two variables.

Linear regression requires a pair of observations (X and Y) for each subject. The Y variable is usually designated as the dependent variable (DV), and the X variable is designated as the independent variable (IV). Our goal, then, is to predict Y from a given value of X. In our LOS (X) and total charges (Y) correlation problem discussed previously, the Pearson r is equal to .88, and the coefficient of determination, r^2, is equal to .774, indicating that 77.4% of the variation in total charges is explained by the variable LOS. Thus, there is a strong relationship between the two variables, and it is appropriate to develop a regression model that predicts total charges from LOS.

Just as with the Pearson r, in linear regression, a major assumption is that the two variables under consideration are linearly related. That is, a straight line can be used to describe the relationship between the two variables. A scatter diagram should be constructed to assess the relationship between the two variables. If the relationship appears to be linear, it can be described by a straight line. From your high school algebra, you may recall that the general form for a straight line is

$$Y = a + bX$$

where b is the slope of the line and a is the point where the line intercepts the y axis. The slope represents the average change in Y that is associated with a change in X. The steeper the slope, the greater the change in Y that is associated with a change in X, and the stronger the relationship between the two variables of interest. The point at which a intercepts or crosses the Y axis is an estimate of the average value of Y when X is equal to zero.

For any two points, it is easy to determine the equation for the straight line. However, if there are three or more points, it is not possible to find a straight line that goes through all points simultaneously unless the correlation is a perfect ±1.0. Thus, in linear regression we find the line that "best fits" all the points. The **line of best fit** is called the **regression line**.

The equation for the straight line indicates that for each observation of X, only one Y value is possible. This indicates that the measurement is precise—that is, without error. However, in reality, most relationship studies are inexact. And as you may recall from Chapter 3, error is integral to the measurement process. So the regression equation is more realistically expressed as

$$Y = a + bX + e$$

where e represents error. The error term acknowledges that the prediction equation does not perfectly predict Y. Thus, for a given X, there may be more than one Y. So the slope (b) indicates the average change in Y associated with X.

To illustrate these principles, consider the following data set for X and Y:

X	Y
0	5
1	7
2	9
3	11
4	13
5	15

In this data set, for each value of X, there is only one value for Y. The relationship between the two variables is perfect, as shown in the scatter diagram in Figure 8–4. The regression line perfectly fits the X, Y data points. And the corresponding regression equation is $Y = 5 + 2X$. Note that the regression line crosses the y axis at 5—the average value of Y when X is equal to zero.

Figure 8–4 Scatter Diagram, X and Y

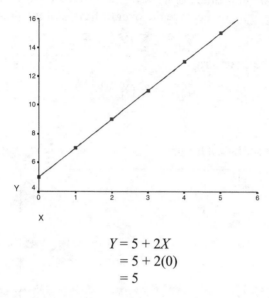

$$Y = 5 + 2X$$
$$= 5 + 2(0)$$
$$= 5$$

However, such perfection is rarely encountered in health care data analysis. Most often, we find the line that "best fits" all the points in the regression problems. The line of best fit is called the regression line. As an example, consider the following data set in the following table:

X	Y	X	Y
0	4	3	10
0	5	3	11
0	6	3	12
1	6	4	12
1	7	4	13
1	8	4	14
2	8	5	14
2	9	5	15
2	10	5	16

In examining the data set, you can see that a given X variable does not take on the same value for Y each time. Therefore, the regression line will not perfectly fit all of the (X, Y) data points. The regression line that appears in the scatter diagram in Figure 8–5 is the line that best fits all of the data points. The distance between the data points and the regression line represents the error term in the regression equation. The distances of the observations from the line of best fit are represented as

$$d_i = Y_i - \hat{Y}$$

where $\hat{Y}$ (pronounced "y-hat") is the predicted value of Y from X. Since the distance from the regression line may be either positive or negative, we compute the sum of the squared deviations from the regression line to measure the overall fitness of the line:

$$\sum d_i^2 = \sum (Y_i - \hat{Y})^2$$

or, when expressed as the error term,

$$\text{SSE} = \sum (Y_i - \hat{Y})^2$$

Figure 8–5 Scatter Diagram and Line of Best Fit

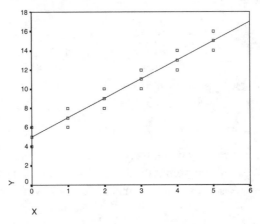

Error is the difference between the observed value of Y and the predicted value of $Y(\hat{Y})$. It is the amount of variation that cannot be accounted for in the regression model. The predicted value of $Y(\hat{Y})$ is the mean of the population of possible Y's for a given X. In Figure 8–5, you can see that the regression line falls through the means of the observed values of Y for a given X. Exhibit 8–6 shows the descriptive statistics and correlations for X and Y.

Exhibit 8–6 Pearson r Correlation Coefficients for X and Y (SPSS Output)

Descriptive Statistics				Correlations		
	X	Y			X	Y
			X	Pearson Correlation	1.000	.973*
Mean	2.50000	10.0000		Sig. (2-tailed)	.	.000
Std. Deviation	1.7573	3.6137		N	18	18
N	18	18	Y	Pearson Correlation	.973*	1.000
				Sig. (2-tailed)	.000	.
				N	18	18

*Correlation is significant at the 0.01 level (2-tailed).

For some cases, we can set up the regression equation to predict either Y from X or X from Y. In other cases, it makes more sense to designate one variable as the independent variable (X) and the other variable as the dependent variable (Y). By convention, the DV is plotted on the y axis and the IV on the x axis. The equation for the sample regression line is written as

$$\hat{Y} = \hat{\beta}_0 + \hat{\beta}_1 X$$

where $\hat{Y}$ is the estimated value of Y given by the population regression line, $\hat{\beta}_0$ (pronounced "beta naught") is a constant that indicates where the regression line "intercepts" the y axis and that estimates the average value of Y when $X = 0$, and $\hat{\beta}_1$ (pronounced "beta sub one") is the slope estimate that indicates the average change in Y associated with a change in X. Both $\hat{\beta}_0$ and $\hat{\beta}_1$ are referred to as the population regression coefficients and may vary from sample to sample.

The **slope** of the regression line ($\hat{\beta}_1$) indicates how steeply the regression line rises or falls. If the slope has an upward slant, the slope is positive and indicates that the correlation between X and Y is positive. If the slope has a downward slant, the slope is negative and indicates that the correlation between X and Y is negative (Figure 8–1).

To develop the regression equation, we need to find the values for the regression coefficients, $\hat{\beta}_0$ and $\hat{\beta}_1$. As stated earlier, we can either regress Y from X or X from Y. To solve for $\hat{\beta}_0$ and $\hat{\beta}_1$ when Y is regressed from X, we have:

$$\beta_{1yx} = \sum xy \, / \sum x^2$$

and

$$\beta_{0yx} = \overline{Y} - \beta_1 \overline{X}$$

and to regress X from Y, we have

$$\beta_{1xy} = \sum xy \, / \sum y^2$$

and

$$\beta_{0xy} = \overline{X} - \beta_1 \overline{Y}$$

To illustrate, we will use some hypothetical height and weight data of nine patients. These data appear in Table 8–2. The scatter diagram and the descriptive statistics and correlations for height and weight appear in Figure 8–6 and Exhibit 8–7 respectively. The scatter diagram indicates a positive linear relationship.

Table 8–2 Height and Weight Measurements for Nine Patients

Patient	Height (X) (in inches)	Weight (Y)	X^2	Y^2	XY
1	60	135	3,600	18,225	8,100
2	60	120	3,600	14,400	7,200
3	62	140	3,844	19,600	8,680
4	62	130	3,844	16,900	8,060
5	62	135	3,844	18,225	8,370
6	64	145	4,096	21,025	9,280
7	66	150	4,356	22,500	9,900
8	68	150	4,624	22,500	10,200
9	68	160	4,624	25,600	10,880
	572	1,265	$\sum X^2 = 36,432$	$\sum Y^2 = 178,975$	$\sum XY = 80,670$
	$\overline{X} = 63.6$	$\overline{Y} = 140.6$	$\sum x^2 = 78.2$	$\sum y^2 = 1172.2$	$\sum xy = 272.2$
	$s_x = 3.13$	$s_y = 12.10$			

Figure 8–6 Scatter Diagram, Height and Weight

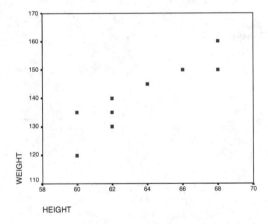

Exhibit 8–7 Descriptive Statistics and Correlation for Height and Weight (SPSS Output)

Descriptive Statistics

	Height	Weight
Mean	63.5556	140.5556
Std. Deviation	3.1269	12.1049
N	9	9

Correlations

		Height	Weight
HEIGHT	Pearson Correlation	1.000	.899*
	Sig. (2-tailed)	.	.001
	N	9	9
WEIGHT	Pearson Correlation	.899*	1.000
	Sig. (2-tailed)	.001	.
	N	9	9

*Correlation is significant at the 0.01 level (2-tailed).

Using the data in Table 8–2, we will regress Y (weight) from X (height):

$$\beta_{1yx} = \sum xy / \sum x^2$$
$$= 272.2 / 78.2$$
$$= 3.48$$

$$\beta_{0yx} = \bar{Y} - \beta_1 \bar{X}$$
$$= 140.6 - 3.48(63.6)$$
$$= 140.6 - 221.328$$
$$= -80.7$$

Thus, to predict weight from height, our regression equation is

$$\hat{Y} = -80.7 + 3.48X$$

Alternatively, we can also regress X from Y as follows:

$$\beta_{1xy} = \sum xy / \sum y^2$$
$$= 272.2 / 1,172.2$$
$$= .23$$

$$\beta_{0xy} = \bar{X} - \beta_1 \bar{Y}$$
$$= 63.6 - (.23)140.6$$
$$= 31.3$$

So, to predict height from weight, the regression equation is

$$\hat{X} = 31.3 + 23Y$$

We will now reproduce the scatter diagram that appears in Figure 8–6 with the addition of the regression line (Figure 8–7).

Figure 8–7 Scatter Diagram and Regression Line—Height and Weight

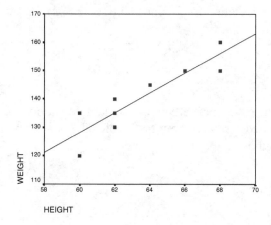

As we have already discussed, because regression deals with prediction, there is error. It is unlikely that the predicted value of Y will correspond exactly to the actual value of Y for a given value of X. Not all of the (X, Y) plots in Figure 8–7 fall on the regression line. For example, if a woman is $5'5''$ (65 inches), we do not expect that her weight will be exactly 145.5 pounds, as predicted by the regression equation

$$\hat{Y} = -80.7 + 3.48X$$
$$= -80.7 + 3.48(65)$$
$$= 145.5$$

The predicted value is an estimate of the average weight of individuals who are of that height. As you may recall, the average is the best estimate or the most typical value in a distribution. In this case, it is the best estimate of a person's weight. If the correlation between the two variables is low, there will be considerable variation of the actual values around the predicted values, and if the correlation is high, the actual values will cluster more closely around the predicted values. Only when the correlation is a perfect ± 1.0 (termed *unity*) will the actual value match the predicted values.

If there is a great deal of scatter in the observed values of Y around the regression line, the predicted values of Y based on the regression equation will not be very close to the observed values of Y. The standard error of the estimate is a measure of scatter or spread of the observed values of Y around the corresponding values estimated from the regression equation.

Just as we calculate the standard error of the mean, we can calculate the **standard error of the estimate**, designated s_{yx}. The standard error of the estimate measures the scatter of the observed values of Y around the predicted values of Y. To calculate the standard error of the estimate,

$$s_{yx} = \sqrt{\text{SSE} / n - 2}$$

where we have already seen that

$$\text{SSE} = \sum (Y_i - \hat{Y})^2$$

But since it is rather cumbersome to calculate the SSE using this formula, we will use the alternative (the standard deviation for Y appears in Table 8–2):

$$s_{yx} = s_y \sqrt{1 - r^2}$$
$$= 12.1\sqrt{1 - .808}$$
$$= 5.30$$

The standard error of the estimate is a type of standard deviation, the standard deviation of the distribution of obtained Y scores about the predicted Y score, and it is used to develop a confidence interval around $\hat{Y}$.

INTERPRETATION OF THE STANDARD ERROR OF THE ESTIMATE

Recall from our discussion of the normal curve and standard deviation in Chapter 5 that

68% of the scores fall within the limits $\overline{X} \pm 1s$
95% of the scores fall within the limits $\overline{X} \pm 1.96s$
99% of the scores fall within the limits $\overline{X} \pm 2.58s$

Since the standard error of the estimate is a kind of standard deviation, we can make a similar interpretation regarding $\hat{Y}$ in that the obtained scores (Y) are normally distributed around $\hat{Y}$. Thus:

68% of the obtained values of Y fall within the limits $\hat{Y} \pm s_{yx}$
95% of the obtained values of Y fall within the limits $\hat{Y} \pm 1.96s_{yx}$
99% of the obtained values of Y fall within the limits $\hat{Y} \pm 2.58s_{yx}$

For example, suppose we have 10 students and we ask each his or her height and predict his or her weight on the basis of the regression equation.

$$\hat{Y} = -80.7 + 3.48X$$

We then go back and determine the actual weight of each of these 10 students and compare their actual weight to their predicted weight. The difference between their actual weight (Y) and their predicted weight ($\hat{Y}$) is error and describes how scores vary around the regression line that follows a normal distribution. Using the standard error of the estimate, we can develop 95% confidence interval for $\hat{Y}$. For small sample sizes, the t distribution for the appropriate number of degrees of freedom is used to calculate the confidence interval rather than the normal distribution.

$$CI_{95} = \hat{Y} \pm t_{.05}(s_{yx})$$

For the predicted weight of 145.5, the standard error of estimate is 5.30. For seven degrees of freedom ($n - 2$), $\alpha = .05$, the critical t is 2.365. The 95% confidence interval is calculated:

$$CI_{95} = \hat{Y} \pm 2.365(s_{yx})$$
$$= 145.5 \pm 2.365(5.30)$$
$$= 145.5 \pm 12.53$$
$$[132.97, 158.03]$$

The interpretation is that for a height of 65 inches, 95% of the obtained weights will fall within a range of 132.97 to 158.03 pounds.

Caution must be exercised when predicting Y beyond the range of the actual observations upon which the data analysis is based. In our current problem where we are predicting weight from height, the relationship described by the straight line may hold for a height of 70 inches, which is not too far beyond the range of observations in our data set. But as we move to greater heights such as 75 inches or to lesser heights such as 36 inches, the same linear relationship may no longer continue.

Also, notice that in the regression equation for predicting weight from height, the constant is –80.7. A negative value indicates that the regression line **intercepts** the y axis at a point below zero. The literal interpretation would be that for certain heights, the predicted weight was less than zero. But we know that this is not possible. The constant is a fixed value that ensures that the predicted value "comes out right."

An example that illustrates both of these points is the case of a newborn whose length at birth is 20 inches. According to our regression equation, the predicted weight is –11.1 pounds.

$$\hat{Y} = -80.7 + 3.48X$$
$$= -80.7 + 3.48(20)$$
$$= -80.7 + 69.6$$
$$= -11.1$$

We know that this result is impossible. In this example, the newborn's length is considerably outside the range of observations upon which our regression equation was modeled, and the negative constant brings the predicted weight to less than zero. This demonstrates the importance of the researcher's judgment when using statistics. Empirical data together with the judgment of the researcher are required in the decision-making process.

HYPOTHESIS TESTING

Before using the regression model for actual predictions, we must conduct a statistical test to determine that the predicted slope does not equal zero. In regression, the hypothesis test is for the regression coefficient for the slope of the line ($\hat{\beta}_1$), which is indicative of the correlation between X and Y. The slope is defined as

$$\text{Slope} = \frac{\text{change in } X}{\text{change in } Y}$$

If the slope equals zero, Y will be a constant that does not change with changes in X. The null hypothesis is that the true slope of $\hat{\beta}_1$ of the population regression line is equal to zero:

$$H_0: \beta = 0$$
$$H_A: \beta \neq 0$$

The t distribution where df $= n - 2$ is used to test the null hypothesis, where

$$t = \hat{\beta}_1 / \left(s_{yx} / \sqrt{\sum x^2} \right)$$

For our example of height and weight, $\hat{\beta} = 3.48, \sum x^2 = 78.2$, and $s_{yx} = 5.30$. So,

$$t = 3.48 / (5.30 / \sqrt{78.2})$$
$$= 3.48 / .60$$
$$= 5.84$$

For $\alpha = .05$, the tabled t for 7 degrees of freedom is 2.365. Since the calculated t is greater than the critical t, we reject the null hypothesis of no linear relationship between X and Y.

To construct a 95% confidence interval around the regression coefficient, we have

$$CI_{95} = \hat{\beta}_1 \pm t_{.05}\left(s_{yx} / \sqrt{\sum x^2} \right)$$
$$= 3.48 \pm 2.365\,(530 \,/ \sqrt{78.2}\,)$$
$$= 3.48 \pm 2.365(.60)$$
$$= 3.48 \pm 1.42$$
$$= [2.06, \ 4.90]$$

Thus, we are 95% confident that the population regression coefficient (β) falls between 2.06 and 4.90.

COEFFICIENT OF DETERMINATION

We previously encountered the coefficient of determination (r^2) in our discussion of correlation. The r^2 indicates the explanatory power of our linear model. The range of r^2 is 0 to +1. The r^2 indicates the amount of variation in the dependent variable that is explained by the independent variable. When $r^2 = +1.0$, the independent variable accounts for 100% of the variation in the dependent variable, and all of the observations fall on the regression line. When r^2 equals zero, the IV accounts for no variation in Y and is not helpful in predicting Y. The closer the r^2 is to 1, the better the fit of the regression line to the data points. When r^2 is close to zero, the two variables are said to be independent of each other—that is, they do not vary together in any systematic way. A high value for r^2 is necessary if our predictions are to be accurate. We know that for the height and weight problem, $r = .899$ and $r^2 = .808$. Thus, 80.8% of the variation in weight is explained by an individual's height.

F TEST

SPSS provides an analysis of variance (ANOVA) model for the regression equation that indicates the significance of the regression model. The components of the model are

Total variation = regression + residual (Error)

The variation that can be explained by the regression model is represented in the "regression" component of the model, and the unexplained variance (error) is represented in the "residual" component of the model. Thus, the model may be expressed as:

Total variation = explained variation + unexplained variation

These terms are explained below:

Variation in the ANOVA Model

Source of Variation	Explanation
Total variation $\sum (Y - \bar{Y})^2$	The sum of the squares of the differences between the observed value of Y and the mean value of Y
Explained variation $\sum (Y_c - \bar{Y})^2$	The sum of the squares of the differences between the calculated value of Y and the mean value of Y
Unexplained variation $\sum (Y - \bar{Y}_c)^2$	The sum of the squares for the differences between observed value of Y and the calculated value of Y for a given X

We will now use SPSS to verify our hand calculations. With slight differences due to rounding, the SPSS output in Exhibit 8–8 matches our hand calculations—for example, our hand-calculated standard error of the estimate is 5.3, and that provided by SPSS is 5.67. This is because the SPSS-provided standard error was based on the adjusted r^2 of .781 rather than the r^2 of .808 used in our calculations. The ANOVA indicates that the regression mode is significant ($F = 29.492$, df $= 1, 7, p = .001$). We obtain the formula for the regression model from the coefficients table in Exhibit 8–8. The constant is –80.625, and the β_1 coefficient for the slope is 3.48; the calculated t for the slope is significant. Our hand-calculated t is slightly different from the t provided by SPSS because of the slight difference in the standard error. As before, our regression model is

$$\hat{Y} = -80.625 + 3.48X$$

Exhibit 8–8 SPSS Output for Regression Model, Height and Weight

Model Summary

Model	R	R Square	Adjusted R Square	Std. Error of the Estimate
1	.899[a]	.808	.781	5.6677

[a] Predictors: (Constant), HEIGHT

ANOVA[a]

Model		Sum of Squares	df	Mean Square	F	Sig.
1	Regression	947.364	1	947.364	29.492	.001[b]
	Residual	224.858	7	32.123		
	Total	1172.222	8			

[a] Dependent Variable: WEIGHT
[b] Predictors: (Constant), HEIGHT

Coefficients[a]

Model		Unstandardized Coefficients B	Std. Error	Standardized Coefficients Beta	t	Sig.
1	(Constant)	−80.625	40.772		−1.977	.089
	HEIGHT	3.480	.641	.899	5.431	.001

[a] Dependent Variable: WEIGHT

The Excel output for the regression model appears in Exhibit 8–9. The Excel output is similar to that for SPSS.

Exhibit 8–9 Excel Output for Regression Model, Height and Weight

SUMMARY OUTPUT

Regression Statistics

Multiple R	0.899
R Square	0.808
Adjusted R Square	0.781
Standard Error	5.668
Observations	9

ANOVA

	df	SS	MS	F	Significance F
Regression	1	947.364	947.364	29.492	0.001
Residual	7	224.858	32.123		
Total	8	1172.222			

	Coefficients	Standard Error	t Stat	P Value	Lower 95%	Upper 95%
Intercept	−80.625	40.772	−1.977	0.089	−177.035	15.785
Height	3.480	0.641	5.431	0.001	1.965	4.995

REGRESSION MODEL FOR LENGTH OF STAY AND TOTAL CHARGES

Now let's return to the problem of LOS and total charges for DRG 087. We will construct a scatter diagram that includes the regression line (Figure 8–8).

Figure 8–8 Scatter Diagram, Length of Stay (LOS) and Total Charges (TOTCHG), DRG 087

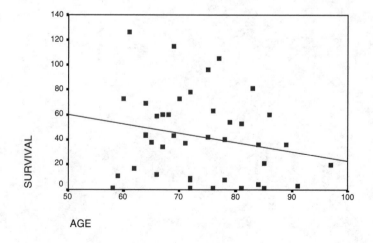

In this example, the means and standard deviations are provided for both LOS and total charges. The SPSS model summary displayed in Exhibit 8–10 indicates a fairly strong relationship between LOS and total charges that is statistically significant ($r = .880, p < .01$). In the model summary, the investigator can find r^2, the coefficient of determination, which in this example is .775, indicating that LOS accounts for approximately 77.5% of the variation

Exhibit 8–10 SPSS Output for Linear Regression, Length of Stay (LOS) and Total Charges (TOTCHG), DRG 087

Descriptive Statistics

	TOTCHG	LOS
Mean	13454.18	5.0882
Std. Deviation	7305.2037	2.7233
N	34	34

Model Summary

Model	R	R Square	Adjusted R Square	Std. Error of the Estimate
1	.880[a]	.775	.768	3522.1820

[a] Predictors: (Constant), LOS

ANOVA[a]

Model		Sum of Squares	df	Mean Square	F	Sig.
1	Regression	1.4E+09	1	1.4E+09	109.956	.000[b]
	Residual	4.0E+08	32	1.2E+07		
	Total	1.8E+09	33			

[a] Dependent Variable: TOTCHG
[b] Predictors: (Constant), LOS

Coefficients[a]

Model		Unstandardized Coefficients		Standardized Coefficients			95% Confidence Interval for B	
		B	Std. Error	Beta	t	Sig.	Lower Bound	Upper Bound
1	(Constant)	1441.467	1295.091		1.113	.274	−1196.547	4079.482
	LOS	2360.879	225.146	.880	10.486	.000	1902.273	2819.486

[a] Dependent Variable: TOTCHG

in total charges. The standard error of the estimate is 3,522.182. The Excel regression statistics for LOS and total charges for DRG 087 are displayed in Exhibit 8–11.

Exhibit 8–11 Excel Output for Linear Regression, Length of Stay (LOS) and Total Charges, DRG 087

SUMMARY OUTPUT

Regression Statistics

Multiple R	0.880
R Square	0.775
Adjusted R Square	0.768
Standard Error	3522.182
Observations	34

ANOVA

	df	SS	MS	F	Significance F
Regression	1	1364093516	1364093516	109.956	7.00993E-12
Residual	32	396984516.7	12405766.15		
Total	33	1761078033			

	Coefficients	Standard Error	t Stat	P-value	Lower 95%	Upper 95%
Intercept	1441.467	1295.091	1.113	0.274	–1196.544	4079.479
Length of Stay	2360.879	225.146	10.486	0.000	1902.273	2819.48

In the "Coefficients" section, we find the regression coefficients, LOS or $\hat{\beta}_1 = 2{,}360.879$, and the constant, $\hat{\beta}_0 = 1{,}441.467$. SPSS also provides the 95% confidence interval and standard error for both coefficients. The calculated t values for both coefficients are also provided, along with their precise level of statistical significance, indicating that β_1 (slope) is statistically significant. The ANOVA regression model indicates that the regression model is statistically significant ($F = 109.956$, df $= 1, 32, p < .01$). The regression model for predicting charges from LOS for DRG 087 is

$$\hat{Y} = 1{,}441.467 + 2{,}360.879\,X$$

We will now look at several applications for linear regression.

✓ To Obtain Linear Regression Using SPSS:

- From the menus choose:
  - →Analyze
    - →Regression
      - →Linear
- In the "Linear Regression" dialog box, select a numeric dependent variable.
- Select one or more numeric independent variables.

Example 1: Predicting Cancer Deaths from Age

As researchers for a statewide cancer registry, we have been asked to build a regression model for predicting colon cancer survival time based on the age of the patient at time of diagnosis. The raw data for cancer survival time appear in Table 8–3. In building the regression model, we have designated "Age at Diagnosis" as the independent variable (X), and "Survival Time in Months" as the dependent variable (Y).

Table 8–3 Age at Diagnosis and Survival Time in Months, for Cases of Colon Cancer, Your Hospital, 19AA

Age at Diagnosis	Survival Time in Months	Age at Diagnosis	Survival Time in Months
61	126	89	36
78	8	75	96
69	115	84	36
62	17	64	69
77	105	72	78
81	53	67	60
81	1	60	73
83	81	70	73
72	1	76	63
85	21	86	60
58	1	66	59
64	43	69	43
68	60	85	1
79	54	76	1
75	42	64	44
78	40	65	38
67	34	71	37
97	20	72	9
72	8	91	3
84	4	59	11
66	12		

Source: Data from *Self-Instructional Manual for Cancer Registries, Book 7: Statistics and Epidemiology for Cancer Registries*, p. 121, U.S. Department of Health and Human Services, Public Health Service, National Institutes of Health, National Cancer Institute.

The first step is to prepare a scatter diagram, which appears in Figure 8–9. The plots are widely scattered, indicating that the relationship between age at diagnosis and survival time may not be linear and that the correlation between the two variables may be small. The regression line, which is somewhat flat, indicates a negative relationship between age and survival time.

Figure 8–9 Scatter Diagram—Age at Diagnosis of Colon Cancer and Survival Time (in Months). *Source:* Data from *Self-Instructional Manual for Cancer Registries, Book 7: Statistics and Epidemiology for Cancer Registries*, p. 121, U.S. Department of Health and Human Services, Public Health Service, National Institutes of Health, National Cancer Institute.

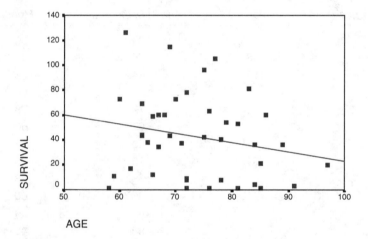

The null and alternative hypotheses are

$$H_0: \beta_1 = 0$$
$$H_1: \beta_1 \neq 0$$
$$\alpha = .05$$

Analysis of the SPSS output in Exhibit 8–12 does verify our suspicion that the relationship between the two variables is slight and that the relationship is negative and not statistically significant ($r = -.210$, $p = .187$). The r^2 indicates that the age variable accounts for only 4% of the variance in survival time. The regression model for predicting survival time from age at diagnosis is

$$Y = 97.063 - .743X$$

Exhibit 8–12 SPSS Output for Pearson r Correlation, Age at Diagnosis of Colon Cancer and Survival Time in Months

		Age	Survival Time in Months
Age	Pearson Correlation	1.000	−.210
	Sig. (2-tailed)	.	.187
	N	41	41
Survival Time in Months	Pearson Correlation	−.210	1.000
	Sig. (2-tailed)	.187	.
	N	41	41

Source: Data from *Self-Instructional Manual for Cancer Registries, Book 7: Statistics and Epidemiology for Cancer Registries*, p. 121, U.S. Department of Health and Human Services, Public Health Service, National Institutes of Health, National Cancer Institute.

As expected, the calculated t for the regression coefficient, β_1, is not significant ($t = -1.337$, $p = .187$). So we fail to reject the null hypothesis and conclude that the regression coefficient, β_1, equals zero. The ANOVA model (see Exhibit 8–13) also indicates that the regression model is not statistically significant. In this case, age at diagnosis is not an important indicator in predicting patient survival time. We therefore conclude that we cannot predict survival time from age at diagnosis. The β_1 coefficient indicates that there is not much change in Y associated with a change in X.

Exhibit 8–13 SPSS Output for Linear Regression, Age at Diagnosis of Colon Cancer and Survival Time in Months

Descriptive Statistics

	Mean	Std. Deviation	N
Survival Time in Months	42.3415	33.5668	41
Age	73.6098	9.4891	41

Model Summary

Model	R	R Square	Adjusted R Square	Std. Error of the Estimate
1	.210[a]	.044	.020	33.2353

[a] Predictors: (Constant), Age

ANOVA[a]

Model		Sum of Squares	df	Mean Square	F	Sig.
1	Regression	1990.474	1	1990.474	1.802	.187[b]
	Residual	43078.745	39	1104.583		
	Total	45069.220	40			

[a] Dependent Variable: Survival Time in Months
[b] Predictors: (Constant), Age

Coefficients[a]

Model		Unstandardized Coefficients		Standardized Coefficients			95% Confidence Interval for B	
		B	Std. Error	Beta	t	Sig.	Lower Bound	Upper Bound
1	(Constant)	97.063	41.093		2.362	.023	13.944	180.182
	LOS	−.743	.554	−.210	−1.342	.187	−1.864	.377

[a] Dependent Variable: Survival Time in Months
Source: Data from *Self-Instructional Manual for Cancer Registries, Book 7: Statistics and Epidemiology for Cancer Registries*, p. 121, U.S. Department of Health and Human Services, Public Health Service, National Institutes of Health, National Cancer Institute.

Example 2: Predicting Total Charges from Age

Earlier, we had an example where the total charges appeared to decrease with the age of the patient. We will now examine this phenomenon in more detail for DRG 336, Transurethral Prostatectomy with CC. The number of patients discharged from DRG 336 is 28. The descriptive statistics for total charges and age appear in Exhibit 8–1, and the scatter diagram with fitted regression line appears in Figure 8–10.

Figure 8–10 Scatter Diagram with Fitted Regression Line, Age and Total Charges (TOTCHG)

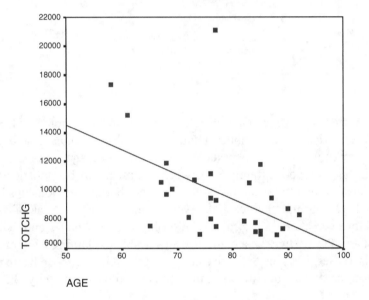

The Pearson *r* for age and total charges appears in Exhibit 8–14. The Pearson *r* is $-.471$, $p = .011$. Even though the correlation appears to be moderate, age is accounting for only 22.2% of the variation in total charges. There must be something else at work that is causing this to occur. Another variable that affects total charges is LOS, as we have already demonstrated. The correlation matrix in Exhibit 8–14 provides the correlations between total charges and length of stay ($r = .838$) and total charges and age ($r = -.471$).

Exhibit 8–14 Pearson r Correlation Coefficients for Total Charges (TOTCHG) by Age and Length of Stay (LOS) (SPSS Output)

		TOTCHG	AGE	LOS
TOTCHG	Pearson Correlation	1.000	−.471*	.838**
	Sig. (2-tailed)	.	.011	.000
	N	28	28	28
AGE	Pearson Correlation	−.471*	1.000	−.310
	Sig. (2-tailed)	.011	.	.108
	N	28	28	28
LOS	Pearson Correlation	.838**	−.310	1.000
	Sig. (2-tailed)	.000	.108	.
	N	28	28	28

* Correlation is significant at the 0.05 level (2-tailed).
** Correlation is significant at the 0.01 level (2-tailed).

For DRG 336, there are two third-party payers—Medicare and commercial. Since "Payer" is a nominal-level variable, we cannot correlate payer with total charges, age, or LOS using the Pearson r. However, if we compare the mean total charges, age, and LOS by third-party payer, we find the observed differences between the means to be statistically significant (Table 8–4). Substituting eta for the Pearson r, we find that the relationships between LOS and payer and between total charges and payer are moderate, with etas of .428 and .538, respectively. However, there is a strong relationship between payer and age, eta = .708. Thus, "Third-Party Payer" may be a confounding variable explaining why total charges decrease as age increases. In Table 8–4, we can see that the ALOS for Medicare patients, 1.82 days, is less than the ALOS for patients in the commercial payer category, 3.27 days.

Table 8–4 Mean Age, Length of Stay (LOS), and Total Charges by Third-Party Payer, DRG 336

	Payer				
	Medicare Mean	Commercial Mean	F	p	eta
Age	82.5	69.5	26.16	<.001	.708
LOS	1.82	3.27	5.82	.023	.428
Total charges	$8,389.35	$11,989.64	10.61	.003	.538

Since these variables, including payer, correlate well with total charges, we can develop a simple regression model for each of these independent variables separately. (Linear regression allows us to use nominal-level variables in which there are two categories.) The regression models for LOS, age, and payer appear in Exhibits 8–15 through Exhibit 8–17. Each of the three models below is statistically significant:

Predictor	Model	r^2
Length of stay	$Y = 5,845.578 + 1,654.162X$	.702
Age	$Y = 23,111 + -171.878X$	.222
Payer	$Y = 7,489.282 + 900.071X$	.290

The strongest model is the one produced by the independent variable, LOS. This is evidenced by the β_1 coefficient and the r^2, which indicates that 70.2% of the variation in total charges is accounted for by LOS. Does this mean that we can sum the r^2 for the other two

Exhibit 8–15 SPSS Regression Statistics, Total Charges (TOTCHG) and Length of Stay (LOS), DRG 336

Model Summary

Model	R	R Square	Adjusted R Square	Std. Error of the Estimate
1	.838[a]	.702	.691	1850.0794

[a] Predictors (Constant), LOS

ANOVA[a]

Model		Sum of Squares	df	Mean Square	F	Sig.
1	Regression	2.1E+08	1	2.1E+08	61.298	.000[b]
	Residual	8.9E+07	26	3422794		
	Total	3.0E+08	27			

[a] Dependent Variable: TOTCHG
[b] Predictors (Constant), LOS

Coefficients[a]

Model		Unstandardized Coefficients		Standardized Coefficients			95% Confidence Interval for B	
		B	Std. Error	Beta	t	Sig.	Lower Bound	Upper Bound
1	(Constant)	5845.578	614.679		9.510	.000	4582.086	7109.069
	LOS	1654.162	211.278	.838	7.829	.000	1219.874	2088.449

[a] Dependent Variable: TOTCHG

Exhibit 8–16 SPSS Regression Statistics for Total Charges (TOTCHG) and Age, DRG 336

Model Summary

Model	R	R Square	Adjusted R Square	Std. Error of the Estimate
1	.471[a]	.222	.192	2990.2852

[a] Predictors: (Constant), AGE

ANOVA[a]

Model		Sum of Squares	df	Mean Square	F	Sig.
1	Regression	6.6E+07	1	6.6E+07	7.417	.011[b]
	Residual	2.3E+08	26	8941806		
	Total	3.0E+08	27			

[a] Dependent Variable: TOTCHG
[b] Predictors: (Constant), AGE

Coefficients[a]

Model		Unstandardized Coefficients		Standardized Coefficients			95% Confidence Interval for B	
		B	Std. Error	Beta	t	Sig.	Lower Bound	Upper Bound
1	(Constant)	23111.999	4919.310		4.698	.000	13000.213	33223.785
	AGE	−171.878	63.113	−.471	−2.723	.011	−301.608	−42.147

[a] Dependent Variable: TOTCHG

variables to determine the total amount of variation in total charges? The answer is no. This is because each variable was analyzed separately—not in relation to how they act together. In addition, by looking at each variable separately, we increase the probability of making a type I error.

Adjusted r^2 in SPSS:
The sample r^2 tends to optimistically estimate how well the models fit the population. The model usually does not fit the population as well as it fits the sample from which it is derived. Adjusted r^2 attempts to correct r^2 to more closely reflect the goodness of fit of the model in the population.

Source: Data from SPSS 9.0 for Windows, Copyright SPSS Inc. 1998, Chicago, Illinois, USA.

Exhibit 8–17 SPSS Regression Statistics for Total Charges (TOTCHG) and Payer, DRG 336

Model Summary

Model	R	R Square	Adjusted R Square	Std. Error of the Estimate
1	.538[a]	.290	.262	2857.0865

[a] Predictors: (Constant) Payer

ANOVA[a]

Model		Sum of Squares	df	Mean Square	F	Sig.
1	Regression	8.7E+07	1	8.7E+07	10.605	.003[b]
	Residual	2.1E+08	26	8162943		
	Total	3.0E+08	27			

[a] Dependent Variable: TOTCHG
[b] Predictors: (Constant), Payer

Coefficients[a]

Model		Unstandardized Coefficients B	Unstandardized Coefficients Std. Error	Standardized Coefficients Beta	t	Sig.	95% Confidence Interval for B Lower Bound	95% Confidence Interval for B Upper Bound
1	(Constant)	7489.282	892.553		8.391	.000	5654.613	9323.951
	Payer	900.071	276.390	.538	3.257	.003	331.944	1468.198

[a] Dependent Variable: TOTCHG

To determine the effect of the three independent variables together on the dependent variable, total charges, we can develop a **multiple regression** model. This discussion will serve only as a brief introduction to multiple regression.

Basically, in multiple regression we are incorporating more than one independent variable into the model. This procedure usually provides a fuller explanation of the effects on the dependent variable. Also, the effect of a single variable is made more certain. The multiple regression model is an extension of the bivariate model and is symbolized as

$$Y = \beta_0 + \beta_1 X_1 + \beta_2 X_2 + \beta_3 X_3 ... + \beta_k X_k + e$$

The interpretation of the constant in the above model is the same as that for simple regression—the average value of Y when each of the independent values equals zero. The interpretation for slope is slightly different. In the multiple-regression situation, the slope is interpreted as the average change in Y associated with a unit change in X when the other independent variables are held constant. Thus, we are able to separate out the effect of any independent variable (X_k) from any distorting influences of the other independent variables. This is sometimes referred to as partial slope or partial regression coefficient.

Now let us develop the regression model using the three independent variables together. SPSS provides several methods for entering the independent variables into the regression model: enter, where all variables appear in the model whether or not they are significant, and forward, backward, and stepwise. In the other methods, a variable is entered into the model on the basis of certain entry or removal criteria. We will use the stepwise multiple-regression procedure, which examines each variable in the model in a block (together) at each step for entry or removal of each independent variable. The stepwise method produces two regression models—one with LOS as the sole predictor variable and the other adding age as a second predictor variable. "Payer" does not enter the regression model.

Upon examination of the two models (Exhibit 8–18), we see that in model 1, the variable LOS alone accounts for 70.2% of the variance in total charges. If we add age to the model, the amount of variance accounted for by the two variables together improves to 75.1%. The model may help explain the variation in charges, but it still does not help us answer why charges decrease with age. This illustrates a problem that occurs with multiple regression: two of the independent variables are highly correlated with one another. In this example, payer and age are highly correlated (eta = .708). Since payer is highly correlated with age, the resultant statistics in the regression model become unstable. When two independent variables are highly correlated with each other, a phenomenon often termed **multicollinearity**, it is difficult to separate the effects of each independent variable on the dependent variable.

In this DRG, there are only two payers—Medicare and commercial PPO. The Medicare group has a smaller LOS (Table 8–5), and hence lower total charges than the commercial payer, even though the average age of Medicare patients is 82.53 versus 69.55 for the commercial payer group. Even though the payer variable does not appear in the multiple-regression model, this could be an explanation for the decrease in total charges by either age or LOS because these two variables are so closely related to the payer variable. This may also suggest that the third-party payer has a strong influence on a patient's LOS.

CONCLUSION

In this chapter, we explored correlation and linear regression. We can use the Pearson r correlation coefficient to determine whether there is a relationship between two variables, X and Y. For the Pearson r, the variables must be at least at the interval scale of measurement; furthermore, it is assumed that the relationship between the two variables is linear. The Pearson r correlation coefficient ranges from -1.00, indicating a perfect negative correlation, to $+1.00$, indicating a perfect positive correlation. A correlation coefficient of 0.00 indicates no linear relationship. Prior to calculating the Pearson r, a scatter diagram should be constructed to determine if the relationship between the two variables is linear.

If two variables have a high correlation with one another and the relationship is linear, it may be possible to predict one (Y) from our knowledge of the other (X). When predicting Y

Exhibit 8–18 SPSS Regression Statistics, Total Charges (TOTCHG) from Length of Stay (LOS), Age, and Payer, DRG 336

Model Summary

Model	R	R Square	Adjusted R Square	Std. Error of the Estimate	Change Statistics R Square Change	F Change	df1	df2	Sig. F Change
1	.838[a]	.702	.691	1850.0794	.702	61.298	1	26	.000
2	.867[b]	.751	.732	1723.4038	.049	4.963	1	25	.035

[a] Predictors: (Constant), LOS
[b] Predictors: (Constant), LOS, AGE

ANOVA[a]

Model		Sum of Squares	df	Mean Square	F	Sig.
1	Regression	2.1E+08	1	2.1E+08	61.298	.000[b]
	Residual	8.9E+07	26	3422794		
	Total	3.0E+08	27			
2	Residual	2.2E+08	2	1.1E+08	37.802	.000[c]
	Residual	7.4E+07	25	2970121		
	Total	3.0E+08	27			

[c] Dependent Variable: TOTCHG
[b] Predictors: (Constant), LOS
[c] Predictors: (Constant), LOS, AGE

Coefficients[a]

Model		Unstandardized Coefficients B	Std. Error	Standardized Coefficients Beta	t	Sig.	95% Confidence Interval for B Lower Bound	Upper Bound
1	(Constant)	5845.578	614.679		9.510	.000	4582.086	7109.069
	LOS	1654.162	211.278	.838	7.829	.000	1219.874	2088.449
2	(Constant)	12787.664	3168.430		4.036	.000	6262.161	19313.167
	LOS	1511.082	207.026	.765	7.299	.000	1084.704	1937.461
	AGE	−85.236	38.262	−.234	−2.228	.035	−164.038	−6.434

[a] Dependent Variable: TOTCHG

Excluded Variables[a]

Model		Beta In	t	Sig.	Partial Correlation	Collinearity Statistics Tolerance
1	Payer	.220[b]	1.958	.062	.365	.817
	AGE	−.234[b]	−2.228	.035	−.407	.904
2	Payer	.101[c]	.671	.509	.136	.451

[a] Dependent Variable: TOTCHG
[b] Predictors in the Model: (Constant), LOS
[c] Predictors in the Model: (Constant), LOS, AGE

Table 8–5 Means of Total Charges (TOTCHG) and Length of Stay (LOS) by Payer (SPSS Output)

Payer		TOTCHG	AGE	LOS
Medicare	Mean	8389.3529	82.5294	1.8235
	N	17	17	17
	Std. Deviation	1376.6135	6.6060	.9510
Commercial PPO	Mean	11989.64	69.5455	3.2727
	N	11	11	11
	Std. Deviation	4265.1551	6.4863	2.1950
Total	Mean	9803.7500	77.4286	2.3929
	N	28	28	28
	Std. Deviation	3326.6847	9.1183	1.6852

from X, we are constructing a regression model. The components of the regression model are $Y = a + BX$ where a is the intercept and B is the regression coefficient. The intercept is the average of Y when X is equal to zero; the regression coefficient represents the average change in Y that is associated with a unit change in X. In making predictions from regression models, we must be careful to limit the range of X to the observations that were used to develop the model.

In both the Pearson r correlation and linear regression, we can request the coefficient of determination, r^2. The r^2 can help us determine the power of the model; it tells us how much of the variation in the dependent variable can be explained by the independent variable.

ADDITIONAL RESOURCES

Duncan, R.C., et al. 1983. *Introductory biostatistics for the health sciences.* Albany, NY: Delmar Publishers.

Edwards, A.L. 1966. *Statistical methods for the behavioral sciences.* New York: Holt, Rinehart & Winston.

Lewis-Beck, M.S. 1986. *Applied regression: An introduction.* Beverly Hills, CA: Sage Publications.

Minium, E.W. 1978. *Statistical reasoning in psychology and education.* New York: John Wiley & Sons.

Phillips, D.S. 1978. *Basic statistics for health science students.* San Francisco: W.H. Freeman & Co.

Appendix 8–A

Exercises for Solving Problems

KNOWLEDGE QUESTIONS

1. Define the key terms listed at the beginning of this chapter.

2. What is the Pearson r? At what level(s) of measurement must the variables be in order to use the Pearson r?

3. What is the range for the Pearson r? How is the Pearson r statistic interpreted? Explain the concepts of positive linear relationship and negative linear relationship.

4. Describe the relationship between the Pearson r and the coefficient of determination.

5. What is the interpretation of the regression line in a scatter diagram?

6. Explain simple linear regression and multiple regression. Give an example for each.

MULTIPLE CHOICE

1. To calculate the Pearson r, the two variables should be:
   a. normally distributed
   b. linearly related
   c. random
   d. all of the above

2. In the scatter diagram below, the Pearson r can be described as:
   a. equal to 0.0
   b. equal to +1.0
   c. negative
   d. positive

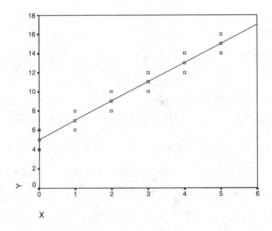

3. If the Pearson r is equal to +1.0, we can say that:
   a. x causes y
   b. y causes x
   c. there is a perfect positive relationship between x and y
   d. x and y are negatively correlated

4. Which of the following values for the Pearson r indicates the strongest relationship?
   a. +.85
   b. +.76
   c. 0.0
   d. −.89

5. Which of the following values for the Pearson r indicates the weakest relationship?
   a. +.85
   b. +.76
   c. 0.0
   d. −.89

6. If we cannot predict *y* from *x*, we would conclude that the Pearson *r* is:
   a. 0.0
   b. negative
   c. positive
   d. cannot determine from information provided

7. We have calculated a Pearson *r* for length of stay (*y*) and age (*x*). Our result is $r = -1.16$. We therefore conclude that:
   a. as age increases, the length of stay decreases
   b. as age increases, the length of stay increases
   c. we cannot predict length of stay from age
   d. we have made an error in our calculations

8. We have calculated the Pearson *r* for length of stay (*x*) and total charges (*y*). Our result is $r = +0.64$. We therefore conclude that:
   a. as length of stay increases, total charges decrease
   b. as length of stay increases, total charges increase
   c. we cannot predict total charges from length of stay
   d. we have made an error in our calculations

PROBLEMS

1. You are studying DRG 395, Red Blood Cell Disorders, Age > 17, for Critical Care Hospital. Using the data provided in Table 8–A–1, calculate the Pearson *r* for each of the following pairs:
   • Age and length of stay
   • Total charges and length of stay
   • Age and total charges
   a. State the null and alternative hypotheses and alpha level for each.
   b. Construct a scatter diagram with regression line for each.
   c. State your conclusions for each.

2. Construct a regression model for predicting total charges from length of stay for DRG 395.
   a. State the null and alternative hypotheses and alpha level.
   b. Prepare a scatter diagram with the regression line for the two variables.
   c. What are the *r* and r^2? What is the importance of the *r* and r^2 results?
   d. What is the regression equation?
   e. What are your conclusions?

Table 8–A–1 Case Summaries for DRG 395, Red Blood Cell Disorders, Age > 17

	Race	Sex	Age	LOS	Total Charges	Payer
1	White	Female	51.00	1.00	4,497.00	Commercial PPO
2	White Hispanic	Female	88.00	10.00	21,769.00	Medicare
3	White	Female	68.00	5.00	16,754.00	Medicare
4	White	Female	49.00	1.00	5,565.00	Medicare
5	White	Female	77.00	6.00	18,752.00	Medicare
6	White	Male	82.00	1.00	4,214.00	Commercial PPO
7	White	Female	72.00	4.00	9,817.00	Commercial PPO
8	Black	Male	20.00	7.00	19,350.00	Self-pay
9	White	Female	63.00	5.00	14,681.00	Commercial
10	Black	Male	29.00	1.00	4,200.00	Commercial
11	Black	Female	85.00	1.00	2,347.00	Commercial PPO
12	Black	Male	20.00	4.00	6,834.00	Self-pay
13	White	Female	60.00	1.00	3,445.00	Commercial PPO
14	White	Male	72.00	6.00	20,906.00	Commercial PPO
15	White	Female	78.00	2.00	5,458.00	Commercial PPO
16	White	Male	82.00	1.00	4,834.00	Medicare
17	Black	Male	21.00	2.00	3,483.00	Self-pay
18	White	Female	87.00	3.00	11,775.00	Medicare
19	White	Female	85.00	3.00	9,752.00	Commercial PPO
20	White	Female	85.00	2.00	4,494.00	Medicare
21	White	Female	77.00	1.00	4,334.00	Commercial PPO
22	Black	Male	21.00	1.00	2,856.00	Self-pay
23	White	Female	75.00	8.00	24,545.00	Medicare
24	Black	Female	47.00	5.00	8,372.00	Medicare
25	Black Hispanic	Female	76.00	8.00	26,144.00	Commercial PPO
26	White	Female	76.00	8.00	17,245.00	Commercial PPO
27	White	Female	61.00	1.00	3,916.00	Commercial
28	White	Female	55.00	1.00	4,847.00	Commercial PPO
29	White	Female	71.00	3.00	8,888.00	Medicare
Total N	29	29	29	29	29	29

CHAPTER 9

Chi Square

KEY TERMS   Contingency tables χ^2 goodness-of-fit test
                χ^2 test of independence   McNemar test
                Standardized residuals
                Yates correction for continuity
                Phi coefficient
                Contingency coefficient
                Cramer's V
                Fisher's exact test

LEARNING   Upon completion of this chapter, you should be able to:
OBJECTIVES
1. Define key terms
2. Differentiate between parametric and nonparametric statistical procedures.
3. Outline the assumptions for nonparametric procedures.
4. Conduct the χ^2 test of independence for given situations.
5. Explain the concept of standardized residuals.
6. Analyze results of the χ^2 test of independence using standardized residuals.
7. Conduct the McNemar test for given situations.
8. Use microcomputer statistical software to solve nonparametric problems.

The statistical procedures discussed thus far are called *parametric statistics*. Parametric statistical procedures require certain assumptions about the underlying population, most particularly that the underlying population is normally distributed, that measures are at the interval or ratio level of measurement, and that the samples are randomly drawn and independent. In contrast, nonparametric procedures have less restrictive assumptions. There are no assumptions that the underlying population distribution is normal, and the distributions may take on any shape, so they are not limited to the bell shape of the normal distribution. Thus, nonparametric statistical procedures are often referred to as *distribution-free statistics*.

Nonparametric procedures may be used to analyze data about populations that consist of nominal, ordinal, interval, and/or ratio data. Many nonparametric tests analyze the ranks or orders of the data set rather than the numerical values of the observations. Nonparametric procedures also are used when sample sizes are small (≤ 30) or when there are extreme values in the data set so that the median rather than the mean is more representative of the distribution. Also, when the shape of the distributions is either unknown or non-normal, nonparametric procedures may be more powerful, reducing the chance of committing a type II error.

Nonparametric methods may be used for testing hypotheses regarding

- relationships between variables
- relationships between variables in paired samples
- relationships between variables in two independent samples
- relationships between variables in three or more independent samples

There are, however, disadvantages associated with the use of nonparametric tests, especially when it is possible to use a corresponding parametric procedure. Since nonparametric procedures involve testing orders or ranks rather than interval/ratio data that are continuous, some information is lost. Consequently, we have a conflict because nonparametric procedures may be considered less powerful than their parametric counterparts, also increasing the probability of committing a type II error. It is therefore imperative that the researcher select the appropriate test in view of the level of measurement used in the data collection process and the sample size. Table 9–1 provides a listing of tests that may be used in relation to the variables' levels of measurement.

Table 9–1 Parametric/Nonparametric Procedures by Level of Measurement

Variable 2	Variable 1		
	Nominal	Ordinal	Interval/Ratio
Nominal	χ^2 test Fisher's exact test McNemar χ^2 test (paired) Phi coefficient Cramer's V Kappa coefficient		
Ordinal	Sign test Wilcoxon signed ranks test (paired) Mann-Whitney Wilcoxon test Kruskal-Wallis test	Spearman rho	
Interval/ratio	Student's paired t test Student's t test for two independent samples One-way ANOVA	Spearman rho	Pearson r Simple regression

Source: Adapted with permission from M.A. Pett, *Nonparametric Statistics for Health Care Research: Statistics for Small Samples and Unusual Distributions*, p. 274, copyright © 1997, Sage Publications, Inc.

The power of nonparametric tests can be improved by increasing the sample size. Less powerful tests are less likely to detect a small difference between groups when one exists. If it is important to the researcher to detect small differences, a parametric procedure should be used if possible. Parametric and nonparametric procedures are compared in Table 9–2.

Table 9–2 Comparison of Parametric and Nonparametric Procedures

Parametric Procedures	*Nonparametric Procedures*
For Data on Sample or Paired Samples	
Student's *t* test for two independent samples ANOVA	Fisher's exact test Mann-Whitney Wilcoxon *U* test χ^2 test for two independent samples
For Three or More Independent Samples	
ANOVA	Kruskal-Wallis analysis of ranks χ^2 test for *k* independent samples
For Relationships between Variables	
Pearson *r* (bivariate)	Spearman rho (bivariate) χ^2 test Cramer's V Phi coefficient Fisher's exact test

Source: Data from M.A. Pett, *Nonparametric Statistics for Health Care Research: Statistics for Small Samples and Unusual Distributions*, p. 278, © 1997, Sage Publications.

In this chapter, we will discuss the various forms of the chi-square test. In Chapter 10, we review other nonparametric procedures.

CHI-SQUARE (χ^2) TESTS

One of the more commonly used nonparametric tests is the chi-square (χ^2) test. The χ^2 distribution is a positive distribution based on the number of degrees of freedom. There is more than one type of χ^2 test that can be used to analyze frequency data; however, all are based on comparing actual observations with expected frequencies. With frequency data, we are reporting the percentages or frequencies of an independent variable on the characteristic of interest. **Contingency tables** are used to display frequency data. A two-by-two (2×2) contingency table is the simplest form.

In a 2×2 table, the distribution of one variable is conditionally dependent, or contingent, upon the other. The table is made up of cells, which are specific locations in the matrix created by the two variables under study. Each cell represents the joint frequencies for the categories on each variable. The categories that make up each variable are dichotomous and must be mutually exclusive. The sums of the rows and columns are placed in the margins and are thus called marginal frequencies. The total for the row and column marginals is the cell in the lower right-hand corner (grand total); this sum is equal to N. The basic shell for a 2×2 contingency table is presented in Exhibit 9–1.

Exhibit 9–1 Shell for a 2×2 Contingency Table

		Variable 1		
		Category 1	Category 2	Total
Variable 2	Category 1	a	b	$a + b$
	Category 2	c	d	$c + d$
		$a + c$	$b + d$	$a + b + c + d$

Source: Adapted from *Principles of Epidemiology: An Introduction to Applied Epidemiology and Biostatistics*, p. 210, 1992, U.S. Department of Health and Human Services, Public Health Service.

Contingency tables may be larger than 2×2. If there are more than two categories for a given variable, the table is referred to as an $R \times C$ table (R = rows, C = columns).

We will now use data collected by Osborn to construct a two-by-two contingency table. Osborn[1] conducted a survey in which data were collected on two variables: professional credential and geographic location. "Credential" had two categories, accredited record technician (ART) and registered record administrator (RRA), and geographic location was classified into two categories: urban/suburban and rural. The question of interest was whether there is a relationship between professional credential and geographic practice location—urban/suburban or rural. The results of the classification appear in Table 9–3. When we read a 2×2 contingency table or $R \times C$ table, the percentages that appear in the cells represent the percentages of the column totals.

We will now conduct the χ^2 test of independence on these data.

Table 9–3 Contingency Table of Professional Credential and Geographic Location

Location	Credential		
	ART	RRA	Total
Urban/suburban	31	77	108
	(36.5%)	(68.1%)	(54.5%)
Rural	54	36	90
	(63.5%)	(31.9%)	(45.5%)
Total	85	113	198

Source: Reprinted with permission from C.E. Osborn, *Benchmarks in HIM Practice*, 1998 AHIMA National Convention Proceedings Book, p. 381, © 1998, American Health Information Management Association.

THE χ^2 TEST OF INDEPENDENCE

In the χ^2 **test of independence**, we can determine whether a relationship exists between two variables in a 2 × 2 contingency table or R × C table. It is one of the most widely used statistics in health care. The question that we are trying to answer is whether the categories of the row variable are distributed differentially across the column variables—that is, how one variable relates to another. If the variables are independent, a change in one variable does not have any effect on the other. We will use the data in Table 9–3 to calculate χ^2.

The null hypothesis is that the two variables, credential and geographic location, are independent of each other—in other words, that there is no relationship between the two variables. If the null is true, we would expect that geographic location would appear in the same proportions in both the ART population and the RRA population. The alternative hypothesis is nondirectional and states that there is an association between the two variables of interest.

> H_0: There is no association between credential and geographic location.
> H_A: There is an association between credential and geographic location.
> $\alpha = .05$

Exhibit 9–2 summarizes the important aspects of the χ^2 test of independence.

Exhibit 9–2 χ^2 Test of Independence—Points To Remember

1. The χ^2 statistic is used when both the independent variable and the dependent variable are at the nominal level of measurement and the categories of each variable are mutually exclusive.
2. Data contained in the contingency table or R × C table are frequencies, not scores.
3. Observations must be independent of each other (except for McNemar's χ^2).
4. The total number of observations (N) should be greater than 20, and the expected frequency per cell should be equal to or greater than 5. For large tables, 20% of the expected frequencies may be less than 5, but should not be less than 2.

The χ^2 test involves comparing observed frequencies with expected frequencies. In a contingency table, the expected frequencies are the proportion of each category that we would expect to find in each cell by chance over the long run. In our example, there are 198 total observations. Of these 198, 108, or 54.5%, practice in urban/suburban areas, and 90, or 45.5%, practice in rural areas. Therefore, in the long run, we would expect these frequencies to occur in each group. In our contingency table, there are 85 ARTs and 113 RRAs. Therefore, we would expect that 54.5% in each group would be practicing in urban/suburban locations—46.4 ARTs and 61.6 RRAs. The expected frequencies are generated on this assumption. An easy way to generate the expected frequencies is given by the following formula:

$$\text{Expected frequency} = \frac{\text{row marginal} \times \text{column marginal}}{\text{grand total } (N)}$$

The next step is to subtract the expected cell frequency (E) from the observed cell frequency (O). This gives the amount of deviation in each cell. The sum of the deviates for both rows and columns is equal to zero. The deviates in each cell are then squared, $(O - E)^2$, and divided by the expected value for each cell, $(O - E)^2/E$. This is similar to the numerator of the variance, $(X - \bar{X})^2$, where $\bar{X}$ is the expected value. But where the denominator for the variance is divided by the degrees of freedom, $n - 1$, the denominator for χ^2 is the expected (E) frequency. Therefore, the basic statistical method for measuring variation in a data set, the total sum of squares (TSS), is rewritten for χ^2 as the sum of $(O - E)^2$.

The formula for calculating the χ^2 statistic is:

$$\chi^2_{\text{calc}} = \sum [(O - E)^2]/E$$

which is defined as the sum of the squared deviations divided by the expected frequency for each cell. To calculate the expected frequency for the first cell, ART × urban/suburban, we multiply the column marginal by the row marginal (Table 9–3) and divide by the grand total: $(85 \times 108)/198 = 46.36$. We proceed in the same manner for each cell. The expected frequency for each cell is subtracted from the observed frequency, squared, and divided by the expected frequency. The results for each cell are then summed. For the data in Table 9–4, χ^2 is calculated as:

$$\chi^2_{\text{calc}} = \sum [(O - E)^2]/E$$
$$= 5.09 + 6.10 + 3.83 + 4.60$$
$$= 19.62$$

Table 9–4 χ^2 Test of Independence for Credential and Geographic Location

	Credential					
	ART			RRA		
Location	O	E	$(O - E)^2/E$	O	E	$(O - E)^2/E$
Urban/suburban	31	46.36	5.09	77 4	61.64	3.83
Rural	54	38.64	6.10	36 6	51.36	4.60
Total	85	85		113	113	

Source: Data from C.E. Osborn, *Benchmarks in HIM Practice*, 1998 AHIMA National Convention Proceedings Book, p. 381, © 1998, American Health Information Management Association.

In our example, the calculated χ^2 is fairly large, indicating that the observed frequencies do differ markedly from the theoretical or expected frequencies. This is verified by comparing the calculated χ^2 with the critical value of χ^2 in Appendix B, Table B–6. In a 2×2 contingency table, degrees of freedom are equal to 1 (df = 1). In larger tables, the number of degrees of freedom is determined by

$$df = (R - 1) \times (C - 1).$$

Conceptual models for degrees of freedom in contingency tables and R × C tables are displayed in Exhibit 9–3.

Exhibit 9–3 Degrees of Freedom

In a 2×2 contingency table, the best estimate of the expected counts in a distribution is given in the row and column totals. Therefore, the row and column totals are considered fixed. Once an observed count is entered into a cell in a 2×2 table, no other cells are free to vary.

	Column 1	*Column 2*	*Total*
Row 1	Degree of freedom a	Fixed b	Fixed $a + b$
Row 2	Fixed c	Fixed d	Fixed $c + d$
Total	Fixed $a + c$	Fixed $b + d$	Fixed $a + b + c + d$ (N)

We can extend this idea to R × C tables. As above, the row and column totals are fixed. Now assume that the last column and the bottom row are never free to vary because they must consist of numbers to make the totals come out right. This is illustrated in the 4×3 table below (4 rows, 3 columns):

	Column 1	*Column 2*	*Column 3*	*Total*
Row 1	Degree of freedom	Degree of freedom	Fixed	Fixed row total
Row 2	Degree of freedom	Degree of freedom	Fixed	Fixed row total
Row 3	Degree of freedom	Degree of freedom	Fixed	Fixed row total
Row 4	Fixed	Fixed	Fixed	Fixed row total
Total	Fixed column total	Fixed column total	Fixed column total	Fixed grand total

Source: Adapted with permission from J.F. Jekel et al., *Epidemiology, Biostatistics and Preventive Medicine*, p. 148, © 1996, W.B. Saunders Company.

From Table B–6 in Appendix B, the χ^2 critical for $\alpha = .05$ and for one degree of freedom is 3.841. Since the calculated χ^2 is greater than the critical χ^2, we reject the null and conclude that the variables, credential and geographic location, are related or that they vary together in some systematic way.

There are several points to remember when calculating χ^2 from a contingency table or the larger R × C table. First, the expected counts for each cell should be 5 or more. For larger tables, 20% of the expected counts could be less than 5 but should not be less than 2. When expected cell counts are less than 5, consider collapsing the number of categories.

The χ^2 test of independence is an example of statistical modeling. Statistical modeling is a process by which a model is developed to predict the relationship of one or more dependent variables with an independent variable. We have already had experience with statistical modeling with linear regression. On the basis of our results in the previous example, we would expect that for any sample drawn from a population of ARTs and RRAs, RRAs would be more likely to practice in urban areas than ARTs.

EXAMINATION OF RESIDUALS

A large χ^2 often results in statistical significance, indicating an association between the two variables under study. However, this does not always tell us which levels of the variable are contributing the most to the χ^2 statistic. By examining the χ^2 residuals, we can determine which cells are contributing the most to the calculated χ^2.

A residual is defined as the difference between the actual frequencies and the expected frequencies in each cell $(O - E)$. SPSS provides unstandardized, standardized, and adjusted residuals for each cell. We most often use the **standardized residuals**, which are obtained by

$$\text{Standardized residual} = \frac{O - E}{\sqrt{E}}$$

If the value of the obtained standardized residual is greater than +2 or less than –2 in any cell, we can conclude that the cell in question is an important contributor to the significance of χ^2. In the SPSS output in Exhibit 9–4, the ART cells for geographic location are contributing the most to the calculated χ^2, indicating that the observed frequencies deviate most from the expected frequencies.

Exhibit 9–4 SPSS Output for Chi-Square Procedure, Credential and Geographic Location

GEOGRAPHIC LOCATION * CREDENTIAL Crosstabulation

			CREDENTIAL		
			ART	RRA	Total
GEOGRAPHIC LOCATION	URBAN/SUBURBAN	Count	31	77	108
		Expected Count	46.4	61.6	108.0
		Std. Residual	−2.3	2.0	
	RURAL	Count	54	36	90
		Expected Count	38.6	51.4	90.0
		Std. Residual	2.5	−2.1	
Total		Count	85	113	198
		Expected Count	85.0	113.0	198.0

Chi-Square Tests

	Value	df	Asymp. Sig. (2-sided)	Exact Sig. (2-sided)	Exact Sig. (1-sided)
Pearson Chi-Square	19.625[a]	1	.000		
Continuity Correction[b]	18.369	1	.000		
Likelihood Ratio	19.884	1	.000		
Fisher's Exact Test				.000	.000
Linear-by-Linear Association	19.526	1	.000		
N of Valid Cases	198				

[a] 0 cells (.0%) have expected count less than 5. The minimum expected count is 38.64.
[b] Computed only for a 2 × 2 table.

Symmetric Measures

		Value	Approx. Sig.
Nominal by Nominal	Phi	−.315	.000
	Cramer's V	.315	.000
	Contingency Coefficient	.300	.000
N of Valid Cases		198	

Source: Data from C.E. Osborn, *Benchmarks in HIM Practice*, 1998 AHIMA National Convention Proceedings Book, p. 381, © 1998, American Health Information Management Association.

YATES CORRECTION FOR CONTINUITY

Because the χ^2 test is based on comparing the calculated values of χ^2, which form a discontinuous distribution with the theoretical values of χ^2, which form a continuous distribution, many recommend that the Yates continuity correction be used when the table numbers are small and df = 1. The only difference in the χ^2 formula is that the 0.5 is subtracted from the absolute value of $(O - E)$ in each cell.

$$\text{Yates } \chi^2 = \sum \left[\left(|O - E| - 0.5 \right)^2 \right] / E$$

Obviously, this will reduce the size of the calculated χ^2, thus reducing the chance of finding statistical significance and increasing the probability of making a type II error—failing to reject the null hypothesis when it is false. Recalculating our credential and geographic location data using the **Yates correction for continuity** reduces chi square slightly, $\chi^2 = 18.37$, but it still remains statistically significant.

PHI COEFFICIENT

Chi square tells us if there is an association between two variables, but it does not tell us the degree of association, as does the Pearson r correlation coefficient. Also, we cannot compare values of χ^2 across samples because the calculated χ^2 is a function of sample size. The **phi coefficient** corrects for sample size and measures the degree of association between the two variables under study. The formula for phi is

$$\varphi = \sqrt{\chi^2 / n}$$

The phi coefficient is interpreted in the same way as the Pearson r, but the range of phi is 0 to 1. As a general rule of thumb, a value less than .30 may be interpreted as a trivial association. The phi coefficient for the data in Table 9–4 is calculated as

$$\varphi = \sqrt{\chi^2 / n}$$
$$= \sqrt{19.63 / 198}$$
$$= .315$$

Therefore, the relationship between credential and geographic location is not very strong. We can see that phi provides us with more knowledge about our sample profile than χ^2 alone.

CONTINGENCY COEFFICIENT

The **contingency coefficient** (C) is an alternative to the phi coefficient when one dimension of the contingency table is greater than two ($2 \times k$). The contingency coefficient is calculated as

$$C = \sqrt{\chi^2 / \chi^2 + N}$$

The value of the contingency coefficient ranges from 0 to 1.0. However, its maximum value depends on the number of rows and columns in the table.

CRAMER'S V

The phi coefficient is a useful statistic when working with large samples where statistical significance can be easily achieved. Phi adjusts for sample size and can be considered the correlation coefficient for data in 2×2 tables. **Cramer's V** is used when the table is larger than 2×2.

$$\text{Cramer's } V = \sqrt{\chi^2 / N(m-1)}$$

where m is the smaller of the number of the rows or columns in the R x C table. The range for Cramer's V is 0 to 1.0, and the significance level will be the same as that for the χ^2.

SPSS will perform the procedures described: chi square, Yates correction for continuity, phi coefficient, and Cramer's V. When categorical variables are used, they must be coded for correct entry onto the data sheet. For the variables in Table 9–3, credential was coded as ART $= 1$ and RRA $= 2$. Geographic location was coded as urban/suburban $= 1$ and rural $= 2$.

✓ To Obtain a Chi-Square Test Using SPSS:

- From the "Analyze" menu, choose:
  →Descriptive statistics
    →crosstabs
- Select one or more row variables and one or more column variables.
  →Click "Statistics" for tests and measures of association (chi square, phi coefficient, Cramer's V, etc.).
    →Click "Cells" for observed and expected values, percentages, and residuals.

The results of the SPSS calculations appear in Exhibit 9–4. The Pearson χ^2 provided by SPSS is 19.625, and the continuity correction is 18.369. Rounding accounts for the differences between our hand-calculated results and the SPSS results. SPSS provides the same results for the phi coefficient and Cramer's V. Note that SPSS reports the phi coefficient as a negative value—an idiosyncrasy of the program, as a square root cannot be negative. The standardized residuals indicate that the ART cells are contributing the most to the calculated χ^2 statistic.

The likelihood ratio, **Fisher's exact test**, and "Linear × Linear Association" appear by default. The likelihood ratio is a goodness-of-fit statistic similar to the χ^2 goodness of fit, which we will discuss later in this chapter. For large sample sizes, they are identical. The advantage of the likelihood ratio is that it can be subdivided into interpretable parts that sum to the total. The significance level of the likelihood ratio is of more interest than the actual value of the statistic itself.

The χ^2 test for linear association tells us whether the relationship between the two variables under study is a linear one. That is, the observations on both variables increase in the same direction. Although SPSS reports the χ^2 test for linearity by default, it is not appropriate for nominal-level data.

FISHER'S EXACT TEST

There may be times that we have nominal level data on two variables but the sample size is too small, usually defined as less than or equal to 20, for the χ^2 test of independence. In these cases, **Fisher's exact test** is a useful procedure. The purpose of Fisher's exact test is to examine whether two populations differ from each other in the proportion of subjects who fall into one of two classifications of the variables. In the most common form of Fisher's exact test, there are usually two levels for each variable and the collected data are classified into a 2×2 table, as in Table 9–5. However, Fisher's exact test may be extended to larger tables. The null and alternative hypotheses are

H_0: There is no association between the two variables of interest.
H_A: There is an association between the two variables of interest.

Table 9–5 Contingency Table of Smoking by Sex

	Sex		
Smoking	Male	Female	Total
Yes	7	2	9
No	3	8	11
Total	10	10	20

We calculate Fisher's exact test by

$$p = \frac{(a+b)!(c+d)!(a+c)!(b+d)!}{N!\,a!\,b!\,c!\,d!}$$

Where p is the probability of obtaining the observed frequencies that appear in the contingency variable. As you might expect, calculating the p for this test with a hand-held calculator is quite tedious. When using SPSS, Fisher's exact test is the default of the χ^2 test of independence when sample sizes are less than 20 or when the expected frequencies for each cell are less than 5. The assumptions for Fisher's exact test are displayed in Exhibit 9–5.

Exhibit 9–5 Assumptions for Fisher's Exact Test

1. Both variables of interest are dichotomous.
2. Assigned categories are mutually exclusive.
3. Data contained within the table are frequencies, not scores.

As an example, let's assume that we are studying the relatedness of smoking and sex; we will limit the sample size to 20. The null and alternative hypotheses are

H_0: There is no association between smoking and sex.
H_A: There is an association between smoking and sex.
$\alpha = .05$

The results of our sampling appear in Table 9–5.
Given these data, p would be calculated as

$$p = \frac{(a+b)!(c+d)!(a+c)!(b+d)!}{N!a!b!c!d!}$$

$$p = \frac{(9)!(11)!(10)!(10)!}{(20)!(7)!(2)!(3)!(8)!}$$

$$= .032$$

In this case, the resulting p is the actual probability of obtaining this sampling result. The calculation of $p = .032$ is a one-tailed test result. Since our null is nondirectional (i.e., two tailed), we double the obtained p value of .032, which results in a two-tailed p value of .064. Since $p > .05$, we fail to reject the null and conclude that the two variables, smoking and sex, are independent.

To calculate Fisher's exact test using SPSS, we must first code the dichotomous variables to be used in the analysis. The sex variable will be coded as male = 1 and female = 2. The smoking variable will be coded as smoking = 1 and no smoking = 2. Fisher's exact test is provided by default. The SPSS results for Fisher's exact test appear in Exhibit 9–6. SPSS provides both the one- and two-tailed p values. The two-tailed p value is .070. SPSS adjusts the p value because the row margin totals are not equal: that is, $(a + b) \neq (c + d)$.

Exhibit 9–6 SPSS Output for Fisher's Exact Test

SMOKING * SEX Crosstabulation

SEX

			MALE	FEMALE	Total
SMOKING	SMOKING	Count	7	2	9
		Expected Count	4.5	4.5	9.0
		Std. Residual	1.2	−1.2	
	NO SMOKING	Count	3	8	11
		Expected Count	5.5	5.5	11.0
		Std. Residual	−1.1	1.1	
Total		Count	10	10	20
		Expected Count	10.0	10.0	20.0

Chi-Square Tests

	Value	df	Asymp. Sig. (2-sided)	Exact Sig. (2-sided)	Exact Sig. 1-sided)
Pearson Chi-Square	5.051[a]	1	.025		
Continuity of Correction[b]	3.232	1	.072		
Likelihood Ratio	5.300	1	.021		
Fisher's Exact Test				.070	.035
Linear-by-Linear Association	4.798	1	.028		
N of Valid Cases	20				

[a] 2 cells (50.0%) have expected count less than 5. The minimum expected count is 4.50.

[b] Computed only for a 2 × 2 table.

χ^2 GOODNESS OF FIT

In the χ^2 **goodness-of-fit test**, we are also comparing actual frequencies with expected or theoretical frequencies in a distribution. However, the expected counts instead of being based on the collected data, as in Table 9–3, are based on our knowledge of the population under study. For example, if 75% of the physicians practicing in our hospital are men and 25% are women, we will expect to draw a sample composed of 75% men and 25% women. We know that the drawn sample will not precisely match the proportions in the population, but we want to be assured that the sample proportions are not significantly different from the underlying population proportions. In this procedure, the goal is to determine how well the observed counts in our sample fit the expected counts based on the model—that is, how well the observed count matches a theoretical frequency distribution.

As an example, Osborn[2] received 355 responses to a survey that was mailed to directors of health information management (HIM) centers in acute care facilities across the United

States. A χ^2 goodness-of-fit test was conducted to ensure that the respondent profile matched that of the distribution of practitioners in the general HIM population. A variable used to compare the respondent profile to the general population was the hospital bed size in which professionals practiced. The obtained frequency distribution of HIM respondents is compared to the respondent profile in Table 9–6.

Table 9–6 HIM Population Distribution and Respondent Profile by Hospital Size

Hospital Size	HIM Population % 1990	Respondent %
<100 beds	20.1	21.7
101–300 beds	38.9	41.4
301–500 beds	21.9	22.3
501+ beds	19.0	14.6

Source: Reprinted from C.E. Osborn, *Roles and Functions of Accredited Record Technicians and Registered Record Administrators,* p. 87, 1990, Dissertation, The Ohio State University.

The null hypothesis, based on the actual HIM frequency distribution, is

H_0: $p_1 = .201, p_2 = .389, p_3 = .219, p_4 = .190$
H_A: At least one of the hypothesized proportions is different from the expected.

The expected frequencies are generated on the basis of the actual frequency distribution of the characteristic of interest in the general population. In the example, 20.1% of the HIM professionals practice in hospitals with fewer than 100 beds; therefore, the expected frequency count for the actual respondents for this category is 71.4 ($355 \times .201 = 71.4$). Table 9–7 displays the observed and expected frequencies. If the calculated χ^2 is small, there is close agreement between the observed and expected frequencies. As the discrepancy between the observed and expected frequencies increases, the calculated χ^2 increases, and the more likely we are to reject the null hypothesis and conclude that the population proportions are significantly different from the expected population proportions.

Table 9–7 Observed (*O*) and Expected (*E*) Frequencies of Respondents by Hospital Bed Size

Hospital Bed Size	O	E	(O–E)	(O–E)²	(O–E)²/E
<100 beds	77	71.4	5.6	31.36	.44
101–300 beds	147	138.2	8.8	77.4	.56
301–500 beds	79	77.8	1.2	1.44	.02
501+ beds	52	67.5	–15.5	240.25	3.56
	355				4.58

Source: Data from C.E. Osborn, *Roles and Functions of Accredited Record Technicians and Registered Record Administrators,* p. 87, 1990, Dissertation, The Ohio State University.

In this example, we are comparing observed frequencies with the expected frequencies across four categories (rows) on the variable hospital bed size. In the one-variable case, degrees of freedom are based on the number of categories (k) and are equal to the number of categories minus 1 (i.e., $k - 1$). In this example, $k - 1 = 3$, and for 3 df, the critical value of χ^2, $\alpha = .05$, is 7.82. Since the calculated χ^2 does not equal or exceed the critical value of χ^2, we fail to reject the null hypothesis and conclude that the respondent profile "fits" the population profile. Even though we can generalize our results to our population of interest, it is important to note that the category "501+ beds" contributes the most to the χ^2 statistic. It is this category that deviates the most from the expected frequencies.

The SPSS calculations for the data in Table 9–7 appear in Exhibit 9–7. SPSS reports the χ^2 as 4.575, $p = .206$. SPSS requires that the expected frequencies for each category be entered into the dialog box. The expected frequencies may be specified as proportions, percentages, or actual values. The assumptions for the χ^2 goodness-of-fit test are summarized in Exhibit 9–8.

Exhibit 9–7 SPSS Output for Chi-Square Goodness of Fit

HOSPITAL SIZE

	Observed N	Expected N	Residual
6–100 BEDS	77	71.4	5.6
101–300 BEDS	147	138.2	8.8
301–500 BEDS	79	77.8	1.2
501+ BEDS	52	67.5	–15.5
Total	355		

Test Statistics

	HOSPITAL SIZE
Chi-Square[a]	4.576
df	3
Asymp. Sig.	.206

[a] 0 cells (.0%) have expected frequencies less than 5. The minimum expected cell frequency is 67.5.

Source: Data from C.E. Osborn, *Roles and Functions of Accredited Record Technicians and Registered Record Administrators*, p. 87, 1990, Dissertation, The Ohio State University.

Exhibit 9–8 Assumptions for χ^2 Goodness of Fit

1. Select a criterion upon which to compare the selected sample with the underlying population, such as sex, level of education, or certification.
2. Select the null and alternative hypotheses and the significance level for rejection of the null.
3. The criterion variable must have two or more categories, and the categories must be mutually exclusive and exhaustive.
4. The data contained within the cells are frequencies, not scores.
5. Determine the expected or theoretical frequencies under the assumption that the null hypothesis is true. The expected frequencies are obtained by the researcher's knowledge of the target population. Frequencies must be specified in advance.
6. If categories are dichotomous, the expected frequencies for each cell should be at least 5. If there are more than two categories, no more than 20% of the cells should have frequencies less than 5. If this requirement cannot be met, consider collapsing the categories.
7. Compare the observed frequencies to the expected frequencies for each cell.
8. If the aggregate discrepancy (χ^2_{calc}) between the observed and expected frequencies is too great to attribute to chance at the selected significance level, reject the null.

✓ To Obtain a Chi-Square Test Using SPSS:

- From the "Analyze" menu, choose:
  →Nonparametric
   →chi square
- Select one or more test variables. Each variable produces a separate test.
- Click "Options" for descriptive statistics, etc.

χ^2 TEST FOR PAIRED DATA—McNEMAR TEST

When we previously discussed identifying differences between paired data, we reviewed the paired *t* test. In the paired *t* test, the dependent variable is continuous and the independent variable is categorical. The **McNemar test** is used when we have paired data and the variable under study is nominal. The McNemar test is a modified χ^2 with one degree of freedom. If the resultant χ^2 is significant, the conclusion is that there was a change from the pretest condition to the posttest condition, or that there is an association between the treatment and the effect. Exhibit 9–9 outlines the assumptions for the McNemar test.

Exhibit 9–9 Assumptions for McNemar Test

1. Observations are dichotomous.
2. Dichotomous measures are paired observations of the same subjects or matched pairs.
3. Dichotomous categories are mutually exclusive.
4. Data that are contained in the cells of the table are the number of pairs.

As an example, we are interested in comparing student attitudes before enrollment in a professional HIM baccalaureate degree program and after graduation. Fifty students were asked to complete an attitude survey prior to formal program enrollment and one week post-graduation. Responses were recorded as either positive or negative—a dichotomous response. The subjects (students) are serving as their own controls, as it is their pre-enrollment and postgraduation scores that are being compared.

For the McNemar test, we first prepare a 2 × 2 contingency table. The pre-enrollment attitudes appear on the left, and postgraduation attitudes appear across the top (Table 9–8).

Table 9–8 Pre-Enrollment and Postgraduation Attitudes of HIM Students

| | Postgraduation | | |
Pre-Enrollment	Positive	Negative	Total
Positive	38	5	43
	a	b	a + b
Negative	2	5	7
	c	d	c + d
Total	40	10	50
	a + c	b + d	a + b + c + d

Each cell in the table represents one of the four following combinations:

a = positive before and after—no change
b = change from positive to negative
c = change from negative to positive
d = negative before and after—no change

Only the b and c cells are used in the analysis because they represent change—if it occurred. Cells a and d do not contribute anything to the analysis, since the cell frequencies remain the same before enrollment in the baccalaureate program and after graduation.

The null and alternative hypotheses are

H_0: pre-enrollment attitude = postgraduation attitude
H_A: pre-enrollment attitude ≠ postgraduation attitude

The formula for the McNemar χ^2 is

$$
\begin{aligned}
\text{McNemar } \chi^2 &= (|b - c| - 1)^2/(b + c) \\
&= (|5 - 2| - 1)^2/(5 + 2) \\
&= 0.57
\end{aligned}
$$

The critical value for χ^2, $\alpha = .05$, with one degree of freedom, is 3.841. Since the calculated χ^2 does not equal or exceed the critical value, the McNemar test result is not statistically significant. So even though there were observed changes in attitudes, in that three students changed their attitudes from positive to negative, the changes are not statistically significant. But even though these results are not statistically significant, it would be worthwhile to investigate the reasons for change in student attitudes.

The SPSS calculations for the McNemar test appear in Exhibit 9–10. The two paired variables for analysis are the pre-enrollment attitudes and the postgraduation attitudes. Positive attitudes were coded as "1," and negative attitudes were coded as "2." SPSS does not display the actual McNemar statistic, and it uses the binomial distribution (see Chapter 10) to calculate the level of significance ($p = .453$).

Exhibit 9–10 SPSS Output for McNemar Test

Pre-Enrollment * Postgraduation Crosstabulation

Count

		Postgraduation		
		Positive	Negative	Total
Pre-enrollment	positive	38	5	43
	negative	2	5	7
Total		40	10	50

Chi-Square Tests

	Value	Exact Sig. (2-sided)
McNemar Test		.453[a]
N of Valid Cases	50	

[a] Binomial distribution used.

✓ **To Obtain McNemar's Test Using SPSS:**

- From the "Analyze" menu, choose:
    →descriptive statistics
        →crosstabs
- Select one or more row variables and one or more column variables.
    →Click "statistics for McNemar test"

CONCLUSION

In this chapter, we were introduced to the various forms of the chi-square test, which is a nonparametric procedure. Nonparametric procedures are less restrictive than their parametric counterparts. Nonparametric procedures do not make assumptions regarding the underlying population distribution; nor do they require large sample sizes. Nonparametric methods may also be used for analyzing frequencies for nominal- and ordinal-level data.

We can use the chi-square test to measure the relationship between two variables. This is called the chi-square test of independence. Other frequency measures of association based on chi square include Cramer's V, the phi coefficient, and Fisher's exact test. These tests use frequencies rather than the values of observations in the calculations.

If we are interested in making comparisons between two independent samples, the forms of chi square to be used are Fisher's exact test and the chi-square test for two independent samples. If we are interested in making comparisons between paired samples, we can use McNemar's chi square.

NOTES

1. C.E. Osborn, *Benchmarks in HIM practice*. Proceedings of the 1998 AHIMA Annual Convention, New Orleans, LA, 1998.

2. C.E. Osborn, *Roles and functions of accredited record technicians and registered record administrators*. Dissertation. The Ohio State University, Columbus, Ohio, 1990.

ADDITIONAL RESOURCES

Besag, F.P., and P.L. Besag. 1985. *Statistics for the helping professions*. Beverly Hills, CA: Sage Publications.

Fleiss, J.L. 1981. *Statistical methods for rates and proportions*. New York: John Wiley & Sons.

Gibbon, J.D. 1993. *Non-parametric statistics: An introduction*. Newbury Park, CA: Sage Publications.

Hollander, M., and D. Wolfe. 1973. *Non-parametric statistical methods*. New York: John Wiley & Sons.

Jekel, J.F., et al. 1996. *Epidemiology, biostatistics and preventive medicine*. Philadelphia: W.B. Saunders.

Pett, M.A. 1997. *Nonparametric statistics for health care research: Statistics for small samples and unusual distributions*. Thousand Oaks, CA: Sage Publications.

Statsoft Electronic Textbook. 1998. www.statsoft.com/textbook

Appendix 9–A

Exercises for Solving Problems

KNOWLEDGE QUESTIONS

1. Define the key terms listed at the beginning of this chapter.

2. Describe the major differences between parametric and nonparametric procedures.

3. Describe the circumstances under which it would be appropriate to use the chi-square test.

4. What questions would a researcher be attempting to answer when using the chi-square goodness-of-fit test?

MULTIPLE CHOICE

1. We use the chi-square test to test for differences between:
   a. means
   b. variances
   c. frequencies
   d. proportions
   e. c and d
   f. all of the above

2. You want to compare the number of male and female patients discharged by service at Critical Care Hospital. There are 10 services. For the chi-square test, the number of degrees of freedom is:
   a. 1
   b. 2
   c. 9
   d. 10

3. In the chi-square test, if the result is *not* significant, the:
   a. observed frequencies are similar to the expected frequencies
   b. observed frequencies do not match the expected frequencies
   c. expected frequencies are greater than the observed frequencies
   d. observed frequencies are greater than the expected frequencies

For questions 4 through 9, refer to the following R × C table:

	Phys A	Phys B	Phys C	Total
Male				50
Female	20	50		150
Total	40	60	100	200

4. The observed number of male patients discharged by physician C is:
   a. 10
   b. 20
   c. 30
   d. not enough information provided

5. The expected number of male patients discharged by physician B is:
   a. 10
   b. 15
   c. 20
   d. not enough information provided

6. The observed number of males discharged by physician A is:
   a. 10
   b. 20
   c. 30
   d. not enough information provided

7. The expected number of females discharged by physician A is:
   a. 20
   b. 25
   c. 30
   d. not enough information provided

8. The number of degrees of freedom for this problem is equal to:
   a. 2
   b. 4
   c. 6
   d. 199

9. For the above problem, χ^2_{calc} is equal to 16.87; χ^2_{crit} is equal to 5.99. We therefore:
   a. reject the null hypothesis
   b. fail to reject the null hypothesis
   c. conclude that these physicians have the same number of discharges
   d. conclude that these physicians prefer to treat men over women

10. The phi coefficient is used to measure the:
    a. correlation of two ordered variables
    b. correlation of interval-level variables
    c. strength of the association between variables in a 2×2 table
    d. all of the above

PROBLEMS

1. You are assisting Dr. Hartman in studying the number of deaths due to acute myocardial infarctions (AMIs). Dr. Hartman is particularly interested in knowing if more men died from AMIs than women. To answer this question, you review discharges by sex for DRG 123, Circulatory Disorders with AMI, Expired. Use the nonparametric procedure for chi square to determine if there is an association between sex and deaths due to AMI at Critical Care Hospital. A frequency distribution of discharges by sex and age from DRG 123 appears in Table 9–A–1.

   a. State the null and alternative hypotheses.
   b. State the alpha level.
   c. What is the result of the chi-square test?
   d. State your conclusions.

Table 9–A–1 Frequency Distribution of Discharges by Age and Sex, DRG 123 (SPSS Output)

AGE * SEX Crosstabulation

Count

		SEX		
		Male	Female	Total
AGE	48.00		1	1
	68.00		1	1
	69.00	2		2
	71.00	1		1
	76.00		1	1
	78.00		1	1
	79.00	1		1
	81.00	1		1
	83.00		1	1
	85.00	1		1
	87.00		1	1
	88.00		1	1
	89.00	1	2	3
	91.00		1	1
	94.00		1	1
	95.00	2		2
Total		9	11	20

2. Using the same information in Table 9–A–1, use the chi-square test to determine if there is an association between age and sex for discharges from DRG 123. Calculate the phi coefficient.

   a. State the null and alternative hypotheses.
   b. State the alpha level.
   c. What is the result of the chi-square test?
   d. What does the phi coefficient indicate?
   e. State your conclusions.

CHAPTER 10

Nonparametric Methods

KEY TERMS	Spearman rho	Mann-Whitney Wilcoxon test
	Sign test	Kruskall-Wallis test
	Wilcoxon signed ranks test	

LEARNING OBJECTIVES

Upon completion of this chapter, you should be able to:

1. Define key terms.
2. Conduct the following tests for given situations: Spearman rho, Sign test, Wilcoxon signed ranks test, Mann-Whitney Wilcoxon test, and the Kruskall-Wallis test.
3. Distinguish between the Pearson r correlation coefficient and the Spearman rho correlation coefficient.
4. Use microcomputer statistical software to solve nonparametric problems.

In Chapter 9, we discussed the various forms of chi square and their respective applications. In this chapter, we will discuss some of the other commonly used nonparametric procedures. We will first discuss the Spearman rho rank order correlation coefficient. This test is the nonparametric counterpart of the Pearson r correlation coefficient.

THE SPEARMAN RHO RANK ORDER CORRELATION COEFFICIENT

An alternative to the Pearson r correlation coefficient that we previously discussed is the Spearman rho rank order correlation coefficient. The Spearman rho is used when at least one of the two variables under study falls on the ordinal scale of measurement. The correlation coefficient obtained from the **Spearman rho** procedure is the result of the rankings of the observations, not the actual values of the observations.

To calculate the Spearman rho, we rank the observations on each variable from lowest to highest. Tied observations are assigned the average of the ranks. If two observations are tied for second position, they actually occupy positions 2 and 3, and both are assigned the average rank of $(2+3)/2$, or 2.5. For example, consider the following data set:

Observed score	2	5	5	5	7
Rank	1	2	3	4	5

The total number of possible ranks is five, but three subjects have the same observation of "5," and it is incorrect to assign them different ranks. To obtain the average rank, we sum the ranks 2, 3, and 4 and divide by 3 to obtain the average rank of 3. The assigned ranks become

Observed score	2	5	5	5	7
Rank	1	3	3	3	5

Once the ranks have been assigned, the differences between the ranks on the X and Y variables are obtained, summed, and squared (Table 10–1). The resulting values are substituted into the following formula:

$$r_{rho} = 1 - [(6\Sigma D^2) / n(n^2 - 1)]$$

The range for the Spearman rho is the same as that for the Pearson r, -1.0 to $+1.0$, and has the same interpretation.

Table 10–1 Patient Ranks by Smoking and Severity of Illness

Patient	No. of Cigarettes Smoked R_1	Severity of Illness R_2	Difference in Ranks $D (R_1-R_2)$	D^2
1	1	2	−1	1
2	2	4	−2	4
3	3	3	0	0
4	4	1	3	9
5	5	7	−2	4
6	6	5	1	1
7	7	8	−1	1
8	8	6	2	4
			0	24

As an example, let's consider a hypothetical case of eight subjects who smoke. The R_1 column (Table 10–1) indicates the rank for each patient in terms of number of cigarettes smoked, from lowest (rank = 1) to highest (rank = 8). The R_2 column indicates the rank for each patient in terms of severity of illness, from least severe (rank = 1) to most severe (rank = 8). To complete the table, R_2 is subtracted from R_1, and the difference is squared. The null and alternative hypotheses are

H_0: There is no relationship between number of cigarettes smoked and severity of illness.
H_A: There is a relationship between number of cigarettes smoked and severity of illness.

Notice that the D column sums to zero. This column does not need to be summed, but it does serve as a check on our calculations. The difference between the ranks column should always sum to zero. Substituting our obtained values into the formula:

$$r_{rho} = 1 - [(6\Sigma D^2) / n(n^2 - 1)]$$
$$= 1 - [6(24)] / [8(64 - 1)]$$
$$= .71$$

To test the significance of rho, we use the Pearson r table (Appendix B, Table B–5), where df = $n - 2$. However, when the sample size is less than 10, we must use the t distribution where df = $n - 2$ (Appendix B, Table B–2). The formula for calculating t is

$$t = rho \sqrt{n-2} / \sqrt{1 - rho^2}$$

substituting in the formula

$$t = .71\sqrt{6} / \sqrt{1 - .71^2}$$
$$= 1.74 / .7$$
$$= 2.49$$

For six degrees of freedom, $\alpha = .05$, $t_{crit} = 2.447$; since the calculated t, 2.49, is greater than the critical t, it falls in the region of rejection. We therefore reject the null hypothesis and conclude that there is a statistically significant positive relationship between the number of cigarettes smoked and severity of illness.

The Spearman rho can also be calculated when one of the variables falls on the interval scale of measurement, but it is first necessary to convert the observations to ranks. As an example, we will calculate the Spearman rho for a data set in which variable X falls on the ordinal scale of measurement and variable Y falls on the interval scale, as in Table 10–2. Variable Y must be converted to ranks. The null and alternative hypotheses are

H_0: There is no relationship between variables X and Y.
H_A: There is a relationship between variables X and Y.
$\alpha = .05$

Table 10–2 Spearman rho for Ordinal and Interval-Level Data

Patient	X R₁	Y	R₂	Difference in Ranks D (R₁–R₂)	D²
1	8.5	135	6.5	2	4
4	8.5	120	9	−.5	.25
3	6	140	5	1	1
4	6	130	8	−2	4
5	6	135	6.5	−.5	.25
6	4	145	4	0	0
7	3	150	2.5	.5	.25
8	1.5	150	2.5	−1	1
9	1.5	160	1	.5	.25
				0	11

The calculations for the Spearman rho are

$$r_{\text{rho}} = 1 - \left(6\sum D^2\right) / n(n^2 - 1)$$
$$= 1 - [6(11)] / [9(81 - 1)]$$
$$= .91$$

Since we have a sample size that is less than 10, we evaluate the significance of rho by using *t*:

$$t = \text{rho } \sqrt{n-2} / \sqrt{1 - \text{rho}^2}$$

substituting in the formula

$$t = .91 \sqrt{7} / \sqrt{1 - .91^2}$$
$$= 2.41 / .41$$
$$= 5.88$$

The critical value of *t*, for seven degrees of freedom, $\alpha = .05$, is 2.365. Since the calculated *t* is greater than the critical *t*, it falls in the region of rejection. We reject the null hypothesis and conclude that there is a strong positive relationship between variables *X* and *Y*.

✓ To Obtain the Spearman Rho Using SPSS:

- From the "Analyze" menu, choose:
    →correlate
        →bivariate
- Select two numeric variables.
    →Select options.
        →Click "Spearman rho."

The SPSS output for the Spearman rho appears in Exhibit 10–1. SPSS does not require that interval-level data be recorded for the Spearman rho.

Exhibit 10-1 SPSS Output for Spearman rho

			X	*Y*
Spearman's rho	X	Correlation Coefficient	1.000	−.91*
		Sig. (2-tailed)	.	.001
		N	9	9
	Y	Correlation Coefficient	−.91*	1.000
		Sig. (2-tailed)	.001	.
		N	9	9

*Correlation is significant at the .01 level (2-tailed).

LOCATION TESTS FOR SINGLE AND PAIRED SAMPLES

The **sign test** and the **Wilcoxon signed ranks test** are used for analyzing data from single data sets or data collected in pairs. The results of these tests are inferences concerned with the median of a population (M) and the median (M_D) of the population differences for paired samples. These are examples of location tests. In a location test, we are concerned with the value of a measure of central tendency, or central location, and its associated confidence intervals. The parametric counterpart of these tests is the paired t test.

Sign Test

The sign test is used to test hypotheses about the location of a population distribution. The test is often used when evaluating data in the form of matched pairs—that is, "before" and "after" data such as pretests and posttests that are in the form of a single sample. In this case, the test is for a median difference of zero between the matched pairs rather than a mean difference of zero, as in the paired sample t test. The sign test does not require that the underlying population be normally distributed. In the sign test, the null hypothesis is stated as

$$H_0: M = M_0$$

As you recall, the median is the value that divides the area under the curve in half. In a normal distribution, the mean and median are equal. If the null hypothesis is true, M_0 is the central value—one-half of the observations in the sample should be larger than M_0, and one-half should be smaller. To evaluate the null, the sign statistic, S, is defined as

S = number of plus signs among the differences $X_1 - M_0, X_2 - M_0 \ldots X_n - M_0$.

The null distribution of S is the binomial distribution, with n and $p = 0.5$.

$$p(S = x) = \binom{n}{x}(.5)^x (.5)^{n-x}$$

The binomial distribution describes the possible number of times that an event will occur in a given number of trials. When using the binomial distribution, the variables of interest are at the nominal level of measurement and are dichotomous. We use the binomial distribution when we are interested in the frequency of occurrence of an event—for example, how many patients survived/did not survive a particular cancer treatment.

In using the binomial distribution, there must only be two possible mutually exclusive outcomes, such as survived/did not survive, yes/no, or success/failure. Each observation must be independent, and the outcome of one trial must not influence another. The two possible outcomes are designated as

p = probability that a successful event (x) will occur in a single trial
$1 - p$ = probability that a successful event (x) will not occur in a single trial

To determine the value of p or $1 - p$, it is necessary to know the number of ways in which success or failure can occur in a specified number of trials (n). This is obtained from the binomial coefficient $\binom{n}{x}$ where n equals the number of trials and x is the number of times a successful outcome will occur.

As an example, let's consider the probability of drawing a delinquent medical record from the incomplete file. We know that 10% of the records are delinquent at any one time. If we randomly select five records from the incomplete file, what is the probability that one will be delinquent? The binomial coefficient is $\binom{5}{1}$: that is, the number of possible combinations of an event where five records are randomly drawn with the probability of one delinquent record. This is illustrated as

$$D\ N\ N\ N\ N$$
$$N\ D\ N\ N\ N$$
$$N\ N\ D\ N\ N$$
$$N\ N\ N\ D\ N$$
$$N\ N\ N\ N\ D$$

(where D = delinquent record and N = nondelinquent record)

The formula for determining the probability of a designated number of successes $p(x)$ in n trials equals the number of possible combinations of the event multiplied by the probability of success, 10%, and failure.

$$p(x) = \binom{n}{x}(p)^x (1-p)^{n-x}$$

The probability of drawing one delinquent record in five trials is

$$p(1) = \binom{5}{1}(.10)^1 (1-.10)^{5-1}$$
$$= 5(.10)(.90)^4$$
$$= 5(.10)(.6561)$$
$$= 0.32805, \text{ or } .33$$

Thus, the probability that one delinquent record will be drawn in five trials is .33%, or 33%.

For sample sizes greater than 20, we can use the normal approximation to the binomial distribution with the test statistic z:

$$z = \frac{S - .5n \pm .5}{.5\sqrt{n}}$$

where $\pm .5$ is a continuity correction to improve the normal approximation to the binomial distribution. If the calculated sign statistic, S, is less than $.5n$, $+.5$ is used in the above formula; if S is greater than $.5n$, $-.5$ is used.

When calculating S, any difference between X_i and X_0 that is equal to zero is called zero. As long as zero differences are few, ignore them, and reduce the size of n accordingly.

Under the previously stated null hypothesis, there are two one-sided alternatives and one two-sided:

$$H_{A+}: M > M_0$$
$$H_{A-}: M < M_0$$
$$H_A: M \neq M_0$$

In the positive-sided alternative, we expect that the number of observations greater than M_0 will be large and that the calculated S will be large. Conversely, in the negative-sided alternative, we expect that the number of observations less than M_0 will be large and that the calculated S will be small.

We will now look at a hypothetical example for calculating the S statistic. In a health information management (HIM) coding class, the students have been reluctant to use encoding software to code ICD-9-CM diagnoses and procedures. The instructor believes that if the students used the computer program just once they would have a more positive attitude toward using it. To test this hypothesis, the instructor administers a pre- and postuse attitude assessment on the use of the computerized software. The assessment consisted of 20 questions, all stated in positive terms regarding computerized encoders. The null and alternative hypotheses are

$$H_0: M = M_0$$
$$H_A: M > M_0.$$

To test the hypothesis in the single-sample sign test, the average preuse assessment score for each item is subtracted from the average postuse assessment score for each item. The differences are recorded as either plus (greater posttest score) or minus (greater pretest score). The average difference for each item appears in Table 10–3.

Table 10–3 Pretest and Posttest Coding Results, Sign Test

Item	Average Pretest Posttest Difference	Sign	Item	Average Pretest Posttest Difference	Sign
1	+.3	+	11	−.3	−
2	+.1	+	12	+.5	+
3	−.4	−	13	+.1	+
4	+.2	+	14	+.2	+
5	+.5	+	15	−.5	−
6	+.3	+	16	+.4	+
7	−.2	−	17	+.1	+
8	+.6	+	18	+.3	+
9	+.4	+	19	+.2	+
10	−.1	−	20	+.1	+
					$S = 15$

Our calculations result in $S = 15$; that is, 15 plus signs. Conclusions for nonparametric tests are often reported in terms of the p value, and we use the binomial table, where $p = .50$, to determine the value of p when $n \leq 20$ (Appendix B, Table B–7). For a given n, the entry in the column labeled "p" is the left-tail cumulative probability for the corresponding number in the column labeled "Left S," and this same p value is the right-tail probability for the corresponding number in the column labeled "Right S." A partial table for the binomial distribution for $n = 20$ is presented in Exhibit 10–2.

Exhibit 10–2 Partial Binomial Distribution, $p = 0.50$

n	Left S	p	Right S
20	0	.0000	20
	1	.0000	19
	2	.0002	18
	3	.0013	17
	4	.0059	16
	5	.0207	15
	6	.0577	14
	7	.1316	13
	8	.2517	12
	9	.4119	11
	10	.5881	10

Source: Reprinted from National Bureau of Standards.

For our example, $n = 20$, the $\Pr(S \geq 15) = .0207$. Thus, we reject the null and conclude that students had a more positive attitude regarding computerized encoders after actually using the computer programs.

Using the same data, we can also calculate the corresponding large sample approximation (the continuity correction, -0.5, is used because $S > \frac{1}{2} n$):

$$z = \frac{S - .5n \pm .5}{.5\sqrt{n}}$$
$$= 15 - 10 - .5 / .5\sqrt{20}$$
$$= 4.5 / 2.24$$
$$= 2.01$$

The corresponding p value for $z = 2.01$ is .0222 (Appendix B, Table B–1).

The p value can also be calculated using the binomial test available on SPSS. From the "Analyze" menu, select "Nonparametric" and then select "Binomial." The p value must be set at .50 to correspond to the sign test. The results of the SPSS output appear in Exhibit 10–3. Note that the p value for the SPSS binomial test is .041—this is for a two-tailed test.

Exhibit 10–3 SPSS Output for Sign Test

| | Binomial Test | | |
| | PRE-, POSTTEST DIFFERENCES | | |
	Group 1	Group 2	Total
Category	positive	negative	
N	15	5	20
Observed Prop.	.75	.25	1.00
Test Prop.	.50		
Exact Sig. (2-tailed)	.041		

Dividing the p value in half, we obtain $p = .0205$, which is very close to the p value for the binomial distribution that appears in Exhibit 10–2.

The Wilcoxon Signed Ranks Test

In the sign test, the only information we used to calculate S was the signs of the differences between the pre- and posttest scores. Information regarding the size of the differences between the pre- and posttest scores was not considered. As we shall see, the Wilcoxon signed ranks test uses more information in its calculations and thus is a more powerful test. The Wilcoxon signed ranks test assumes that the observations are symmetric about the median M. If the underlying population is extremely nonsymmetric, the Wilcoxon signed ranks test should not be used. The assumptions for the Wilcoxon signed ranks test are summarized in Exhibit 10–4.

Exhibit 10–4 Assumptions for the Wilcoxon Signed Ranks Test

1. Data are paired observations from a single random sample either constructed as matched pairs or using subjects as controls.
2. Data are continuous and at least at the ordinal level of measurement.
3. There is symmetry of the difference scores about the true median for the population.

In the sign test discussed previously, we looked at the average differences for each item. We will now consider the differences in pre- and posttest scores for 15 students in the class. Here we will view the pre- and posttest scores as matched pairs—similar to the t test for matched pairs. What we want to know is whether there is a significant difference in the pre- and posttest medians. In the Wilcoxon signed ranks test, we calculate T where T_+ is the sum of the positive ranks and T_- is the sum of the negative ranks. To calculate T, we take the absolute values of the differences between the pre- and posttest scores, keeping track of the original positive and negative signs, and assign ranks from lowest to highest. In the example, the rankings will range from 1 to 15. If there are observations that are tied, we assign the average or the midpoint of the ranks they would have if they were not tied. The absolute values of the differences between pre- and posttest scores and their corresponding ranks appear in Table 10–4. The null and alternative hypotheses are the same as for the sign test:

$$H_0: M = M_0$$
$$H_{A+}: M > M_0$$

Table 10–4 The Sign Test of Pretest and Posttest Coding Results

Coder	Pretest Score	Posttest Score	Difference D	Sign	|D|	Rank
1	13	20	+7	+	7	11.5
2	15	16	+1	+	1	1
3	15	11	−4	−	4	5.5
4	12	16	+4	+	4	5.5
5	10	15	+5	+	5	7
6	8	11	+3	+	3	3.5
7	12	10	−2	−	2	2
8	9	15	+6	+	6	9
9	9	18	+9	+	9	14
10	5	12	+7	+	7	11.5
11	10	20	+10	+	10	15
12	7	1	−6	−	6	9
13	5	13	+8	+	8	13
14	16	10	−6	−	6	9
15	10	7	−3	−	3	3.5

$$S = 10$$
$$\Sigma T_+ = 91 \qquad \Sigma T_- = 29$$

Under the null hypothesis, we would expect that the sum of the positive rankings, T_+, would be similar to the sum of T_-. In our example, the sum of T_+ equals 91, and the sum of T_- equals 29—a wide difference in values. To determine the significance of T, we use the Wilcoxon signed ranks distribution of T. For $T_+ = 91$, $n = 15$, we obtain a p value of 0.042. We therefore reject the null and conclude that $M > 0$; thus, students' use of computerized encoders did have a positive impact on attitude.

Tables for the critical values of T are often not large enough for sample sizes greater than 15. When the sample size is greater than 15, the normal approximation must be used to calculate T, where

$$z = \frac{T - n(n+1)/4}{\sqrt{n(n+1)(2n+1)/24}}$$

where T is the sum of the positive or negative ranks, depending on the proposed alternative hypotheses, and n is the number of positive and negative ranks, excluding ties.

We can use SPSS to calculate the sign test and the Wilcoxon signed ranks test (Exhibit 10–5). For comparison purposes, the Student's t for matched pairs is also calculated (Exhibit 10–6). The p value for the Wilcoxon signed ranks test is given for the normal approximation of T. Since the p value is for a two-tailed test, we divide the given p value of .078 by 2, and the significance level becomes .039. Also, the p value for the Student's t test is for the two-sided alternative. For the one-sided alternative, where $t = 1.818$ and df = 14, the p value is .0455 (.091/2).

Exhibit 10–5 SPSS Output for Wilcoxon Signed Ranks Test

Ranks

POSTTEST–PRETEST

	Negative Ranks	Positive Ranks	Ties	Total
N	5[a]	10[b]	0[c]	15
Mean Rank	5.80	9.10		
Sum of Ranks	29.00	91.00		

[a] POSTTEST < PRETEST
[b] POSTTEST > PRETEST
[c] PRETEST = POSTTEST

Test Statistics[a]

	POSTTEST–PRETEST
Z	−1.763[b]
Asymp. Sig. (2-tailed)	.078

[a] Wilcoxon signed ranks test.
[b] Based on negative ranks.

Exhibit 10-6 SPSS Output for Student's *t* Test for Matched Pairs

Paired Samples Statistics

		Mean	*N*	*Std. Deviation*	*Std. Error Mean*
Pair 1	PRETEST	10.4000	15	3.4393	.8880
	POSTTEST	13.0000	15	5.0427	1.3020

Paired Samples Test

			Pair 1 PRETEST–POSTTEST
Paired Differences	Mean		−2.6000
	Std. Deviation		5.5395
	Std. Error Mean		1.4303
	95% Confidence Interval of the Difference	Lower	−5.6677
		Upper	.4677
t			−1.818
df			14
Sig. (2-tailed)			.091

✓ **To Obtain Wilcoxon Signed Ranks Test Using SPSS:**

- From the menus, choose:
  →statistics
  →nonparametric
  →2 related samples
- Select one or more pairs of variables.

MANN-WHITNEY WILCOXON TEST

When two independent samples violate the assumptions associated with the independent samples *t* test, the **Mann-Whitney Wilcoxon test**, also known as the Mann-Whitney *U* test (*U*) and the Wilcoxon rank sum test (*T* or *W*), may be used in its place. In this test, we are interested in comparing the medians of two independent samples, X and Y. The Mann-Whitney Wilcoxon test is based on the ranks of observations, with the two independent samples treated as one. Because the test takes into account the rankings of measurements in each sample, it uses more information than the previously discussed sign test.

For the Mann-Whitney Wilcoxon test, the null hypothesis is

$$H_0: M_X = M_Y$$

and the alternative hypotheses are

$$H_{T+}: M_X > M_Y$$
$$H_{T-}: M_X < M_Y$$
$$H_A: M_X \neq M_Y$$

The Mann-Whitney Wilcoxon statistic provides a measurement of the difference between the ranked observations of the two samples and provides evidence of the difference of the medians between the two populations. If the null was true, we would expect the average of the two summed ranks to be about the same. The total possible sum or all the ranks is determined by $N(N+1)/2$. In the example in Table 10–5, the sum of all the ranks is equal to 300; therefore, we would expect the ranks for each group to average 150 (300/2). If the average rank for hospital sample X is greater than the average rank for hospital sample Y, most of the physician satisfaction scores for hospital sample X will be greater than the physician satisfaction scores from sample Y, and vice versa. The procedure for calculating the Mann-Whitney Wilcoxon statistic is outlined in Exhibit 10–7.

Table 10–5 Calculation on Mann-Whitney Wilcoxon Statistic for Physician Satisfaction Levels in Hospital X and Hospital Y

	Hospital X			Hospital Y	
Doctor	Score	$Rank_X$	Doctor	Score	$Rank_Y$
1	7	7	13	15	17.5
2	6	5.5	14	14	15
3	4	2.5	15	15	17.5
4	11	10.5	16	16	21
5	16	21	17	16	21
6	4	2.5	18	16	21
7	10	9	19	14	15
8	6	5.5	20	12	12
9	9	8	21	14	15
10	3	1	22	17	24
11	13	13	23	16	21
12	5	4	24	11	10.5
		$\Sigma R_X = 89.5$			$\Sigma R_Y = 210.5$
		$R_X = 7.5$			$R_Y = 17.5$
		$T = 89.5$			

Exhibit 10–7 Calculation of Mann-Whitney Wilcoxon Statistic

---

1. Designate one sample as X and the other as Y. If the sample sizes are unequal, designate the sample with the fewest observations as sample X.
2. Rank all the observations in order from lowest to highest, without regard to whether the observation is from sample X or sample Y. If ranks are tied, assign the average of the ranks they would have if they were not tied.
3. The observations from the first sample are identified, and their ranks are summed. The result is the T statistic.
4. The calculated value of T is compared to the critical value of T. The critical value is related to the number of observations in sample X (n_1) and sample Y (n_2).

Let's consider an example. The director of HIM distributes a satisfaction survey to 12 physicians in the facility (hospital X) who are consistent users of HIM services. The same survey is distributed to 12 physicians at another hospital (hospital Y) within the corporate group. The lowest score that may be obtained on the instrument is 1, and the highest score is 20. The director wants to determine if there is a difference in the median levels of satisfaction between the two hospitals. The null and alternative hypotheses are

$$H_0: M_X = M_Y$$
$$H_A: M_X \neq M_Y$$

The results appear in Table 10–5.

To assign the ranks, as they appear in Table 10–5, we combine the 24 scores into a single ordered array; we keep track of which sample produced which score by underlining the scores from hospital X:

$$\underline{3}\ 4\ \underline{4}\ \underline{5}\ \underline{6}\ \underline{6}\ \underline{7}\ \underline{9}\ \underline{10}\ \underline{11}\ 11\ 12\ \underline{13}\ 14\ 14\ 14\ 15\ 15\ \underline{16}\ 16\ 16\ 16\ 16\ 17$$

From eyeballing the raw data, it appears that the physicians in hospital Y are more satisfied than physicians in hospital X—the scores from hospital X are generally lower than the scores from hospital Y. In addition, the sum of the ranks for the samples X and Y are markedly different from the expected sum, 150. The Mann-Whitney Wilcoxon statistic, T, is the sum of the ranks assigned to the X observations, or, as in this example, the sum of the ranks for physicians practicing in hospital X.

A large value of T_X supports the alternative hypothesis ($H_{T+}: M_X > M_Y$) and requires a right-tailed p value. A small value of T_X supports $H_{T-}: M_X < M_Y$ and requires a left-tailed p value. For the alternative $H_T: M_X \neq M_Y$, double the smallest p value.

To determine the critical values of T, refer to Appendix B, Table B–8. For $n_1 = 12$ and $n_2 = 12$, $\alpha = .05$, the critical values of X range from 120 to 180. The null is rejected if ΣR_X equals or falls below the lower number (120) or if it equals or exceeds the higher number (180). Since $\Sigma R_X < R_{crit}$ (120), we reject the null and conclude that the median level of physician satisfaction with HIM services is significantly different between the two hospitals.

An alternative to calculating T is the U statistic. U is calculated as

$$U_1 = n_1 n_2 + [n_1(n_1 + 1)/2] - \sum R_1$$
$$U_2 = n_1 n_2 + [n_2(n_2 + 1)/2] - \sum R_2$$

where n_1 is the number of observations in sample 1, n_2 is the number of observations in sample 2, R_1 is the sum of ranks for sample 1, and R_2 is the sum of ranks for sample 2. The null is rejected if the calculated value of U, the smaller of U_1 or U_2, is smaller than the critical value of U at the predetermined alpha level.

In our example, the Mann-Whitney U statistic is calculated as

$$
\begin{aligned}
U_1 &= n_1 n_2 + [n_1(n_1 + 1)/2] - \sum R_1 \\
&= (12)(12) + [12(12 + 1)/2] - 89.5 \\
&= 144 + 78 - 89.5 \\
&= 132.5
\end{aligned}
$$

$$
\begin{aligned}
U_2 &= n_1 n_2 + [n_2(n_2 + 1)/2] - \sum R_2 \\
&= (12)(12) + [12(12 + 1)/2] - 210.5 \\
&= 144 + 78 - 210.5 \\
&= 11.5
\end{aligned}
$$

The calculated U statistic is 11.5, $p < .05$.

The assumptions for the Mann-Whitney Wilcoxon test are summarized in Exhibit 10–8.

Exhibit 10–8 Assumptions for the Mann-Whitney Wilcoxon Test

1. The independent variable is dichotomous, and the scale of measurement for the dependent variable is at least ordinal.
2. Data are collected from a randomly selected sample of independent observations from two independent groups.
3. The categories of the independent variable are mutually exclusive.
4. The population distributions of the two independent samples share a similar unspecified shape but with a possible difference in measures of central tendency.

When sample sizes are too large to use the tables, an alternate method for determining statistical significance between the two groups is to calculate z, where

$$z = \frac{\sum R_1 - .5[n_1(n_1 + n_2 + 1)]}{\sqrt{n_1 n_2 (n_1 + n_2 + 1)/12}}$$

Using the data in Table 8–14, we have

$$z = \frac{89.5 - [.5(12)(12 + 12 + 1]}{\sqrt{(12 \times 12)(12 + 12 + 1)/12}}$$
$$= 89.5 - [150/\sqrt{300}\,]$$
$$= -3.5$$

For $\alpha = .05$, the critical value of z is -1.96. Since our calculated value, -3.5, falls in the region of rejection, we reject the null and conclude that the level of physician satisfaction between hospitals X and Y is significantly different.

The SPSS output for the Mann-Whitney U test appears in Exhibit 10–9. The Wilcoxon W, which is provided by default, is the same as our calculated T in Table 10–5. SPSS provides both the Wilcoxon W, which is the sum of the ranks of the smaller of U_1 and U_2, and the calculated z statistic, -3.514.

Exhibit 10–9 SPSS Output for Mann-Whitney Wilcoxon Test

Ranks

	Hospital	N	Mean Rank	Sum of Ranks
Rank	X	12	7.46	89.50
	Y	12	17.54	210.50
	Total	24		

Test Statistics[a]

	Rank
Mann-Whitney U	11.500
Wilcoxon W	89.500
Z	–3.514
Asymp. Sig. (2-tailed)	.000
Exact Sig. [2*(1-tailed) Sig.)]	.000[b]

[a] Grouping Variable: Hospital.
[b] Not corrected for ties.

✓ **To Obtain the Mann-Whitney U Using SPSS:**

- From the menu, choose "Analyze"
  - →nonparametric
    - →2 independent samples
- Select one or more numeric variables.
  - →Click "Mann-Whitney U."

KRUSKAL-WALLIS TEST

The nonparametric procedure that is comparable to analysis of variance (ANOVA) is the Kruskal-Wallis procedure. The **Kruskal-Wallis test** is used when the populations under study violate the assumptions of normality. The Kruskal-Wallis test does require that the samples be independent and that there be three or more groups ($k \geq 3$). The procedure for calculating the Kruskal-Wallis statistic, which is similar to that for the Mann-Whitney Wilcoxon statistic, is described in Exhibit 10–10.

Exhibit 10–10 Calculation of Kruskal-Wallis Statistic

---

1. Combine the k samples into one single ordered array.
2. Rank-order each observation from lowest to highest, keeping track of the samples. When ranks are tied, assign the average of the ranks that would have been assigned.
3. Sample sizes are noted by $n_1, n_2, \ldots n_k$. The sample sizes do not have to be equal.
4. Calculate the sum and average of the ranks for each sample $R_1, R_2, \ldots R_k$, and $R_1, R_2, \ldots R_k$.
5. Calculate the Kruskal-Wallis statistic Q. Let N be the size of the combined samples ($N = n_1 + n_2 + n_3 \ldots n_i$). Calculate the Q statistic according to

$$Q = 12 / N(N+1) \sum_{i=1}^{k} \frac{R_i^2}{n_i} - 3(N+1)$$

   where R_1 is the sum of the ranks in sample 1, etc.; n_1 is the number of cases in subgroup 1, etc.; and N is the number of cases in all samples.
6. The resulting Q statistic is compared to the critical value of χ^2 for $k - 1$ degrees of freedom.

Like the Mann-Whitney Wilcoxon test, the Kruskal-Wallis test is based on the ranks of the data. The null hypothesis is that all medians are equal:

$$H_0: M_1 = M_2 = M_3$$

The alternative hypothesis is that not all of the medians are the same:

$$H_A: M_1 \neq M_2 \neq M_3$$

Under the null hypothesis, we expect the average of the ranks for each group to be about equal. If the sum of all the ranks is equal to $N(N+1)/2$, we would expect that the sum of the ranks for each group would be the average of the sum of all the ranks $\dfrac{N(N+1)/2}{k}$. In the example in Table 10–6, there are 36 possible ranks, and the total sum of the ranks is (36 [(36+1)]/2), or 666. Therefore, we expect the sum of the ranks for each group to be 222. The Kruskal-Wallis test statistic Q, also referred to as the H statistic, is a function of the weighted

Table 10–6 Calculation of the Kruskal-Wallis Q Statistic for Physician Satisfaction Levels in Hospitals A, B, and C

Hospital A			Hospital B			Hospital C		
Phys	Score	Rank 1	Phys	Score	Rank 2	Phys	Score	Rank 3
1	7	7	13	15	24	25	10	10.5
2	6	5.5	14	14	19.5	26	20	36
3	4	2.5	15	15	24	27	18	35
4	11	12.5	16	16	28.5	28	13	15.5
5	16	28.5	17	16	28.5	29	14	19.5
6	4	2.5	18	16	28.5	30	8	8
7	10	10.5	19	14	19.5	31	17	33
8	6	5.5	20	12	14	32	17	33
9	9	9	21	14	19.5	33	14	19.5
10	3	1	22	17	33	34	14	19.5
11	13	15.5	23	16	28.5	35	15	24
12	5	4	24	11	12.5	36	16	28.5
		$\Sigma R_A = 104$			$\Sigma R_A = 280$			$\Sigma R_C = 282$
		$R_A = 8.67$			$R_A = 23.33$			$R_C = 23.5$

sum of squares of the deviations of the actual rank sums for each group from the expected rank sums for each group:

$$Q = 12 / N(N+1)\sum_{i=1}^{k} \frac{R_i^2}{n_i} - 3(N+1)$$

The value of the Q is a special case of the χ^2 distribution with $k-1$ degrees of freedom.

Referring to the procedure outlined in Exhibit 10–10, and extending the physician satisfaction problem to three samples instead of two, we can calculate the Kruskal-Wallis Q statistic (Table 10–6):

$$Q = 12 / N(N+1)\sum_{i=1}^{k} \frac{R_i^2}{n_i} - 3(N+1)$$

$$= 12 / 36(36+1)[(104^2 / 12) + (280^2 / 12) + (282^2 / 12)] - [3(36+1)]$$

$$= [(12 / 1,332) \times (901.33 + 6,533.33 + 6,627)] - 111$$

$$= (.009 \times 14,061.66) - 111$$

$$= 126.55 - 111$$

$$= 15.85$$

In the Kruskal-Wallis procedure, the degrees of freedom are equal to $k-1$, where k equals the number of groups. In our example, the number of groups is three; therefore, the df is equal to 2 ($k - 1 = 3 - 1 = 2$). With three groups and four or more cases per group, the χ^2 distribution can be used to evaluate the significance of Q_{calc}. For 2 degrees of freedom, $\alpha =$ .05, $\chi^2_{crit} = 5.991$. Since the calculated Q exceeds the critical value, we reject the null and conclude that the physician satisfaction level varies by hospital.

The result of the Kruskal-Wallis procedure indicates that there is a significant difference in the group medians. But which groups are different from each other? Just as with the ANOVA procedure, we can determine where the differences lie by conducting multiple pairwise comparisons. The number of possible comparisons that can be made is determined by $k(k-1)/2$; in our example we have three groups, so the total number of comparisons that can be made is three ($3[3-1]/2 = 3$). We would then compare hospitals A and B, A and C, and B and C. We can determine the value of the difference between the average ranks that must exist in order for the difference to be statistically significant by

$$\left| \overline{R}_i - \overline{R}_j \right| > Z_c \left[\sqrt{[N(N+1)/12][1/n_i + 1/n_j]} \right]$$

where z comes from the standard normal distribution, but not in the normal way. With c pairwise comparisons and an overall level of α, z_c is the critical value that corresponds to a right-tailed p value of $\alpha/2_c$. The value of $c = k(k-1)/2$. Now, what does this mean? Remember that when we use the t test or z, we are comparing two independent samples, and for a two-tailed test, when $\alpha = .05$, we cut 0.025 off each tail to determine significance. In this situation, we are going to make three comparisons, and if we use the same approach, we may be too conservative in our decision making, which could result in a type I error.

A more liberal method for making comparisons in this situation is called the Bonferroni test for inequality. In this method, we set a more liberal alpha—that is, 0.10—to better detect difference between groups. We then have

$$\alpha/k = 0.10/3 = 0.033$$

We then divide $\alpha/2$, as usual for our nondirectional test, which results in $0.033/2 = .017$. The critical value of z, $\alpha = .017$, is 2.128 (from Appendix B, Table B–1). The absolute difference between the average of the ranks that must be achieved is

$$\left| \overline{R}_i - \overline{R}_j \right| > Z_c \left[\sqrt{[N(N+1)/12][1/n_i + 1/n_j]} \right]$$
$$= 2.128\sqrt{[36(36+1)/12][1/12 + 1/12]}$$
$$= 2.128\sqrt{111(.083 + .083)}$$
$$= 2.128(4.3)$$
$$= 9.15$$

Comparing the absolute values of the average ranks, we have

$$\left| \overline{R}_A - \overline{R}_B \right| = \left| 8.67 - 23.33 \right| = 14.66$$
$$\left| \overline{R}_A - \overline{R}_c \right| = \left| 8.67 - 23.50 \right| = 14.83$$
$$\left| \overline{R}_c - \overline{R}_B \right| = \left| 23.50 - 23.33 \right| = 0.17$$

Thus we determine that the median for hospital A is significantly different from the medians for hospitals B and C.

Carrying out these calculations by hand can become quite tedious. We can use SPSS to carry out the calculations for us. From the "Statistics" menu, we select "nonparametric statistics." To conduct the Kruskal-Wallis test, we select the option for "k independent samples." The grouping variable is "hospital," and the test variable is "score." Notice that SPSS (Exhibit 10–11) gives the average rank for each group rather than the sum of the ranks for each group. However, the resulting Kruskal-Wallis χ^2 statistic is 15.851. SPSS does not provide post hoc procedures for the Kruskal-Wallis statistic.

Exhibit 10–11 SPSS Output for Kruskal-Wallis Test

Descriptive Statistics

	N	Mean	Std. Deviation	Minimum	Maximum
SCORE	36	12.3889	4.4994	3.00	20.00
Hospital	36	2.0000	.8281	1.00	3.00

Ranks

	Hospital	N	Mean Rank
SCORE	A	12	8.67
	B	12	23.33
	C	12	23.50
	Total	36	

Test Statistics[a,b]

	SCORE
Chi Square	15.851
df	2
Asymp. Sig.	.000

[a] Kruskal-Wallis Test.
[b] Grouping Variable: Hospital.

✓ To Obtain the Kruskall-Wallis Statistic Using SPSS:

- From the menus, choose "Analyze":
    - → nonparametric
        - →κ independent samples
- Select one or more numeric variables.
- Select a grouping variable.
    - →Click "define range" to specify minimum and maximum integer values for the grouping variable.

CONCLUSION

In this chapter, we have explored nonparametric statistical procedures other than chi square. Nonparametric procedures are less restrictive than their parametric counterparts. Nonparametric procedures do not make assumptions regarding the underlying population distribution nor do they require large sample sizes. Nonparametric methods may also be used for the nominal and ordinal scales of measurement.

For assessing relationships between variables, we can use the Spearman rho correlation coefficient, which is analogous to the Pearson r product moment correlation coefficient. If we are interested in making comparisons between two independent samples, we can use the Mann-Whitney Wilcoxon test as a substitute for the Student's t and ANOVA parametric procedures. For paired samples, nonparametric procedures include the sign test and the Wilcoxon signed ranks test. The corresponding parametric procedure is Student's paired t test. If we are interested in comparing three or more independent samples, the Kruskal-Wallis test is the nonparametric alternative to the ANOVA procedure.

ADDITIONAL RESOURCES

Besag, F.P., and P.L. Besag. 1985. *Statistics for the helping professions*. Beverly Hills, CA: Sage Publications.

Fleiss, J.L. 1981. *Statistical methods for rates and proportions*. New York: John Wiley & Sons.

Gibbon, J.D. 1993. *Nonparametric statistics: An introduction*. Newbury Park, CA: Sage Publications.

Hollander, M., and D. Wolfe. 1973. *Nonparametric statistical methods*. New York: John Wiley & Sons.

Jekel, J.F., et al. 1996. *Epidemiology, biostatistics and preventive medicine*. Philadelphia: W.B. Saunders.

Pett, M.A. 1997. *Nonparametric statistics for health care research: Statistics for small samples and unusual distribution*. Thousand Oaks, CA: Sage Publications.

Statsoft Electronic Textbook. 1998. www.statsoft.com/textbook/

Appendix 10–A

Exercises for Solving Problems

KNOWLEDGE QUESTIONS

1. Define the key terms listed at the beginning of this chapter.

2. Compare the Pearson r with the Spearman rho correlation coefficient.

3. Under what conditions is it appropriate to use the sign test?

4. Under what conditions is it appropriate to use the Wilcoxon signed ranks test?

5. Under what conditions is it appropriate to use the Mann-Whitney Wilcoxon test?

6. Under what conditions is it appropriate to use the Kruskal-Wallis test?

MULTIPLE CHOICE

1. The Spearman rho rank order correlation coefficient:
   a. is used for ordered data
   b. has the same interpretation as the Pearson r
   c. may be used when one sample is ordered and the second sample is at the ratio level of measurement
   d. a and b
   e. all of the above

2. The sign test is an alternative approach to test a hypothesis about:
   a. a single mean
   b. the difference between matched pairs
   c. the difference between two independent samples
   d. the difference between three or more independent samples

3. The sign test is not as likely to detect statistical significance as its parametric counterpart. This means that:
   a. the probability of making a type II error is increased
   b. the sign test is less powerful than its parametric counterpart
   c. the sign test is not as sensitive as its parametric counterpart
   d. all of the above

4. Nonparametric procedures:
   a. are appropriate for ordered data
   b. have less power than their parametric counterparts
   c. have fewer assumptions regarding the underlying population distribution than their parametric counterparts
   d. b and c
   e. all of the above

5. The parametric counterpart of the Kruskal-Wallis procedure is the:
   a. paired t test
   b. independent sample t test
   c. t test for two independent samples
   d. analysis of variance (ANOVA)

6. The sum of a set of ranks may be found by:
   a. $n(n-1)/2$
   b. $n(n+1)/2$
   c. $(n-1)/2$
   d. $(n-1)^2$

PROBLEMS

1. You are analyzing length of stay by physician for DRG 14, Specific Cerebrovascular Disorder except TIA. You are focusing on three physicians that you have coded as 1, 2, and 3. The lengths of stay for the patients of these three physicians appear in Exhibit 10–A–1. Since the sample size for each physician is small, you decide to conduct the Kruskal-Wallis test to compare the mean lengths of stay.

   a. State the null and alternative hypotheses.
   b. State the alpha level.
   c. What is the result of the Kruskal-Wallis test?
   d. State your conclusions.

Exhibit 10–A–1 LOS Physician Crosstabulation (SPSS Output)

Count		Physician			
		1.00	*2.00*	*3.00*	*Total*
LOS	2.00		2		2
	3.00	3	1	2	6
	4.00	1		2	3
	5.00	1	2		3
	6.00			1	1
	8.00			1	1
	9.00			1	1
	17.00	1			1
	18.00	1			1
Total		7	5	7	19

2. You want to determine if more women than men are discharged from DRG 239, Pathological Fractures and Musculoskeletal and Connective Tissue Malignancy. You believe that since more women than men suffer from osteoporosis, that more women should be discharged from this DRG. The frequency distribution of discharges by sex appears in Table 10–A–1. You decide to use the sign test (binomial test) to determine if there is a difference in the proportion of discharges by sex for DRG 239.

   a. State the null and alternative hypotheses.
   b. State the alpha level.
   c. What is the result of the sign test?
   d. State your conclusions.

Table 10–A–1 Frequency Distribution of Discharges from DRG 239 by Sex

	Frequency	%	Valid %	Cumulative %
Male	5	31.3	31.3	31.3
Female	11	68.8	68.8	100.0
Total	16	100.0	100.0	

3. Review Exhibit 10–A–2 for discharges from DRG 82, Respiratory Neoplasms. Use the Mann-Whitney *U* test to determine if there is a difference in age by sex and length of stay by sex for discharges from DRG 82.

   a. State the null and alternative hypotheses.
   b. State the alpha level.
   c. What are the results of the Mann-Whitney *U* tests?
   d. State your conclusions.

Exhibit 10–A–2 Case Summaries for Discharges from DRG 82[a] (SPSS Output)

						PRIM_DX	*DX_1*	*DX–2*	*DX_3*	*LOS*	*AGE*
SEX	Male	DRG	82	1		1972	1629	78609		4.00	66.00
				2		1623	7863	4254	4292	2.00	82.00
				3		1629	49120	4241	4169	5.00	71.00
				4		1629	1977	42731		1.00	55.00
				5		1623	2639	2800	1649	6.00	47.00
				6		1623	7863	5121	3320	11.00	80.00
			Total	N		6	6	6	6	6	6
		Total	N			6	6	6	6	6	6
	Female	DRG	82	1		1620	49320	1971	27800	4.00	63.00
				2		1624	5119			6.00	56.00
				3		1625	1539	5609	1983	4.00	81.00
				4		1951	7895	5119	4019	6.00	74.00
				5		1972	1991	25000		1.00	70.00
				6		2357				1.00	59.00
				7		1972	2765	1991		6.00	94.00
				8		1629	496	2765	5128	7.00	67.00
				9		1972	2761	1991	25000	10.00	70.00
				10		1629	496	5128	4019	4.00	67.00
				11		1970	42731	2765	486	1.00	78.00
				12		1629				1.00	72.00
				13		1972	1629	5640	4019	6.00	80.00
				14		1629	1985	2761	1972	1.00	71.00
				15		1629	1983	490		7.00	55.00
				16		1629	1985	486	5180	4.00	80.00
				17		1629	78609	5183		1.00	83.00
			Total	N		17	17	17	17	17	17
		Total	N			17	17	17	17	17	17
	Total	N				23	23	23	23	23	23

[a] Limited to first 100 cases.

Glossary

Age-adjusted death rate—The crude death rate is adjusted when population proportions by age are different; this adjustment eliminates the effects of different age distributions in different populations; the crude death rate is adjusted when the death rates of two populations are to be compared.

Age-specific death rate (ASDR)—The total number of deaths for a given age group for a certain time frame divided by the estimated population for the same age group and for the same time frame; the ASDR is usually expressed as the number of deaths per 10^n depending on the size of the population.

Alpha error—See **type I error**.

Alpha level—The point at which the null hypothesis will be rejected. The alpha level, which is set prior to conducting the research, is usually set at .05 for small sample sizes and at .01 for larger sample sizes.

Alternative hypothesis—See **hypothesis testing**.

Analysis of variance (ANOVA)—A statistical method for comparing the differences between two or more means for statistical significance; the independent variable is usually nominal, and the dependent variable is at the ratio or interval level of measurement.

Apparent limits—See **class interval**.

Asymptotic curve—A property of the normal distribution in which the tails of the curve approach the x-axis but never touch it.

Attributable risk—A measure of the impact of a disease on a population; measures additional risk of illness as a result of exposure to the risk factor.

Bar chart—A graphic technique for displaying discrete or nominal-level data; one or more variables may be displayed in a bar chart; a bar chart that displays two or more variables is called a grouped bar chart.

Beta error—See **type II error**.

Between-group variance (SSB)—See **sum of squares between**.

Box head—In a table, the box head contains the column headings.

Case fatality rate—The total number of deaths due to a specific illness during a given time period divided by the total number of cases during the same time period.

Cause-specific death rate—The total number of deaths due to a specific cause during a given time interval divided by the estimated mid-interval population.

Cell—In a table, a cell is where the row and column variables intersect.

Central limit theorem—In a repeated number of random samples of size N drawn from a population, the distribution of the sample means approaches the normal distribution as N becomes large. This occurs even when the population distribution is not normal.

Chi-square goodness-of-fit test—See χ^2 **goodness-of-fit test.**

Chi-square test of independence—See χ^2 **test of independence**.

Class interval—A method used to classify interval/ratio level data into categories for analysis; the limits of the class intervals are referred to as either "apparent" or "real." The apparent limits are the upper and lower boundaries of the class interval. For example, the upper and lower limits of two successive intervals may be 18–22 and 23–27. The real limits depict the continuous nature of the frequency distribution, indicating that there are no gaps between successive intervals. For example, the real limits for previously stated intervals are 17.5–22.5 and 22.5–27.5. The upper limit of one class interval is the lower limit for the next class interval.

Cluster sampling—A sampling technique in which the sampling units are groups rather than individuals.

Coefficient alpha—See **Cronbach's alpha**.

Coefficient of determination—The square of the Pearson r. States how much of the variation in the dependent variable Y is explained by the independent variable X.

Confidence interval—Calculated from the standard error of the mean, it is an estimate of the true limits within which the true population mean lies; the range of values that may reasonably contain the true population mean.

Confounding—The relationship between two variables is so close that the effects of either variable cannot be separated from the other.

Confounding factor—See **confounding variable**.

Confounding variable—A factor or variable that contributes differentially across the categories or levels of another variable; confusion of two independent variables so that the effect of one variable cannot be differentiated from the effect of the other.

Construct validity—A type of validity that is the link between a theory and the property being measured; a measurement instrument with construct validity is representative of the property of interest.

Content validity—The adequacy of the sample or number of items used to represent the content area being measured; content validity is a matter of judgment and is evaluated by a panel of experts.

Contingency coefficient—A measure of association between two nominal level variables; it is an alternative to the phi coefficient when one variable has more than two categories; the range of the contingency coefficient is 0 to 1.

Contingency table—A table that displays the relationship between two variables, whether the distribution of one variable is dependent on or related to the distribution of a second variable.

Continuous variable—A measure taken on the interval or ratio level of measurement.

Cramer's V—A statistic used to adjust the χ^2 statistic for sample size. It is a measure of correlation coefficient with a range of 0.0 to 1.0. It is used in place of the phi coefficient when the contingency table is greater than 2×2.

Criterion-related validity—A type of validity in which a measuring instrument correlates with a criterion known to accurately measure the property of interest.

Critical region—In hypothesis testing, the portion of the test statistic distribution that is equal to or beyond the critical value of the test statistic; the region of the z, t, F, or χ^2 distribution that results in rejection of the null hypothesis.

Cronbach's alpha—Also coefficient alpha. A measure of internal consistency. Cronbach's alpha has a range of 0.0 to 1.0; the minimum acceptable criterion for internal consistency is .70.

Crude death rate—The total number of deaths in a given population for a given time period divided by the mid-interval population for the same time period; the crude death rate is usually expressed as the number of deaths per 1,000 population.

Death-to-case ratio—The total number of deaths due to a specific disease during a given time period divided by the number of new cases of the disease reported during the same time period.

Degrees of freedom—The number of observations in a data set that are free to vary after the mean of the distribution has been determined.

Dichotomous variable—A variable that falls on the nominal scale of measurement but is limited to only two categories.

Direct standardization—When mortality rates of two populations are compared, each population is assigned the same standard population proportion for each age group; the standard population proportion is multiplied by the age-specific death rate for each age group in each population; the sum results in the age-adjusted death rate.

Discrete variable—A dichotomous or nominal variable whose values are placed into categories.

Effect—A change in one variable that may be associated with a change in the second variable.

F test—The ratio of the between-group variance (SSB) to the within-group variance (SSW) in the ANOVA procedure. If the F ratio is statistically significant, the observed differences between the group means of the independent variables under study will be significantly different from each other.

Fisher's exact test—A statistical test that is used as a substitute for the χ^2 test of independence when the frequencies in a contingency table are less than or equal to 20.

Footnote—See **note**.

Frequency distribution—A table or graph that displays the number of times (frequency) a particular observation occurs.

Frequency polygon—A line graph of a frequency distribution of interval or ratio level data.

Grouped bar chart—Used to illustrate data from a two- or three-variable table when an outcome variable has only two categories; the bars within a group are adjoining.

Histogram—A graphic technique used to display the frequency distribution of interval or ratio level data; the frequency distribution can be displayed as either numbers or percentages in a series of bars.

Hypothesis testing—A statement regarding the research question to be tested. There are two forms of the hypothesis: the null hypothesis and the alternative hypothesis. The null hypothesis states that there is no difference between the population means or proportions that are being compared; or that there is no association between the two variables that are being compared. The alternative hypothesis states that there is a significant difference in the population means or proportions that are being compared; or that there is an association between the two variables that are being compared. The alternative hypothesis usually states what the researcher believes to be true regarding the problem under study.

Incidence rate—The number of new cases of a particular disease in a population for a given time period divided by the average population for the same time period.

Individuality—For nominal level data, the circumstance in which the number of observations in a given category is limited to one.

Infant mortality rate—The number of deaths of persons under one year of age during a given time period divided by the number of live births reported during the same time period.

Intercept—Represented by a in the regression model. It is the point at which the regression line crosses the y axis. The intercept is the average value of Y when X is equal to zero.

Internal consistency—The extent to which the items on a measuring instrument are consistent with one another; Cronbach's alpha is used to evaluate internal consistency.

Interrater agreement—See **interrater reliability**.

Interrater reliability—The percentage of agreement between raters using the same measuring instrument; the kappa coefficient is used to measure interrater agreement.

Interval scale—Similar to the ratio scale of measurement, but there is no true zero; intervals between successive intervals are equal and continuous.

Kaplan Meier survival analysis—A statistical method used to analyze the survival time of individuals with a specific disease; it is most often used in analyzing the survival time of cancer patients.

Kappa coefficient—A measure of agreement, beyond what would occur by chance, between two raters on the same measuring instrument. The Kappa coefficient ranges from 0.0 to 1.0.

Kruskal-Wallis test—The nonparametric counterpart to the ANOVA procedure; it is used to compare two or more groups of ordinal data.

Kurtosis—The vertical stretching of a frequency distribution.

Level of significance (or significance level)—A cutoff value for evaluating the p value that results from a statistical test; indicates the level of risk that we are willing to take for rejecting the null hypothesis when it is true.

Line graph—A graphic technique that consists of a line connecting a series of points on an arithmetic scale; a line graph is often used to display time trends and survival curves; a line graph does not represent a frequency distribution.

Linear regression—A statistical test used to measure the strength of the linear relationship between two variables; the variables under study are at the interval or ratio level of measurement.

Line of best fit—See **regression line**.

Mann-Whitney *U* test—also known as the **Mann-Whitney Wilcoxon test**. The nonparametric counterpart to the Student's *t* test for two independent samples; used to compare two groups of ordinal-level data.

Mann-Whitney Wilcoxon Test—see **Mann-Whitney *U* Test**.

Maternal mortality rate—The number of deaths assigned to pregnancy-related causes during a given time period divided by the total number of live births during the same period.

McNemar test—The nonparametric test used for paired data; analogous to the paired *t* test.

Mean—A measure of central tendency; arithmetic average of the observations in a frequency distribution; the sum of the values of the observations in a frequency distribution divided by the total number of observations.

Mean square—Also known as the **variance**. The sum of squares divided by the appropriate number of degrees of freedom.

Measurement—The process of measuring an attribute or property of a person, object, or event according to a particular set of rules; the set of rules is used to assign numbers to the attribute or property being measured.

Measures of central tendency—A single value that summarizes a frequency distribution or illustrates the most typical value in a frequency distribution; measures of central tendency are the mean, median, and the mode. The measure selected to represent the data set depends on the characteristics and shape of the distribution.

Measures of variation—Describes how much spread there is in a frequency distribution; measures of variation include the range, standard deviation, and the variance.

Median—A measure of central tendency; midpoint of a frequency distribution when the observations have been arranged in order from lowest to highest; point at which 50% of the observations fall above and 50% of the observations fall below.

Mode—A measure of central tendency; the most frequently occurring observation in a frequency distribution.

Mortality rate—See **crude death rate.**

Multicollinearity—In multiple regression, when two independent variables are highly correlated with one another, and it is difficult to separate the effects of each independent variable on the dependent variable.

Multiple regression—A statistical procedure used to explain the effects of two or more independent variables on a dependent variable; it is an extension of the linear regression model.

Neonatal death rate—The number of deaths of newborns under 28 days of age during a given time period divided by the number of live births during the same time period.

Neonatal mortality rate—See **neonatal death rate**.

Nominal scale—A level of measurement in which the frequencies of observations on variables are placed into categories.

Noncritical region—In hypothesis testing, the area of the test statistic distribution that is between the critical values of the test statistic; if the calculated value of the test statistic falls within this region, we fail to reject the null hypothesis.

Nonparametric statistical tests—Tests used to test for statistical significance when the underlying population distribution does not meet the requirements of the normal distribution or when sample sizes are small.

Normal distribution—A continuous frequency distribution characterized by a bell-shaped curve; a normal distribution is symmetrical with 50% of the values falling above the mean and 50% of the values falling below the mean.

Note—Explanation that appears below a table, chart, or graph to explain symbols or abbreviations that may have been used in the table, chart, or graph.

Null hypothesis—See **hypothesis testing**.

Odds ratio—A relative measure of occurrence of an illness; the odds of exposure in a diseased group divided by the odds of exposure in a nondiseased group.

One-sample *t* test—See *t* **tests**.

100% component bar chart—A variant of the stacked bar chart; all bars in the chart are of the same height; each bar displays the variable categories as percents of the total number; each bar is like its own pie chart.

One-tailed test (directional test)—In hypothesis testing, the researcher is trying to determine if the sample mean is greater than or less than the population parameter.

Ordinal scale—Scale of measurement in which measures are placed into ordered categories or measures are ranked in some predetermined order such as lowest score on a test to highest score on a test; the width between categories or ranks may not be equal.

Outliers—Extreme values in a frequency distribution.

p **value**—The probability that the observed difference could have been obtained by chance alone, given random variation and a single test of the null hypothesis.

Paired *t* test—See *t* **test**.

Parametric statistical tests—Statistical tests of significance used when the underlying population distributions are assumed to be normal.

Pearson *r* correlation coefficient—A measure of the strength of the linear association between two variables that fall on the interval or ratio level of measurement. The Pearson *r* correlation coefficient has a range of -1.0 to $+1.0$; a negative correlation indicates that the variables change in opposite direction to one another, a positive correlation that the variables change in the same direction and a correlation of 0.0 that there is no relationship between the two variables.

Phi coefficient—A measure that indicates the degree of association between two nominal level variables; the range of the phi coefficient is 0 to 1; it has the same interpretation as the Pearson *r* product moment correlation coefficient.

Pie chart—A graphic technique in which the proportions of a nominal variable are displayed as "pieces" of the pie.

Point estimate—The numerical value calculated from a sample that is assumed to best represent the population parameter.

Point prevalence rate—The number of current cases, both new and old, of a specified disease at a given point in time compared to the estimated population at the same point in time; the point prevalence rate is usually expressed as the number of cases per 10^n, depending on the size of the population.

Polarization—The maximum spread or variability in a frequency distribution.

Population—All members of a group that is under study; the group to which the sample results are generalizable; members of the group share some measurable characteristic.

Population parameter—A measure that results from the compilation of data from a population.

Post hoc procedures—Statistical follow-up tests following the ANOVA procedure when three or more means are being compared; the post hoc test indicates whether all means compared are significantly different from each other or if only several are significantly different from each other.

Postneonatal mortality rate—The number of deaths of persons aged 28 days up to and not including one year during a given time period divided by the number of live births for the same time period.

Predictive value—The number of cases correctly identified by a measure out of the total number of cases with the property of interest.

Prevalence rate—The number of cases of a particular disease in a population for a given time period divided by the population for the same time period.

Proportion—A particular type of ratio; in a proportion, the numerator is always included in the denominator.

Proportionate mortality ratio (PMR)—The total number of deaths due to a specific cause during a given time period divided by the number of deaths due to all causes. Proportionate mortality is not a rate because the denominator is the number of deaths during the time period, not the population size during the time period.

Race-specific death rate—The number of deaths in a specific ethnic group for a given time frame compared to the estimated population total for the same ethnic group for the same time frame; the race-specific death rate is usually expressed as the number of deaths per 10^n, depending on the size of the population.

Range—A measure of variability; the difference between the smallest and largest values in a frequency distribution.

Rate—A measure used to compare an event over time; comparison of the number of times an event did happen (numerator) to the number of times an event could have happened (denominator); rates are expressed as the event of interest per 100, 1,000, 10,000, or 100,000 cases.

Ratio—A comparison of categories of dichotomous variables either to each other (e.g., male discharges to female discharges), or of one category to the whole (e.g., male discharges to total discharges).

Ratio scale—The highest level of measurement; intervals between successive intervals are equal and continuous; measurement scale with a true zero.

Real limits—See **class interval**.

Regression line—The slope in the regression model. It is the straight line that best fits all of the data points in the regression problem. If the correlation is perfect, the regression line will go through all of the data points simultaneously.

Relative risk—See **risk ratio**.

Reliability—A characteristic of a measuring instrument that results in consistent measures over repeated trials; measurement results are approximately the same on repeated trials.

Risk ratio—Also called relative risk. A ratio that compares the risk of disease between two groups.

Sample—Items drawn from a population for a study; ideally, members of the sample are drawn randomly and independently from the population of interest; a subset of the population under study.

Sampling method—The process of selecting individuals from a larger group or population in such a way that the resultant sample is representative of the underlying population.

Scales of measurement—Nominal, ordinal, interval, and ratio scales of measurement. The level at which data are collected determines the types of statistics that may be used to describe the population under study.

Sample statistic—The measures that result from analysis of data compiled from samples.

Scatter diagram—A graphic representation of the X and Y variables. The X variable is plotted on the horizontal axis and the Y variable is plotted on the vertical axis. It is used to assess the linearity of the relationship between variables X and Y when conducting either the Pearson r or simple linear regression. If the two variables appear to approximate a straight line, the variables are linearly related.

Scheffé test—A post hoc test used in the analysis of variance procedure when there are three or more sample means being compared. It is a test used to determine which of the means are significantly different from each other.

Sensitivity—An aspect of data accuracy (validity); a measure is sensitive if it identifies the property of interest when that property is truly present.

Sex-specific death rate—The number of male or female deaths for a given time frame compared to the estimated male or female population total for the same time frame; the sex-specific death rate is usually expressed as the number of deaths per 10^n, depending on the size of the population.

Sign test—The nonparametric counterpart to the paired-sample t test; compares whether one group did better than another group.

Simple random sampling—A sampling technique in which each member of a population has an equal chance of being included in the sample.

Skewness—The horizontal stretching of a frequency distribution.

Slope—In the regression model, the slope (b) represents the average change in Y that is associated with X. The greater the slope, the greater the change in Y that is associated with a change in X, and the greater the relationship between X and Y.

Source—A statement following a table, chart, or graph that indicates the resource used to generate the table, chart, or graph.

Spearman rho—The nonparametric counterpart of the Pearson r used when one of the variables is ordered; the interpretation of the Spearman rho is the same as that for the Pearson r.

Specificity—An aspect of data accuracy (validity); a measure that is specific excludes cases when the property of interest is truly absent.

SSB—See **sum of squares between**.

SSW—See **sum of squares within**.

Stability—A type of reliability in which the same or similar results are obtained on repeated measures by administering the same instrument to the same group on two different occasions to obtain a reliability coefficient that ranges from 0.0 (no reliability) to 1.0 (perfect reliability).

Stacked bar chart—A type of bar chart in which the categories of a nominal level variable are stacked like building blocks on top of one another to form a single bar; the bar represents the total number of cases that occurred in the category and the segments represent the frequencies within the category.

Standard deviation—A measure of variability; square root of the variance; describes deviation from the mean in terms of the original unit of measurement (e.g., height, age, blood pressure).

Standard error of the estimate—In linear regression, a measure of the scatter or spread of the observed values of Y around the corresponding values of Y estimated from the regression equation.

Standard error of the mean—A measure of how close the sample mean is to the population mean; it is influenced by the sample size and standard deviation.

Standard mortality rate—See **standard mortality ratio**.

Standard mortality ratio (SMR)—Compares the actual number of deaths in a group or population under study compared to the expected number of deaths based on standard population death rates applied to the study group or population; this measure is always multiplied by 100.

Standard normal deviate—In the standard normal distribution, the distance between the observed value and the mean, μ; it is also referred to as the z score or z value.

Standard normal distribution—A normal distribution with a mean equal to zero and a standard deviation equal to one.

Standardized residuals—In the χ^2 test of independence, a residual is the difference between the observed cell frequencies and the expected cell frequencies. To obtain the standardized residual, the difference between the observed and expected cell frequencies for each cell is divided by the square root of the expected cell frequency. An obtained standardized residual of greater than +2 or less than –2 is an indication that the cell in question is an important contributor to the calculated χ^2.

Statistical power analysis—Statistical power analysis assists the researcher in determining the appropriate sample size for conducting a statistical test while controlling for both type I and type II error.

Statistical significance—In hypothesis testing, when a statistical test results in a p value that is less than or equal to the preset alpha level; this is usually set at .05 for small samples and .01 for large samples. The interpretation of the p value is that the result obtained would occur by chance no more than 5 out of 100 times when $p = .05$, or 1 out of 100 times when $p = .01$.

Stratified random sampling—A sampling technique in which each stratum within a population is proportionately represented in the sample.

Stub—The row captions in a table.

Sum of squares between (SSB)—In the analysis of variance procedure, the SSB is the variation of the sample means around the grand mean.

Sum of squares within (SSW)—In the analysis of variance procedure, the SSW is the variation of the observations in each sample around their respective sample means.

Symmetrical—See **symmetry**.

Symmetry—A property of the normal distribution in which 50% of the observations fall above the mean and 50% of the observations fall below the mean.

Systematic sampling—A sampling technique in which every kth member of a population is selected for inclusion in the sample.

t **statistic**—A statistic that follows the t distribution; see *t* **test.**

t **test**—A parametric statistical test that compares the difference between the means of two groups; the t test may be used when comparing a single sample mean to a known population parameter (independent sample t test), when comparing the means of two independent samples (*t* test for two independent samples), or when comparing the means of matched pairs (paired *t* test).

***t* test for comparing two independent sample means**—See *t* test.

Table—A set of data arranged in rows and columns.

Table shell—Prepared prior to collection of data to show how the data will be organized and displayed after data collection; table shells are complete except for the actual data; table shells show titles, headings, and categories.

Test-retest reliability—See **stability**.

Timeliness—The collection, analysis, and reporting of data/information within a time frame useful for decision making.

Total sum of squares (TSS)—In the analysis of variance procedure, the TSS is the variation of all the observations (combined into one sample) around the grand mean.

Trimmed mean—The calculation of the mean or a frequency distribution after the elimination (trimming) of outliers from the distribution.

TSS—See **total sum of squares**.

Tukey HSD—A post hoc test used in the analysis of variance procedure when there are three or more sample means being compared. It is a test used to determine which of the sample means are significantly different from each other.

Two-tailed test (nondirectional test)—In hypothesis testing, the researcher is interested in determining whether the sample mean and the population parameter are significantly different from each other; the direction of the inequality is not an issue.

Type I error—Also called alpha error; the rejection of the null hypothesis when it is true.

Type II error—Also called beta error; failure to reject the null hypothesis when it is false.

Uniformity—Even distribution of observations in the categories of a nominal variable.

Unimodal—Property of the normal distribution in which there is only one mode.

Validity—Accuracy in measurement; a valid measuring instrument accurately measures what it is intended to measure.

Variable—A characteristic or property that may take on different values.

Variance—A measure of variability; the average of the squared deviations from the mean; measures variability in original units of measurement squared.

Weighted mean—A mean that takes into account differences in sample size; the weighted mean is equal to the sum of the means times the number of observations in each sample divided by the total number of observations in the samples combined.

Wilcoxon signed ranks test—The nonparametric counterpart of the paired *t* test; used when sample sizes are small or when the underlying population distribution is not normally distributed.

Winsorized mean—A type of mean (average) which has been adjusted for extreme values in the frequency distribution; the most extreme values (highest and lowest) in the distribution are changed to the next less extreme values.

Within-group variance (SSW)—Also known as the error term in the ANOVA procedure; a measure of variation within each group that is being compared; it is a measure of the sample observations around the sample mean.

χ^2 **goodness-of-fit test**—A nonparametric test used to determine whether the observed frequencies in a distribution are significantly different from the expected or theoretical frequencies in a distribution, based on the researcher's knowledge of a population under study. The null hypothesis states that there is no difference between the observed and expected frequencies; the alternative hypothesis states that there is a difference between the observed and expected frequencies. The χ^2 goodness-of-fit test is often used to determine whether proportions in a randomly drawn sample are significantly different from the underlying or theoretical population proportions.

χ^2 **test of independence**—A nonparametric test used to determine whether a relationship exists between two variables in a 2×2 contingency table or a $R \times C$ table. Measures for the variables are nominal or dichotomous. The test uses frequencies of the variables, not the actual observations. The null hypothesis states that there is no relationship between the two variables; thus, they are independent of each other. The alternative hypothesis states that there is a relationship between the two variables.

Yates correction for continuity—An adjustment made to the chi-square procedures when the counts in a contingency table are small or when any expected cell count is less than five.

z **score**—In the standard normal distribution, the number of standard deviation units that the observed value is away from the mean, μ.

z **statistic**—The critical value of z; the calculated value of z is compared to the z statistic in order to determine statistical significance.

z **test for comparing two independent population means**—See *z* **tests**.

z **test for comparing two population proportions**—See *z* **tests**.

z **tests**—A parametric test of statistical significance; test is used to make comparisons for two independent population means or two independent population proportions or for comparing a sample mean to a population mean when population parameters are known. It is assumed that the population distributions are normal. In a one-tailed or directional *z* test, the researcher is trying to determine if the sample mean is significantly less or significantly greater than the population parameter μ. In a two-tailed or nondirectional *z* test, the researcher is trying to determine if the sample mean is significantly different (either greater than or less) from the population parameter μ.

z-**value**—See *z*-**score**.

APPENDIX B

Statistical Tables

Table B–1 Areas under the Normal Curve

z	Cum p	Tail p	z	Cum p	Tail p	z	Cum p	Tail p
0.00	0.5000	0.5000	0.32	0.6255	0.3745	0.64	0.7389	0.2611
0.01	0.5040	0.4960	0.33	0.6293	0.3707	0.65	0.7422	0.2578
0.02	0.5080	0.4920	0.34	0.6331	0.3669	0.66	0.7454	0.2546
0.03	0.5120	0.4880	0.35	0.6368	0.3632	0.67	0.7486	0.2514
0.04	0.5160	0.4840	0.36	0.6406	0.3594	0.68	0.7517	0.2483
0.05	0.5199	0.4801	0.37	0.6443	0.3557	0.69	0.7549	0.2451
0.06	0.5239	0.4761	0.38	0.6480	0.3520	0.70	0.7580	0.2420
0.07	0.5279	0.4721	0.39	0.6517	0.3483	0.71	0.7611	0.2389
0.08	0.5319	0.4681	0.40	0.6554	0.3446	0.72	0.7642	0.2358
0.09	0.5359	0.4641	0.41	0.6591	0.3409	0.73	0.7673	0.2327
0.10	0.5398	0.4602	0.42	0.6628	0.3372	0.74	0.7704	0.2296
0.11	0.5438	0.4562	0.43	0.6664	0.3336	0.75	0.7734	0.2266
0.12	0.5478	0.4522	0.44	0.6700	0.3300	0.76	0.7764	0.2236
0.13	0.5517	0.4483	0.45	0.6736	0.3264	0.77	0.7794	0.2206
0.14	0.5557	0.4443	0.46	0.6772	0.3228	0.78	0.7823	0.2177
0.15	0.5596	0.4404	0.47	0.6808	0.3192	0.79	0.7852	0.2148
0.16	0.5636	0.4364	0.48	0.6844	0.3156	0.80	0.7881	0.2119
0.17	0.5675	0.4325	0.49	0.6879	0.3121	0.81	0.7910	0.2090
0.18	0.5714	0.4286	0.50	0.6915	0.3085	0.82	0.7939	0.2061
0.19	0.5753	0.4247	0.51	0.6950	0.3050	0.83	0.7967	0.2033
0.20	0.5793	0.4207	0.52	0.6985	0.3015	0.84	0.7995	0.2005
0.21	0.5832	0.4168	0.53	0.7019	0.2981	0.85	0.8023	0.1977
0.22	0.5871	0.4129	0.54	0.7054	0.2946	0.86	0.8051	0.1949
0.23	0.5910	0.4090	0.55	0.7088	0.2912	0.87	0.8078	0.1922
0.24	0.5948	0.4052	0.56	0.7123	0.2877	0.88	0.8106	0.1894
0.25	0.5987	0.4013	0.57	0.7157	0.2843	0.89	0.8133	0.1867
0.26	0.6026	0.3974	0.58	0.7190	0.2810	0.90	0.8159	0.1841
0.27	0.6064	0.3936	0.59	0.7224	0.2776	0.91	0.8186	0.1814
0.28	0.6103	0.3897	0.60	0.7257	0.2743	0.92	0.8212	0.1788
0.29	0.6141	0.3859	0.61	0.7291	0.2709	0.93	0.8238	0.1762
0.30	0.6179	0.3821	0.62	0.7324	0.2676	0.94	0.8264	0.1736
0.31	0.6217	0.3783	0.63	0.7357	0.2643	0.95	0.8289	0.1711

continues

Table B–1 continued

z	Cum p	Tail p	z	Cum p	Tail p	z	Cum p	Tail p
0.96	0.8315	0.1685	1.45	0.9265	0.0735	1.94	0.9738	0.0262
0.97	0.8340	0.1660	1.46	0.9279	0.0721	1.95	0.9744	0.0256
0.98	0.8365	0.1635	1.47	0.9292	0.0708	**1.96**	**0.9750**	**0.0250**
0.99	0.8389	0.1611	1.48	0.9306	0.0694	1.97	0.9756	0.0244
1.00	0.8413	0.1587	1.49	0.9319	0.0681	1.98	0.9761	0.0239
1.01	0.8438	0.1562	1.50	0.9332	0.0668	1.99	0.9767	0.0233
1.02	0.8461	0.1539	1.51	0.9345	0.0655	2.00	0.9772	0.0228
1.03	0.8485	0.1515	1.52	0.9357	0.0643	2.01	0.9778	0.0222
1.04	0.8508	0.1492	1.53	0.9370	0.0630	2.02	0.9783	0.0217
1.05	0.8531	0.1469	1.54	0.9382	0.0618	2.03	0.9788	0.0212
1.06	0.8554	0.1446	1.55	0.9394	0.0606	2.04	0.9793	0.0207
1.07	0.8577	0.1423	1.56	0.9406	0.0594	2.05	0.9798	0.0202
1.08	0.8599	0.1401	1.57	0.9418	0.0582	2.06	0.9803	0.0197
1.09	0.8621	0.1379	1.58	0.9429	0.0571	2.07	09808	0.0192
1.10	0.8643	0.1357	1.59	0.9441	0.0559	2.08	0.9812	0.0188
1.11	0.8665	0.1335	1.60	0.9452	0.0548	2.09	0.9817	0.0183
1.12	0.8686	0.1314	1.61	0.9463	0.0537	2.10	0.9821	0.0179
1.13	0.8708	0.1292	1.62	0.9474	0.0526	2.11	0.9826	0.0174
1.14	0.8729	0.1271	1.63	0.9484	0.0516	2.12	0.9830	0.0170
1.15	0.8749	0.1251	**1.64**	**0.9495**	**0.0505**	2.13	0.9834	0.0166
1.16	0.8770	0.1230	1.65	0.9505	0.0495	2.14	0.9838	0.0162
1.17	0.8790	0.1210	1.66	0.9515	0.0485	2.15	0.9842	0.0158
1.18	0.8810	0.1190	1.67	0.9525	0.0475	2.16	0.9846	0.0154
1.19	0.8830	0.1170	1.68	0.9535	0.0465	2.17	0.9850	0.0150
1.20	0.8849	0.1151	1.69	0.9545	0.0455	2.18	0.9854	0.0146
1.21	0.8869	0.1131	1.70	0.9554	0.0446	2.19	0.9857	0.0143
1.22	0.8888	0.1112	1.71	0.9564	0.0436	2.20	0.9861	0.0139
1.23	0.8907	0.1093	1.72	0.9573	0.0427	2.21	0.9864	0.0136
1.24	0.8925	0.1075	1.73	0.9582	0.0418	2.22	0.9868	0.0132
1.25	0.8944	0.1056	1.74	0.9591	0.0409	2.23	0.9871	0.0129
1.26	0.8962	0.1038	1.75	0.9599	0.0401	2.24	0.9875	0.0125
1.27	0.8980	0.1020	1.76	0.9608	0.0392	2.25	0.9878	0.0122
1.28	0.8997	0.1003	1.77	0.9616	0.0384	2.26	0.9881	0.0119
1.29	0.9015	0.0985	1.78	0.9625	0.0375	2.27	0.9884	0.0116
1.30	0.9032	0.0968	1.79	0.9633	0.0367	2.28	0.9887	0.0113
1.31	0.9049	0.0951	1.80	0.9641	0.0359	2.29	0.9890	0.0110
1.32	0.9066	0.0934	1.81	0.9649	0.0351	2.30	0.9893	0.0107
1.33	0.9082	0.0918	1.82	0.9656	0.0344	2.31	0.9896	0.0104
1.34	0.9099	0.0901	1.83	0.9664	0.0336	2.32	0.9898	0.0102
1.35	0.9115	0.0885	1.84	0.9671	0.0329	**2.33**	**0.9901**	**0.0099**
1.36	0.9131	0.0869	1.85	0.9678	0.0322	2.34	0.9904	0.0096
1.37	0.9147	0.0853	1.86	0.9686	0.0314	2.35	0.9906	0.0094
1.38	0.9162	0.0838	1.87	0.9693	0.0307	2.36	0.9909	0.0091
1.39	0.9177	0.0823	1.88	0.9699	0.0301	2.37	0.9911	0.0089
1.40	0.9192	0.0808	1.89	0.9706	0.0294	2.38	0.9913	0.0087
1.41	0.9207	0.0793	1.90	0.9713	0.0287	2.39	0.9916	0.0084
1.42	0.9222	0.0778	1.91	0.9719	0.0281	2.40	0.9918	0.0082
1.43	0.9236	0.0764	1.92	0.9726	0.0274	2.41	0.9920	0.0080
1.44	0.9251	0.0749	1.93	0.9732	0.0268	2.42	0.9922	0.0078

continues

Table B–1 continued

z	Cum p	Tail p	z	Cum p	Tail p	z	Cum p	Tail p
2.43	0.9925	0.0075	2.82	0.9976	0.0024	3.21	0.9933	0.0007
2.44	0.9927	0.0073	2.83	0.9977	0.0023	3.22	0.9994	0.0006
2.45	0.9929	0.0071	2.84	0.9977	0.0023	3.23	0.9994	0.0006
2.46	0.9931	0.0069	2.85	0.9978	0.0022	3.24	0.9994	0.0006
2.47	0.9932	0.0068	2.86	0.9979	0.0021	3.25	0.9994	0.0006
2.48	0.9934	0.0066	2.87	0.9979	0.0021	3.26	0.9994	0.0006
2.49	0.9936	0.0064	2.88	0.9980	0.0020	3.27	0.9995	0.0005
2.50	0.9938	0.0062	2.89	0.9981	0.0019	3.28	0.9995	0.0005
2.51	0.9940	0.0060	2.90	0.9981	0.0019	3.29	0.9995	0.0005
2.52	0.9941	0.0059	2.91	0.9982	0.0018	3.30	0.9995	0.0005
2.53	0.9943	0.0057	2.92	0.9982	0.0018	3.31	0.9995	0.0005
2.54	0.9945	0.0055	2.93	0.9983	0.0017	3.32	0.9995	0.0005
2.55	0.9946	0.0054	2.94	0.9984	0.0016	3.33	0.9996	0.0004
2.56	0.9948	0.0052	2.95	0.9984	0.0016	3.34	0.9996	0.0004
2.57	**0.9949**	**0.0051**	2.96	0.9985	0.0015	3.35	0.9996	0.0004
2.58	0.9951	0.0049	2.97	0.9985	0.0015	3.36	0.9996	0.0004
2.59	0.9952	0.0048	2.98	0.9986	0.0014	3.37	0.9996	0.0004
2.60	0.9953	0.0047	2.99	0.9986	0.0014	3.38	0.9996	0.0004
2.61	0.9955	0.0045	3.00	0.9987	0.0013	3.39	0.9997	0.0003
2.62	09956	0.0044	3.01	0.9987	0.0013	3.40	0.9997	0.0003
2.63	0.9957	0.0043	3.02	0.9987	0.0013	3.41	0.9997	0.0003
2.64	0.9959	0.0041	3.03	0.9988	0.0012	3.42	0.9997	0.0003
2.65	0.9960	0.0040	3.04	0.9988	0.0012	3.43	0.9997	0.0003
2.66	0.9961	0.0039	3.05	0.9989	0.0011	3.44	0.9997	0.0003
2.67	0.9962	0.0038	3.06	0.9989	0.0011	3.45	0.9997	0.0003
2.68	0.9963	0.0037	3.07	0.9989	0.0011	3.46	0.9997	0.0003
2.69	0.9964	0.0036	3.08	0.9990	0.0010	3.47	0.9997	0.0003
2.70	0.9965	0.0035	3.09	0.9900	0.0010	3.48	0.9997	0.0003
2.71	0.9966	0.0034	3.10	0.9900	0.0010	3.49	0.9998	0.0002
2.72	0.9967	0.0033	3.11	0.9991	0.0009	3.50	0.9998	0.0002
2.73	0.9968	0.0032	3.12	0.9991	0.0009			
2.74	0.9969	0.0031	3.13	0.9991	0.0009	3.60	0.9998	0.0002
2.75	0.9970	0.0030	3.14	0.9992	0.0008			
2.76	0.9971	0.0029	3.15	0.9992	0.0008	3.70	0.9999	0.0001
2.77	0.9972	0.0028	3.16	0.9992	0.0008			
2.78	0.9973	0.0027	3.17	0.9992	0.0008	3.80	0.9999	0.0001
2.79	0.9974	0.0026	3.18	0.9993	0.0007	3.90	1.000	0.0000
2.80	0.9974	0.0026	3.19	0.9993	0.0007			
2.81	0.9975	0.0025	3.20	0.9993	0.0007			

Source: Copyright © Dr. Victor Bissonnette.

Table B–2 Critical Values of the *t* Distribution

	Two-Tailed Testing/(One-Tailed Testing)					
df	0.2 (0.01)	0.1 (0.05)	0.05 (0.025)	0.02 (0.01)	0.01 (0.005)	0.001 (0.0005)
5	1.476	2.015	2.571	3.365	4.032	6.869
6	1.440	1.943	2.447	3.143	3.707	5.959
7	1.415	1.895	2.365	2.998	3.499	5.408
8	1.397	1.860	2.306	2.896	3.355	5.041
9	1.383	1.833	2.262	2.821	3.250	4.781
10	1.372	0.812	2.228	2.764	3.169	4.587
11	1.363	1.796	2.201	2.718	3.106	4.437
12	1.356	1.782	2.179	2.681	3.055	4.318
13	1.350	1.771	2.160	2.650	3.012	4.221
14	1.345	1.761	2.145	2.624	2.977	4.140
15	1.341	1.753	2.131	2.602	2.947	4.073
16	1.337	1.746	2.120	2.583	2.921	4.015
17	1.333	1.740	2.110	2.567	2.898	3.965
18	1.330	1.734	2.101	2.552	2.878	3.922
19	1.328	1.729	2.093	2.539	2.861	3.883
20	1.325	1.725	2.086	2.528	2.845	3.850
21	1.323	1.721	2.080	2.518	2.831	3.819
22	1.321	1.717	2.074	2.508	2.819	3.792
23	1.319	1.714	2.069	2.500	2.807	3.768
24	1.318	1.711	2.064	2.492	2.797	3.745
25	1.316	1.708	2.060	2.485	2.787	3.725
26	1.315	1.706	20.56	2.479	2.779	3.707
27	1.314	1.703	20.52	2.473	2.771	3.690
28	1.313	1.701	2.048	2.467	2.763	3.674
29	1.311	1.699	2.045	2.462	2.756	3.659
30	1.310	1.697	2.042	2.457	2.750	3.646
40	1.303	1.684	2.021	2.423	2.704	3.551
50	1.299	1.676	2.009	2.403	2.678	3.496
60	1.296	1.671	2.000	2.390	2.660	3.460
80	1.292	1.664	1.990	2.374	2.639	3.416
100	1.290	1.660	1.984	2.364	2.626	3.390
120	1.289	1.658	1.980	2.358	2.617	3.373
∞	1.282	1.645	1.960	2.327	2.576	3.291

Source: Copyright © Dr. Victor Bissonnette.

Table B–3 Critical Values of the *F* Distribution

df within	\multicolumn{11}{c}{df between}

df within	1	2	3	4	5	6	7	8	12	24	∞
5	6.61	5.79	5.41	5.19	5.05	4.95	4.88	4.82	4.68	4.53	4.37
6	5.99	5.14	4.76	4.53	4.39	4.28	4.21	4.15	4.00	3.84	3.67
7	5.59	4.74	4.35	4.12	3.97	3.87	3.79	3.73	3.57	3.41	3.23
8	5.32	4.46	4.07	3.84	3.69	3.58	3.50	3.44	3.28	3.12	2.93
9	5.12	4.26	3.86	3.63	3.48	3.37	3.29	3.23	3.07	2.90	2.71
10	4.96	4.10	3.71	3.48	3.33	3.22	3.14	3.07	2.91	2.74	2.54
11	4.84	3.98	3.59	3.36	3.20	3.09	3.01	2.95	2.79	2.61	2.41
12	4.75	3.89	3.49	3.26	3.11	3.00	2.91	2.85	2.69	2.51	2.30
13	4.67	3.81	3.41	3.18	3.03	2.92	2.83	2.77	2.60	2.42	2.21
14	4.60	3.74	3.34	3.11	2.96	2.85	2.76	2.70	2.53	2.35	2.13
15	4.54	3.68	3.29	3.06	2.90	2.79	2.71	2.64	2.48	2.29	2.07
16	4.49	3.63	3.24	3.01	2.85	2.74	2.66	2.59	2.42	2.24	2.01
17	4.45	3.59	3.20	2.96	2.81	2.70	2.61	2.55	2.38	2.19	1.96
18	4.41	3.55	3.16	2.93	2.77	2.66	2.58	2.51	2.34	2.15	1.92
19	4.38	3.52	3.13	2.90	2.74	2.63	2.54	2.48	2.31	2.11	1.88
20	4.35	3.49	3.10	2.87	2.71	2.60	2.51	2.45	2.28	2.08	1.84
21	4.32	3.47	3.07	2.84	2.68	2.57	2.49	2.42	2.25	2.05	1.81
22	4.30	3.44	3.05	2.82	2.66	2.55	2.46	2.40	2.23	2.03	1.78
23	4.28	3.42	3.03	2.80	2.64	2.53	2.44	2.37	2.20	2.01	1.76
24	4.26	3.40	3.01	2.78	2.62	2.51	2.42	2.36	2.18	1.98	1.73
25	4.24	3.39	2.99	2.76	2.60	2.49	2.40	2.34	2.16	1.96	1.71
26	4.23	3.37	2.98	2.74	2.59	2.47	2.39	2.32	2.15	1.95	1.69
27	4.21	3.35	2.96	2.73	2.57	2.46	2.37	2.31	2.13	1.93	1.67
28	4.20	3.34	2.95	2.71	2.56	2.45	2.36	2.29	2.12	1.91	1.66
29	4.18	3.33	2.93	2.70	2.55	2.43	2.35	2.28	2.10	1.90	1.64
30	4.17	3.32	2.92	2.69	2.53	2.42	2.33	2.27	2.09	1.89	1.62
40	4.08	3.23	2.84	2.61	2.45	2.34	2.25	2.18	2.00	1.79	1.51
60	4.00	3.15	2.76	2.53	2.37	2.25	2.17	2.10	1.92	1.70	1.39
80	3.96	3.11	2.72	2.49	2.33	2.21	2.13	2.06	1.88	1.65	1.33
100	3.94	3.09	2.70	2.46	2.31	2.19	2.10	2.03	1.85	1.63	1.28
120	3.92	3.07	2.68	2.45	2.29	2.18	2.09	2.02	1.83	1.61	1.26
∞	3.84	3.00	2.61	2.37	2.22	2.10	2.01	1.94	1.75	1.52	1.00

Source: Copyright © Dr. Victor Bissonnette.

Table B–4 Critical Values of the Studentized Range Statistic

df_{WG}	a	No. of Groups								
		2	3	4	5	6	7	8	9	10
5	.05	3.64	4.60	5.22	5.67	6.03	6.33	6.58	6.80	6.99
	.01	5.70	6.98	7.80	8.42	8.91	9.32	9.67	9.97	10.24
6	.05	3.46	4.34	4.90	5.30	5.63	5.90	6.12	6.32	6.49
	.01	5.24	6.33	7.03	7.56	7.97	8.32	8.61	8.87	9.10
7	.05	3.34	4.16	4.68	5.06	5.36	5.61	5.82	6.00	6.16
	.01	4.95	5.92	6.54	7.01	7.37	7.68	7.94	8.17	8.37
8	.05	3.26	4.04	4.53	4.89	5.17	4.50	5.60	5.77	5.92
	.01	4.75	5.64	6.20	6.62	6.96	7.24	7.47	7.68	7.86
9	.05	3.20	3.95	4.41	4.76	5.02	5.24	5.43	5.59	5.74
	.01	4.60	5.43	5.96	6.35	6.66	6.91	7.13	7.33	7.49
10	.05	3.15	3.88	4.33	4.65	4.91	5.12	5.30	5.46	5.60
	.01	4.48	5.27	5.77	6.14	6.43	6.67	6.87	7.05	7.21
11	.05	3.11	3.82	4.26	4.57	4.82	5.03	5.20	5.35	5.49
	.01	4.39	5.15	5.62	5.97	6.25	6.48	6.67	6.84	6.99
12	.05	3.08	3.77	4.20	4.51	4.75	4.95	5.12	5.27	5.39
	.01	4.32	5.05	5.50	5.84	6.10	6.32	6.51	6.67	6.81
13	.05	3.06	3.73	4.15	4.45	4.69	4.88	5.05	5.19	5.32
	.01	4.26	4.96	5.40	5.73	5.98	6.19	6.37	6.53	6.67
14	.05	3.03	3.70	4.11	4.41	4.64	4.83	4.99	5.13	5.25
	.01	4.21	4.89	5.32	5.63	5.88	6.08	6.26	6.41	6.54
15	.05	3.01	3.67	4.08	4.37	4.59	4.78	4.94	5.08	5.20
	.01	4.17	4.84	5.25	5.56	5.80	5.99	6.16	6.31	6.44
16	.05	3.00	3.65	4.05	4.33	4.56	4.74	4.90	5.03	5.15
	.01	4.13	4.79	5.19	5.49	5.72	5.92	6.08	6.22	6.35
17	.05	2.98	3.63	4.02	4.30	4.52	4.70	4.86	4.99	5.11
	.01	4.10	4.74	5.14	5.43	5.66	5.85	6.01	6.15	6.27
18	.05	2.97	3.61	4.00	4.28	4.49	4.67	4.82	4.96	5.07
	.01	4.07	4.70	5.09	5.38	5.60	5.79	5.94	6.08	6.20
19	.05	2.96	3.59	3.98	4.25	4.47	4.65	4.79	4.92	5.04
	.01	4.05	4.67	5.05	5.33	5.55	5.73	5.89	6.02	6.14
20	.05	2.95	3.58	3.96	4.23	4.45	4.62	4.77	4.90	5.01
	.01	4.02	4.64	5.02	5.29	5.51	5.69	5.84	5.97	6.09
24	.05	2.92	3.53	3.90	4.17	4.37	4.54	4.68	4.81	4.92
	.01	3.96	4.55	4.91	5.17	5.37	5.54	5.69	5.81	5.92
30	.05	2.89	3.49	3.85	4.10	4.30	4.46	4.60	4.72	4.82
	.01	3.89	4.45	4.80	5.05	5.24	5.40	5.54	5.65	5.76
40	.05	2.86	3.44	3.79	4.04	4.23	4.39	4.52	4.63	4.73
	.01	3.82	4.37	4.70	4.93	5.11	5.26	5.39	5.50	5.60
60	.05	2.83	3.40	3.74	3.98	4.16	4.31	4.44	4.55	4.65
	.01	3.76	4.28	4.59	4.82	4.99	5.13	5.25	5.36	5.45
120	.05	2.80	3.36	3.68	3.92	4.10	4.24	4.36	4.47	4.56
	.01	3.70	4.20	4.50	4.71	4.87	5.01	5.12	5.21	5.30
∞	.05	2.77	3.31	3.63	3.86	4.03	4.17	4.29	4.39	4.47
	.01	3.64	4.12	4.40	4.60	4.76	4.88	4.99	5.08	5.16

Source: Data from E.S. Pearson and H.O. Hartley, *Biometrika Tables for Statisticians,* © 1966, Cambridge University Press; and Harter, Tables of Range and Studentized Range, *Annals of Mathematical Studies,* Vol. 31, pp. 1122–1147.

Table B–5 Critical Values of *r*

	Two-Tailed Testing/(One-Tailed Testing)					
df	0.2 (0.01)	0.1 (0.05)	0.05 (0.025)	0.02 (0.01)	0.01 (0.005)	0.001 (0.0005)
3	0.687	0.805	0.878	0.934	0.959	0.991
4	0.608	0.729	0.811	0.882	0.917	0.974
5	0.551	0.669	0.754	0.833	0.875	0.951
6	0.507	0.621	0.707	0.789	0.834	0.925
7	0.472	0.582	0.666	0.750	0.798	0.898
8	0.443	0.549	0.632	0.715	0.765	0.872
9	0.419	0.521	0.602	0.685	0.735	0.847
10	0.398	0.497	0.576	0.658	0.708	0.823
11	0.380	0.476	0.553	0.634	0.684	0.801
12	0.365	0.458	0.532	0.612	0.661	0.780
13	0.351	0.441	0.514	0.592	0.641	0.760
14	0.338	0.426	0.497	0.574	0.623	0.742
15	0.327	0.412	0.482	0.558	0.606	0.725
16	0.317	0.400	0.468	0.543	0.590	0.708
17	0.308	0.389	0.456	0.529	0.575	0.693
18	0.299	0.378	0.444	0.516	0.561	0.679
19	0.291	0.369	0.433	0.503	0.549	0.665
20	0.284	0.360	0.423	0.492	0.537	0.652
21	0.277	0.352	0.413	0.482	0.526	0.640
22	0.271	0.344	0.404	0.472	0.515	0.629
23	0.265	0.337	0.396	0.462	0.505	0.618
24	0.260	0.330	0.388	0.453	0.496	0.607
25	0.255	0.323	0.381	0.445	0.487	0.597
26	0.250	0.317	0.374	0.437	0.479	0.588
27	0.245	0.311	0.367	0.430	0.471	0.579
28	0.241	0.306	0.361	0.423	0.463	0.570
29	0.237	0.301	0.355	0.416	0.456	0.562
30	0.233	0.296	0.349	0.409	0.449	0.554
40	0.202	0.257	0.304	0.358	0.393	0.490
50	0.181	0.231	0.273	0.322	0.354	0.443
60	0.165	0.211	0.250	0.295	0.325	0.408
80	0.143	0.183	0.217	0.257	0.283	0.357
100	0.128	1.164	0.195	0.230	0.254	0.321
120	0.117	0.150	0.178	0.210	0.232	0.294
140	0.108	0.139	0.165	0.195	0.216	0.273
160	0.101	0.130	0.154	0.183	0.202	0.256
180	0.095	0.122	0.146	0.172	0.190	0.242
200	0.091	0.116	0.138	0.164	0.181	0.230
300	0.074	0.095	0.113	0.134	0.148	0.188
400	0.064	0.082	0.098	0.116	0.128	0.164
500	0.057	0.073	0.088	0.104	0.115	0.146

Table B–6 Critical Values of χ^2 Distribution

	Area in the Upper Tail					
df	0.99	0.95	0.90	0.10	0.05	0.01
1	0.000	0.004	0.016	2.706	3.841	6.635
2	0.020	0.103	0.211	4.605	5.991	9.210
3	0.115	0.352	0.584	6.251	7.185	11.345
4	0.297	0.711	1.064	7.779	9.488	13.277
5	0.554	1.145	1.610	9.236	11.070	15.086
6	0.872	1.635	2.204	10.645	15.592	16.812
7	1.239	2.167	2.833	12.017	14.067	18.475
8	1.646	2.733	3.490	13.362	15.507	20.090
9	2.088	3.325	4.168	14.684	16.919	21.666
10	2.558	3.940	4.865	15.987	18.307	23.209
11	3.053	4.575	5.578	17.275	19.675	24.725
12	3.571	5.226	6.304	18.549	21.026	26.217
13	4.107	5.892	7.042	19.812	22.362	27.688
14	4.660	6.571	7.790	21.064	23.685	29.141
15	5.229	7.261	8.547	22.307	24.996	30.578
16	5.812	7.962	9.312	23.542	26.296	32.000
17	6.408	8.672	10.085	24.769	27.587	33.409
18	7.015	9.390	10.865	25.989	28.869	34.805
19	7.633	10.117	11.651	27.204	30.144	36.191
20	8.260	10.851	12.443	28.412	31.410	37.566
21	8.897	11.591	13.240	29.615	32.671	38.932
22	9.542	12.338	14.041	30.813	33.924	40.289
23	10.196	13.091	14.848	32.007	35.172	41.638
24	10.856	13.848	15.656	33.196	36.415	42.980
25	11.524	14.611	16.473	34.382	37.652	44.314

Source: Copyright © Dr. Victor Bissonnette.

Table B–7 Binomial Distribution with $p = .50$

N	Left S	P	Right S		N	Left S	P	Right S
1	0	.5000	1			6	.6128	5
2	0	.2500	2		13	0	.0001	13
	1	.7500	1			1	.0017	12
3	0	.1250	3			2	.0112	11
	1	.5000	2			3	.0461	10
4	0	.0625	4			4	.1334	9
	1	.3125	3			5	.2905	6
	2	.6875	2			6	.5000	7
5	0	.0312	5		14	0	.0000	14
	1	.1875	4			1	.0009	13
	2	.5000	3			2	.0065	12
6	0	.0156	6			3	.0287	11
	1	.1094	5			4	.0898	10
	2	.3438	4			5	.2120	9
	3	.6562	3			6	.3953	8
7	0	.0078	7			7	.6047	7
	1	.0625	6		15	0	.0000	15
	2	.2266	5			1	.0005	14
	3	.5000	4			2	.0037	13
8	0	.0039	8			3	.0176	12
	1	.0352	7			4	.0592	11
	2	.1445	6			5	.1509	10
	3	.3633	5			6	.3036	9
	4	.6367	4			7	.5000	8
9	0	.0020	9		16	0	.0000	16
	1	.0195	8			1	.0003	15
	2	.0898	7			2	.0021	14
	3	.2539	6			3	.0106	13
	4	.5000	5			4	.0384	12
10	0	.0010	10			5	.1051	11
	1	.0107	9			6	.2272	10
	2	.0547	8			7	.4018	9
	3	.1719	7			8	.5982	8
	4	.3770	6		17	0	.0000	17
	5	.6230	5			1	.0001	16
11	0	.0005	11			2	.0012	15
	1	.0059	10			3	.0064	14
	2	.0327	9			4	.0245	13
	3	.1133	8			5	.0717	12
	4	.2744	7			6	.1662	11
	5	.5000	6			7	.3145	10
12	0	.0002	11			8	.5000	9
	1	.0032	10		18	0	.0000	18
	2	.0193	9			1	.0001	17
	3	.0730	8			2	.0007	16
	4	.1938	7			3	.0038	15
	5	.3872	6			4	.0154	14

continues

Table B–7 continued

N	Left S	P	Right S		N	Left S	P	Right S
	5	.0481	13			8	.3238	11
	6	.1189	12			9	.5000	10
	7	.2403	11		20	0	.0000	20
	8	.4073	10			1	.0000	19
	9	.5927	9			2	.0002	18
19	0	.0000	19			3	.0013	17
	1	.0000	18			4	.0059	16
	2	.0004	17			5	.0207	15
	3	.0022	16			6	.0577	14
	4	.0096	15			7	.1316	13
	5	.0318	14			8	.2517	12
	6	.0835	13			9	.4119	11
	7	.1796	12			10	.5881	10

Note: Entries labeled *P* in the table are the cumulative probability from each extreme to the value of *S*, for the given *n* when *p* = .5. Left-tail probabilities are given for $S \leq .5n$, and right tail for $S \geq .5n$.

Source: Reprinted from National Bureau of Standards.

Table B–8 Critical Values for $\sum R_X$ for the Mann-Whitney Wilcoxon Rank Sum Test

	$n_1 = 3$					$n_1 = 4$			
n_2	.005	.01	.025	.05	n_2	.005	.01	.025	.05
3				6–15	4			10–26	11–25
4				6–18	5		10–30	11–29	12–28
5			6–21	7–20	6	10–34	11–33	12–32	13–31
6			7–23	8–22	7	10–38	11–37	13–35	14–34
7		6–27	7–26	8–25	8	11–41	12–40	14–38	15–37
8		6–30	8–28	9–27	9	11–45	13–43	14–42	16–40
9	6–33	7–32	8–31	10–29	10	12–48	13–47	15–45	17–43
10	6–36	7–35	9–33	10–32	11	12–52	14–50	16–48	18–46
11	6–39	7–38	9–36	11–34	12	13–55	15–53	17–51	19–49
12	7–41	8–40	10–38	11–37	13	13–59	15–57	18–54	20–52
13	7–44	8–43	10–41	12–39	14	14–62	16–60	19–57	21–55
14	7–47	8–46	11–43	13–41	15	15–65	17–63	20–60	22–58
15	8–49	9–48	11–46	13–44					

	$n_1 = 5$					$n_1 = 6$			
n_2	.005	.01	.025	.05	n_2	.005	.01	.025	.05
5	15–40	16–39	17–38	19–36	6	23–55	24–54	26–52	28–50
6	16–44	17–43	18–42	20–40	7	24–60	25–59	27–57	29–55
7	16–49	18–47	20–45	21–44	8	25–65	27–63	29–61	31–59
8	17–53	19–51	21–49	23–47	9	26–70	28–68	31–65	33–63
9	18–57	20–55	22–53	24–51	10	27–75	2973	32–70	35–67
10	19–61	21–59	23–57	26–54	11	28–80	30–78	34–74	37–71
11	20–65	22–63	24–61	27–58	12	30–84	32–82	35–79	38–76
12	21–69	23–67	24–64	28–62	13	31–89	33–87	37–83	40–80
13	22–73	24–71	27–68	30–65	14	32–94	34–92	38–88	42–84
14	22–78	25–75	28–72	31–69	15	33–99	36–96	40–92	44–88
15	23–82	26–79	29–76	33–72					

	$n_1 = 7$					$n_1 = 8$			
n_2	.005	.01	.025	.05	n_2	.005	.01	.025	.05
7	32–73	34–71	36–69	39–66	8	43–93	45–91	49–87	51–85
8	34–78	35–77	38–74	41–71	9	45–99	47–97	51–93	54–90
9	35–84	37–82	40–79	43–76	10	47–105	49–103	53–99	56–96
10	37–89	39–87	42–84	45–81	11	49–111	51–109	55–105	59–101
11	38–95	40–93	44–89	47–86	12	51–117	53–115	58–110	62–106
12	40–100	42–98	46–94	49–91	13	53–123	56–120	60–116	64–112
13	41–106	44–103	48–99	52–95	14	54–130	58–126	62–122	67–117
14	43–111	45–109	50–104	54–100	15	56–136	60–132	65–127	69–123
15	44–117	47–114	52–109	56–105					

continues

Table B–8 continued

n_2	$n_1 = 9$				n_2	$n_1 = 10$			
	.005	.01	.025	.05		.005	.01	.025	.05
9	56–115	59–112	62–109	66–105	10	71–139	74–136	78–132	82–128
10	58–122	61–119	65–115	69–111	11	73–147	77–143	81–139	86–134
11	61–128	63–126	68–121	72–117	12	76–154	79–151	84–146	89–141
12	63–135	66–132	71–127	75–123	13	79–161	82–158	88–152	92–148
13	65–142	68–139	73–134	78–129	14	81–169	85–165	91–159	96–154
14	67–149	71–145	76–140	81–135	15	84–176	88–172	94–166	99–161
15	69–156	73–152	79–146	84–141					

n_2	$n_1 = 11$				n_2	$n_1 = 12$			
	.005	.01	.025	.05		.005	.01	.025	.05
11	87–166	91–162	96–157	100–153	12	105–195	109–191	115–185	120–180
12	90–174	94–170	99–165	104–160	13	109–203	113–199	119–193	125–187
13	93–182	97–178	103–172	108–167	14	112–212	116–208	123–201	129–195
14	96–190	100–186	106–180	112–174	15	115–221	120–216	127–209	133–203
15	99–198	103–194	110–187	116–181					

n_2	$n_1 = 13$				n_2	$n_1 = 14$			
	.005	.01	.025	.05		.005	.01	.025	.05
13	125–166	130–221	136–215	142–209	14	147–259	152–254	160–246	166–240
14	129–235	134–230	141–223	147–217	15	151–269	156–264	164–256	171–249
15	133–244	138–239	145–232	152–225					

n_2	$n_1 = 15$			
	.005	.01	.025	.05
15	171–294	176–289	184–281	192–273

Source: E.W. Minium, *Statistical Reasoning in Psychology and Education,* pp. 549–550, © 1978. Reprinted by permission of John Wiley & Sons, Inc.

Table B–9 Kruskal-Wallis Distribution

n_1, n_2, n_3	Right-Tail Probability for Q				
	0.100	0.050	0.020	0.010	0.001
2, 2, 2	4.571				
3, 2, 1	4.286				
3, 2, 2	4.500	4.714			
3, 3, 1	4.571	5.143			
3, 3, 2	4.556	5.361	6.250		
3, 3, 3	4.622	5.600	6.489	7.200	
4, 2, 1	4.500				
4, 2, 2	4.458	5.333	6.000		
4, 3, 1	4.056	5.208			
4, 3, 2	4.511	5.444	6.144	6.444	
4, 3, 3	4.709	5.791	6.564	6.745	
4, 4, 1	4.167	4.967	6.667	6.667	
4, 4, 2	4.555	5.455	6.600	7.036	
4, 4, 3	4.545	5.598	6.712	7.144	8.909
4, 4, 4	4.654	5.692	6.962	7.654	9.269
5, 2, 1	4.200	5.000			
5, 2, 2	4.373	5.160	6.000	6.533	
5, 3, 1	4.018	4.960	6.044		
5, 3, 2	4.651	5.251	6.124	6.909	
5, 3, 3	4.533	5.648	6.533	7.079	8.727
5, 4, 1	3.987	4.985	6.431	6.955	
5, 4, 2	4.541	5.273	6.505	7.205	8.591
5, 4, 3	4.549	5.656	6.676	7.445	8.795
5, 4, 4	4.668	5.657	6.953	7.760	9.168
5, 5, 1	4.109	5.127	6.145	7.309	
5, 5, 2	4.623	5.338	6.446	7.338	8.938
5, 5, 3	4.545	5.705	6.866	7.578	9.284
5, 5, 4	4.523	5.666	7.000	7.823	9.606
5, 5, 5	4.560	5.780	7.220	8.000	9.920

Note: Each table entry is the smallest value of the Kruskal-Wallis Q such that its right-tail probability is less than or equal to the value given on the top row for $k = 3$, each sample size less than or equal to 5. For $k > 3$, right-tail probabilities for Q are found from Table B–6 with $k - 1$ degrees of freedom.

Source: Adapted with permission from R.L. Iman, D. Quade, & D.A. Alexander, Exact Probability Levels for the Kruskal-Wallis Test, in *Selected Tables in Mathematical Statistics*, Vol. 3, Institute of Mathematical Statistics, ed., pp. 329–384, © 1975, American Mathematical Society.

Frequency Distribution of Discharges by DRG Critical Care Hospital, 1997: An Index to the Number of Cases per DRG

	DRG					DRG			
	Frequency	%	Valid %	Cumulative %		Frequency	%	Valid %	Cumulative %
1.00	3	.0	.0	.0	66.00	1	.0	.0	5.0
5.00	21	.3	.3	.4	68.00	5	.1	.1	5.1
7.00	2	.0	.0	.4	69.00	4	.1	.1	5.2
8.00	2	.0	.0	.4	70.00	3	.0	.0	5.2
9.00	1	.0	.0	.4	71.00	2	.0	.0	5.2
10.00	11	.2	.2.	.6	73.00	1	.0	.0	5.3
12.00	5	.1	.1	.7	75.00	14	.2	.2	5.5
13.00	3	.0	.0	.7	76.00	9	.1	.1	5.6
14.00	115	1.8	1.8	2.5	78.00	5	.1	.1	5.7
15.00	68	1.1	1.1	3.6	79.00	67	1.0	1.0	6.7
16.00	7	.1	.1	3.7	82.00	23	.4	.4	7.1
17.00	4	.1	.1	3.7	83.00	1	.0	.0	7.1
18.00	5	.1	.1	3.8	85.00	5	.1	.1	7.2
19.00	2	.0	.0	3.8	86.00	2	.0	.0	7.2
20.00	3	.0	.0	3.9	87.00	34	.5	.5	7.7
21.00	2	.0	.0	3.9	88.00	120	1.9	1.9	9.6
23.00	2	.0	.0	4.0	89.00	104	1.6	1.6	11.2
24.00	20	3	.3	4.3	90.00	4	.1	.1	11.3
25.00	19	3	.3	4.6	91.00	14	.2	.2	11.5
26.00	1	.0	.0	4.6	92.00	2	.0	.0	11.5
28.00	3	.0	.0	4.6	94.00	3.	.0	.0	11.5
29.00	1	.0	.0	4.6	95.00	4	.1	.1	11.6
34.00	9	.1	.1	4.8	96.00	21	.3	.3	11.9
35.00	3	.0	.0	4.8	97.00	28	.4	.4	12.4
42.00	1	.0	.0	4.8	98.00	25	.4	.4	12.8
49.00	2	.0	.0	4.9	99.00	12	.2	.2	12.9
55.00	1	.0	.0	4.9	100.00	5	.1	.1	13.0
56.00	1	.0	.0	4.9	101.00	10	.2	.2	13.2
57.00	1	.0	.0	4.9	102.00	7	.1	.1	13.3
64.00	1	.0	.0	4.9	110.00	9	.1	.1	13.4
65.00	5	.1	.1	5.0	111.00	1	.0	.0	13.4

	DRG					DRG		
	Frequency	%	Valid %	Cumulative %		Frequency	%	Valid %	Cumulative %
113.00	13	.2	.2	13.6	167.00	11	.2	.2	32.7
114.00	8	.1	.1	13.8	168.00	1	.0	.0	32.7
115.00	6	.1	.1	13.9	169.00	1	.0	.0	32.7
116.00	26	.4	.4	14.3	170.00	3	.0	.0	32.8
118.00	2	.0	.0	14.3	172.00	20	.3	.3	33.1
119.00	1	.0	.0	14.3	174.00	103	1.6	1.6	34.7
120.00	9	.1	.1	14.4	175.00	5	.1	.1	34.8
121.00	119	1.8	1.8	16.3	176.00	7	.1	.1	34.9
122.00	58	.9	.9	17.2	177.00	4	.1	.1	34.9
123.00	20	.3	.3	17.5	178.00	3	.0	.0	35.0
124.00	35	.5	.5	18.0	179.00	4	.1	.1	35.0
125.00	5	.1	.1	18.1	180.00	59	.9	.9	35.9
126.00	2	.0	.0	18.1	181.00	9	.1	.1	36.1
127.00	287	4.4	4.4	22.6	182.00	60	.9	.9	37.0
128.00	22	.3	.3	22.9	183.00	42	.6	.6	37.7
129.00	1	.0	.0	22.9	184.00	20	.3	.3	38.0
130.00	33	.5	.5	23.4	188.00	46	.7	.7	38.7
131.00	12	.2	.2	23.6	189.00	3	.0	.0	38.7
132.00	119	1.8	1.8	25.5	191.00	4	.1	.1	38.8
133.00	4	.1	.1	25.5	193.00	2	.0	.0	38.8
134.00	21	.3	.3	25.9	197.00	10	.2	.2	39.0
135.00	4	.1	.1	25.9	198.00	3	.0	.0	39.0
138.00	77	1.2	1.2	27.1	199.00	1	.0	.0	39.0
139.00	22	.3	.3	27.4	202.00	17	.3	.3	39.3
140.00	51	.8	.8	28.2	203.00	3	.0	.0	39.3
141.00	34	.5	.5	28.8	204.00	16	.2	.2	39.6
142.00	14	.2	.2	29.0	205.00	6	.1	.1	39.7
143.00	71	1.1	1.1	30.1	206.00	1	.0	.0	39.7
144.00	20	.3	.3	30.4	207.00	19	.3	.3	40.0
145.00	5	.1	.1	30.5	208.00	6	.1	.1	40.1
146.00	2	.0	.0	30.5	209.00	162	2.5	2.5	42.6
147.00	1	.0	.0	30.5	210.00	62	1.0	1.0	43.6
148.00	58	.9	.9	31.4	211.00	11	.2	.2	43.7
149.00	4	.1	.1	31.5	212.00	1	.0	.0	43.7
150.00	14	.2	.2	31.7	213.00	1	.0	.0	43.8
151.00	4	.1	.1	31.7	214.00	12	.2	.2	43.9
152.00	2	.0	.0	31.8	215.00	9	.1	.1	44.1
154.00	11	.2	.2	31.9	217.00	9	.1	.1	44.2
157.00	2	.0	.0	32.0	218.00	7	.1	.1	44.3
158.00	3	.0	.0	32.0	219.00	12	.2	.2	44.5
159.00	4	.1	.1	32.1	220.00	3	.0	.0	44.6
160.00	5	.1	.1	32.2	221.00	3	.0	.0	44.6
161.00	5	.1	.1	32.2	222.00	6	.1	.1	44.7
162.00	5	.1	.1	32.3	223.00	9	.1	.1	44.8
164.00	2	.0	.0	32.3	224.00	8	.1	.1	45.0
165.00	7	.1	.1	32.5	225.00	6	.1	.1	45.1
166.00	5	.1	.1	32.5	226.00	1	.0	.0	45.1

DRG	Frequency	%	Valid %	Cumulative %
227.00	8	.1	.1	45.2
229.00	2	.0	.0	45.2
231.00	8	.1	.1	45.3
232.00	2	.0	.0	45.4
233.00	1	.0	.0	45.4
234.00	3	.0	.0	45.4
235.00	1	.0	.0	45.5
236.00	17	.3	.3	45.7
237.00	1	.0	.0	45.7
238.00	4	.1	.1	45.8
239.00	16	.2	.2	46.0
240.00	4	.1	.1	46.1
241.00	1	.0	.0	46.1
242.00	2	.0	.0	46.2
243.00	32	.5	.5	46.6
244.00	2	.0	.0	46.7
247.00	9	.1	.1	46.8
248.00	8	.1	.1	46.9
249.00	5	.1	.1	47.0
250.00	2	.0	.0	47.0
251.00	1	.0	.0	47.1
253.00	9	.1	.1	47.2
254.00	3	.0	.0	47.2
256.00	4	.1	.1	47.3
257.00	3	.0	.0	47.4
258.00	7	.1	.1	47.5
260.00	2	.0	.0	47.5
262.00	2	.0	.0	47.5
263.00	22	.3	.3	47.9
266.00	1	.0	.0	47.9
268.00	1	.0	.0	47.9
269.00	3	.0	.0	47.9
270.00	1	.0	.0	48.0
271.00	4	.1	.1	48.0
272.00	2	.0	.0	48.1
276.00	2	.0	.0	48.1
277.00	40	.6	.6	48.7
278.00	28	.4	.4	49.1
279.00	1	.0	.0	49.1
280.00	4	.1	.1	49.2
281.00	1	.0	.0	49.2
283.00	2	.0	.0	49.3
284.00	2	.0	.0	49.3
285.00	1	.0	.0	49.3
287.00	2	.0	.0	49.3
290.00	7	.1	.1	49.4

DRG	Frequency	%	Valid %	Cumulative %
292.00	2	.0	.0	49.5
294.00	35	.5	.5	50.0
295.00	8	.1	.1	50.1
296.00	59	.9	.9	51.1
297.00	13	.2	.2	51.3
298.00	1	.0	.0	51.3
300.00	7	.1	.1	51.4
301.00	2	.0	.0	51.4
303.00	8	.1	.1	51.5
304.00	6	.1	.1	51.6
305.00	1	.0	.0	51.6
306.00	5	.1	.1	51.7
307.00	1	.0	.0	51.7
308.00	3	.0	.0	51.8
309.00	2	.0	.0	51.8
310.00	7	.1	.1	51.9
311.00	3	.0	.0	52.0
315.00	3	.0	.0	52.0
316.00	24	.4	.4	52.4
318.00	2	.0	.0	52.4
319.00	1	.0	.0	52.4
320.00	33	.5	.5	52.9
321.00	7	.1	.1	53.0
322.00	4	.1	.1	53.1
323.00	11	.2	.2	53.3
324.00	5	.1	.1	53.4
325.00	3	.0	.0	53.4
329.00	1	.0	.0	53.4
331.00	7	.1	.1	53.5
332.00	1	.0	.0	53.5
334.00	6	.1	.1	53.6
335.00	2	.0	.0	53.7
336.00	28	.4	.4	54.1
337.00	6	.1	.1	54.2
340.00	1	.0	.0	54.2
342.00	1	.0	.0	54.2
344.00	1	.0	.0	54.2
347.00	1	.0	.0	54.3
353.00	3	.0	.0	54.3
354.00	7	.1	.1	54.4
355.00	11	.2	.2	54.6
356.00	14	.2	.2	54.8
357.00	3	.0	.0	54.8
358.00	64	1.0	1.0	55.8
359.00	99	1.5	1.5	57.4
360.00	12	.2	.2	57.5

		DRG					DRG	
	Frequency	*%*	*Valid %*	*Cumulative %*		*Frequency*	*%*	*Valid %*	*Cumulative %*
363.00	1	.0	.0	57.6	422.00	4	.1	.1	87.2
364.00	1	.0	.0	57.6	425.00	7	.1	.1	87.3
365.00	1	.0	.0	57.6	429.00	2	.0	.0	87.4
366.00	1	.0	.0	57.6	430.00	4	.1	.1	87.4
367.00	1	.0	.0	57.6	434.00	7	.1	.1	87.5
368.00	9	.1	.1	57.8	435.00	2	.0	.0	87.6
369.00	8	.1	.1	57.9	439.00	1	.0	.0	87.6
370.00	22	.3	.3	58.2	440.00	1	.0	.0	87.6
371.00	189	2.9	2.9	61.1	441.00	3	.0	.0	87.6
372.00	35	.5	.5	61.7	442.00	5	.1	.1	87.7
373.00	505	7.8	7.8	69.5	443.00	1	.0	.0	87.7
374.00	47	.7	.7	70.2	444.00	1	.0	.0	87.8
376.00	3	.0	.0	70.3	447.00	2	.0	.0	87.8
378.00	13	.2	.2	70.5	449.00	12	.2	.2	88.0
379.00	9	.1	.1	70.6	450.00	5	.1	.1	88.0
380.00	4	.1	.1	70.7	451.00	1	.0	.0	88.1
381.00	5	.1	.1	70.7	452.00	4	.1	.1	88.1
382.00	3	.0	.0	70.8	453.00	4	.1	.1	88.2
383.00	19	.3	.3	71.1	454.00	2	.0	.0	88.2
384.00	10	.2	.2	71.2	461.00	8	.1	.1	88.3
385.00	3	.0	.0	71.3	462.00	542	8.4	8.4	96.7
386.00	3	.0	.0	71.3	463.00	1	.0	.0	96.7
387.00	13	.2	.2	71.5	464.00	2	.0	.0	96.8
388.00	4	.1	.1	71.6	467.00	1	.0	.0	96.8
389.00	76	1.2	1.2	72.8	468.00	11	.2	.2	97.0
390.00	64	1.0	1.0	73.8	471.00	1	.0	.0	97.0
391.00	637	9.8	9.8	83.6	473.00	4	.1	.1	97.0
392.00	1	.0	.0	83.6	475.00	52	.8	.8	97.8
395.00	29	.4	.4	84.1	477.00	4	.1	.1	97.9
396.00	1	.0	.0	84.1	478.00	32	.5	.5	98.4
397.00	6	.1	.1	84.2	479.00	2	.0	.0	98.4
398.00	4	.1	.1	84.2	482.00	5	.1	.1	98.5
399.00	1	.0	.0	84.3	483.00	18	.3	.3	98.8
401.00	1	.0	.0	84.3	485.00	2	.0	.0	98.8
403.00	7	.1	.1	84.4	487.00	2	.0	.0	98.8
404.00	1	.0	.0	84.4	489.00	11	.2	.2	99.0
406.00	1	.0	.0	84.4	490.00	5	.1	.1	99.1
408.00	2	.0	.0	84.4	491.00	3	.0	.0	99.1
410.00	31	.5	.5	84.9	493.00	20	.3	.3	99.4
415.00	18	.3	.3	85.2	494.00	28	.4	.4	99.9
416.00	98	1.5	1.5	86.7	496.00	1	.0	.0	99.9
417.00	7	.1	.1	86.8	497.00	1	.0	.0	99.9
418.00	14	.2	.2	87.0	498.00	4	.1	.1	100.0
419.00	2	.0	.0	87.1	500.00	1	.0	.0	100.0
420.00	1	.0	.0	87.1	503.00	1	.0	.0	100.0
421.00	5	.1	.1	87.2	Total	6468	100.0	100.0	

Index

About the Author

Carol E. Osborn, PhD, RHIA, earned an undergraduate degree in health information management from Mercy College of Detroit, a master's degree in health sciences education and evaluation from the State University of New York at Buffalo, and a PhD in research and evaluation from the Ohio State University.

Dr. Osborn has spent most of her career in the academic setting, teaching at both the University of Illinois at Chicago and currently at the Ohio State University. She has also consulted in a variety of health care settings including acute care, specialty care, and health care-related organizations. She was part of the allied health education consulting team to the Ministry of Health, Saudi Arabia. She has also served as a consultant to HIM baccalaureate degree programs.

Dr. Osborn has been active in professional associations at the state and national levels. She served as secretary, treasurer, and president of the Illinois Medical Record Association. Nationally she has served on the Council of Education, Sub-Panel for Accreditation of Academic Programs, and the Joint Committee on Education. For the past nine years, she has been a member of the Panel of Accreditation Surveyors.